An Introduction to Biomechanics of Sport and Exercise

To Shelagh

For Elsevier:

Commissioning Editor: Dinah Thom
Development Editor: Catherine Jackson
Associate Editor: Claire Wilson
Project Manager: Gail Wright
Senior Designer: George Ajayi
Illustration Manager: Gillian Richards
Illustrator: Ethan Danielson

An Introduction to Biomechanics of Sport and Exercise

By

James Watkins PhD FPEA FBASES

Professor of Sports Science, Swansea University, Swansea, UK

Foreword by

David G Kerwin PhD FBASES

Fellow of the Royal Society of Medicine; Professor of Biomechanics, Cardiff School of Sport, University of Wales Institute, Cardiff, UK

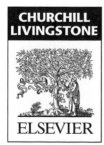

CHURCHILL LIVINGSTONE

ELSEVIER

EDINBURGH LONDON NEW YORK OXFORD PHILADELPHIA ST LOUIS SYDNEY TORONTO 2007

CHURCHILL
LIVINGSTONE
ELSEVIER

First published 2007

ISBN: 978-0-443-10282-0

British Library Cataloguing in Publication Data
A catalogue record for this book is available from the British Library

Library of Congress Cataloging in Publication Data
A catalog record for this book is available from the Library of Congress

ELSEVIER
your source for books,
journals and multimedia
in the health sciences
www.elsevierhealth.com

Working together to grow
libraries in developing countries

www.elsevier.com | www.bookaid.org | www.sabre.org

ELSEVIER | BOOK AID International | Sabre Foundation

The Publisher's policy is to use **paper manufactured from sustainable forests**

Printed in China

Contents

Foreword

Professor James Watkins has been developing courses and writing on the teaching of biomechanics with clarity and purpose for a large part of his academic career. This new book, *An Introduction to Biomechanics of Sport and Exercise*, demonstrates extensive skills in writing about and communicating ideas in biomechanics, while drawing on a wealth of teaching experience.

Professor Watkins (Jim) was Head of Department at the former Scottish School of Physical Education in Glasgow, which later became part of the University of Strathclyde. In 2000 he set up a new Department of Sports Science at Swansea University. Despite the many demands on his time as academic leader and Head of Department, and his work on national and European journals and committees, he has maintained a commitment to the teaching of biomechanics which is reflected in his new book.

This book is directed at students pursuing undergraduate degrees in the sport and exercise sciences. It will also be of interest to physical education teachers and coaches and to anyone seeking an understanding of the mechanics of human movement.

Biomechanics, as applied to sport and exercise, normally focuses on two major themes: improving performance and reducing injury. Both rely on the idea that practitioners understand the mechanics which underpin human movement. This new text by Professor Watkins tackles many of the tricky issues which challenge undergraduate students in sport and exercise science degree programmes, and which

take them outside their comfort zone. The book assumes no prior knowledge in mechanics but instead leads the reader gently from basic principles, and is supported throughout by illustrations and worked examples which neatly complement the explanations being presented.

Jim is the ideal person to write this book. In the UK he is unusual in writing textbooks on biomechanics. This has traditionally been the province of academics based in the USA. Jim has previously produced two main texts on biomechanics. One, *An Introduction to Mechanics of Human Movement*, was written some years ago and can be seen as the forerunner to the current book. The second, *Structure and Function of the Musculoskeletal System*, focused on a different, but related, area. This examined how muscles, bones and joints respond and adapt to the forces exerted on them during training and performance. This 1999 publication received high praise, with excellent sales, and has been translated into Spanish and Chinese. His new book will be eagerly awaited by his current readership. It will also have a ready market in the UK and overseas within the ever-growing community of undergraduate students on programmes where technical and mechanical analyses of human movement feature.

Jim is expert in the fields of sport and exercise sciences and physical education and has been awarded Fellowships by the two leading UK professional bodies, the British Association of Sport and Exercise Sciences (BASES) and the Physical Education Association (PEA). He is an acknowledged expert reviewer of research papers in sport and exercise biomechanics and physical education. He promoted professional aspects of biomechanics during his period of office as Chair of the biomechanics section of BASES, and has twice acted as biomechanics research specialist on the national review panel of UK *Sports Related Subjects* (Higher Education Funding Council of England, Research Assessment Exercise, 1996 and 2001). He thus brings a wealth of experience, expertise and insight to this academic field of study.

This book is constructed in a logical and incremental manner with small steps being taken at each stage. The introduction sets the scene and outlines the scope of the book. It also introduces the main system of units used in all international conferences and publications and employed throughout the book, the International System (SI). There is a brief summary table contrasting SI units with the British imperial system of measurements, which has historical interest and could be useful to modern students when studying old research papers and textbooks or when sourcing comparative data from past studies.

The main body of the book contains sections on *linear motion*, *angular motion* and *work, energy and power*; before moving to the technically demanding, but interesting, section on *fluid mechanics*. There are many references within the text to reflect current knowledge in specialist fields, as illustrated in the chapter on angular motion, where the work of Professor M. R. 'Fred' Yeadon on the mechanics of twisting somersaults has been included. Before moving to the final section of the book, which contains a range of useful laboratory worksheets, there is a chapter on one of Jim's personal favourite topics: the importance of a sound mechanical knowledge to underpin analysis. This chapter, entitled *Biomechanical analysis of human movement*, summarizes a topic that Jim has written on in both physical education and sports sciences contexts. In this chapter he argues strongly for the importance of sound mechanical understanding in qualitative and quantitative analyses of sport and exercise. With this book, students, interested teachers and coaches and allied medical professionals will be able to gain the knowledge and understanding necessary to enhance their skills of analysis.

This new book represents the fruits of 30 years' experience in teaching and communication in the field of sport and exercise biomechanics and will be an invaluable resource for up-and-coming sport and exercise scientists.

David G. Kerwin

Preface

All movements and changes in movement are brought about by the action of forces. The two most common types of force are pushing and pulling, but there are many variations, such as lifting a book from a table, holding a pen, turning a door handle, kicking a ball and throwing a discus. These are all examples of the human body applying a force to an object in order to move it or change the way it is moving, i.e. to change its speed and/or direction of movement.

Human movement is brought about by the musculoskeletal system (skeleton, joints, skeletal muscles) under the control of the nervous system. The muscles pull on the bones in order to control the movements of the joints and, in doing so, control the movement of the body as a whole. Biomechanics of sport and exercise is the study of the forces that act on and within the human body and the effects of these forces on the size, shape, structure and movement of the body.

In sport and exercise, every time a coach, teacher, instructor or therapist attempts to improve an individual's technique (the way that the arms, legs and trunk move in relation to each other during the movement), s/he is trying to improve the mechanics of the individual's movement, i.e. improve the coordination of the forces produced by various muscle groups. In the context of sport and exercise, biomechanics is the science underlying technique. Good technique is characterized by effective performance (the purpose of the movement) and decreased risk of injury (distribution of forces in muscles, bones and joints so that no part is excessively overloaded). Poor technique is characterized by increased risk of injury, even though performance may be effective, at least for a while.

There are basically two ways of analysing technique: qualitative and quantitative. A qualitative analysis is based on observation (directly and/or via film or video). Clearly, knowing what to look for and being able to observe accurately are of prime importance in qualitative analysis. An observer's ability to observe accurately will largely depend upon his/her knowledge and experience and, in particular, his/her ability to identify the mechanical requirements of the movement under consideration. Even then, because of the speed of the movement, it may be difficult to detect faults in technique by observation alone. In these circumstances, a quantitative analysis of technique will be required. A quantitative analysis is based on measurements of the kinematic (distance, speed, acceleration) and kinetic (force) variables that determine performance. For example, stride rate and stride length (obtained from video analysis) and the forces acting on the feet (obtained with the use of a force platform) may be used to evaluate the technique of a runner.

The key to understanding biomechanics is a thorough understanding of the concepts of force, Newton's laws of motion, work and energy. The purpose of this book is to develop knowledge and understanding of these fundamental biomechanical concepts and their application in movement analysis. The book is designed primarily as a course text for undergraduate students of sport and exercise science, but students of physiotherapy, occupational therapy and podiatric medicine will also find the book useful, since an understanding of biomechanics is essential to successful practice in all these professions.

The book has six chapters. Chapter 1 introduces the fundamental concepts of force, mechanics, forms of motion and units of measurement that underlie biomechanics. Chapters 2 and 3 develop the concepts of kinematics (distance, speed, acceleration) and kinetics (the forces responsible for the observed kinematics) in relation to linear and angular motion. Chapter 4 develops the concepts of work, energy, power and mechanical efficiency. Chapter 5 develops the concept of fluid mechanics in relation to air resistance and water resistance. Chapter 6 describes the qualitative and quantitative approaches to movement analysis.

No previous knowledge of mechanics is assumed. All the biomechanical concepts and principles are explained from first principles. To aid learning, the book features a content overview at the start of each chapter, key points highlighted within the text, a large number of applied examples with illustrations, review questions with detailed solutions to all numerical questions, practical worksheets with example results, references to guide further reading, an extensive glossary and an extensive index.

Swansea 2007   James Watkins

Acknowledgements

I thank all of the staff at Elsevier who contributed to the commissioning and production of the book. I also thank my academic colleagues and the large number of undergraduate and graduate students who have helped me, directly and indirectly, over many years, to develop and organize the content of the book.

Chapter 1

Introduction

All movements and changes in movement are brought about by the action of forces. The two most common types of force are pushing and pulling. Human movement is brought about by the musculoskeletal system under the control of the nervous system. The muscles pull on the bones in order to control the movements of the joints and, in doing so, control the movement of the body as a whole. Biomechanics is the study of the forces that act on and within living organisms and the effect of the forces on the size, shape, structure and movement of the organisms. The purpose of this chapter is to introduce the fundamental concepts of force, mechanics, forms of motion and units of measurement that underlie the study of biomechanics.

FORCE

All bodies, animate and inanimate, are continuously acted upon by forces. A force can be defined as that which alters or tends to alter a body's state of rest or type of movement. The forces that act on a body arise from interaction of the body with its environment. There are two types of interaction: contact interaction, which produces contact forces, and attraction interaction, which produces attraction forces.

Contact interaction refers to physical contact between the body and its environment. In contact interactions, the forces exerted by the environment on a body are referred to as contact forces. The environment consists largely of three main types of physical phenomenon: solids, liquids, gases. In sport and exercise, the main sources of contact forces are implements (e.g. balls, rackets), the ground (e.g. walking, running, jumping), water (e.g. swimming, diving), air (e.g. skydiving, ski jumping, downhill skiing) and, of course, the forces exerted by opponents, usually in the form of pushes and pulls.

Attraction interaction refers to naturally occurring forces of attraction between certain bodies that tend to make the bodies move toward each other and to maintain contact with each other after contact is made. For example, electromagnetic attraction force maintains the configuration of atoms in molecules and the configuration of molecules in solids, liquids and gases. Similarly, a magnetized piece of iron attracts other pieces of iron to it by the attraction force of magnetism. The human body is constantly subjected to a very considerable force of attraction, i.e. body weight, the force due to the gravitational pull of the earth. It is body weight that keeps us in contact with the ground and that brings us back to the ground should we leave it, e.g. following a jump into the air.

> All bodies, animate and inanimate, are continuously acted upon by forces that arise from interaction of the body with its environment. The environment exerts two kinds of force, contact forces and attraction forces.

MECHANICS

Forces tend to affect bodies in two ways:

- Forces tend to deform bodies, i.e. to change the shape of the bodies by stretching (pulling force), squashing (pushing force) and twisting (torsion force). For example, squeezing a tube of toothpaste changes the shape of the tube
- Forces determine the movement of bodies, i.e. the forces acting on a body determine whether it moves or remains at rest and determine its speed and direction of movement if it does move.

Mechanics is the study of the forces that act on bodies and the effects of the forces on the size, shape, structure and movement of the bodies (Watkins 2000). The actual effect that a force or combination of forces has on a body, i.e. the amount of deformation and change of movement that occurs, depends upon the size of the force in relation to the mass of the body and the mechanical properties of the body. The mass of a body is the amount of matter (physical substance) that comprises the body. The mass of a body is the product of its volume and its density.

The volume of a body is the amount of space that the mass occupies and its density is the concentration of matter (atoms and molecules) in the mass, i.e. the amount of mass per unit volume. The greater the concentration of mass, the larger the density. For example, the density of iron is greater than that of wood and the density of wood is greater than that of polystyrene. Similarly, with regard to the structure of the human body, bone is more dense than muscle and muscle is more dense than fat.

The mass of a body is a measure of its inertia, i.e. its resistance to start moving if it is at rest and its resistance to change its speed and/or direction if it is already moving. The larger the mass the greater the inertia and, consequently, the larger the force that will be needed to move the mass or change the way it is moving. For example, the inertia of a stationary soccer ball (a small mass) is small in comparison to that of a heavy barbell (a large mass), i.e. much more force will be required to move the barbell than to move the ball.

Whereas the effect of a force on the movement of a body is largely determined by its mass, the amount of deformation that occurs is largely determined by its mechanical properties, in particular, its stiffness (the resistance of the body to deformation) and strength (the amount of force required to break the body). For a given amount of force, the higher the stiffness and the greater the strength of a body, the smaller the deformation that will occur.

> Mechanics is the study of the forces that act on bodies and the effects of the forces on the size, shape, structure and movement of the bodies.

SUBDISCIPLINES OF MECHANICS

The different types and effects of forces are reflected in four overlapping subdisciplines of mechanics: mechanics of materials, fluid mechanics, statics and dynamics. Mechanics of materials is the study of the mechanical properties of materials including, for example, the stiffness and resilience of materials used to make running

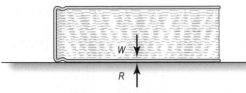

Fig. 1.1   The forces acting on a book resting on a table. W = weight of the book; R = force exerted on the book by the table

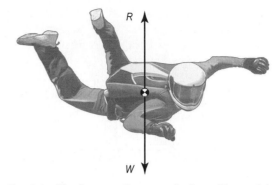

Fig. 1.2   The forces acting on a skydiver. W = weight of the skydiver, clothing and parachute; R = air resistance

tracks and other playing surfaces and the strength of bone, muscle and connective tissues. Fluid mechanics is the study of the movement of liquids and gases, such as blood flow in the cardiovascular system and the effect of liquids and gases on the movement of solids, such as the movement of the human body through water and air.

Statics is the study of bodies under the action of balanced forces, i.e. study of the forces acting on bodies that are at rest or moving with constant speed in a particular direction. In these situations the resultant force (the net effect of all the forces) acting on the body is zero. Figure 1.1 shows a book resting on a table. Since the book is at rest, there are only two forces acting on the book (discounting the force exerted by the surrounding air, which is negligible): the weight of the book W acting downward and the upward reaction force R exerted by the table. The magnitude of W and R is the same but they act in opposite directions and therefore cancel out, such that the resultant force acting on the book is zero.

Figure 1.2 shows a skydiver falling to earth. After jumping out of the aeroplane she is accelerated downward (her downward speed increases) by the force of her weight W. However, as her downward speed increases, so does the upthrust of air on the underside of her body, i.e. the air resistance R. After falling for a few seconds R will be equal in magnitude but opposite in direction to W. Consequently, the resultant force acting on the skydiver will be zero and, provided that she does not alter the orientation or shape of her body, she will continue to fall with constant speed until she opens her parachute.

Dynamics is the study of bodies under the action of unbalanced forces, i.e. bodies moving with non-constant speed. In this situation the resultant force acting on the body will be greater than zero, i.e. the body will be accelerating (speed increasing) or decelerating (speed decreasing) in the direction of the resultant force. For example, Figure 1.3a shows a sprinter in the set position, i.e. when the body is at rest. In this situation the resultant force acting on the sprinter will be zero. However, following the starting signal, the sprinter accelerates away from the blocks under the action of the resultant force acting on his body, i.e. the resultant of his body weight and the forces acting on his feet (Fig. 1.3b).

Kinematics is the branch of dynamics that describes the movement of bodies in relation to space and time (Greek *kinema*, movement). A kinematic analysis describes the movement of a body in terms of distance (change in position), speed (rate of change of position) and acceleration (variability in the rate of change of position). Kinetics is the branch of dynamics that describes the forces acting on bodies, i.e. the cause of the observed kinematics (Greek *kinein*, to move). The main subdisciplines of mechanics are summarized in Figure 1.4.

BIOMECHANICS

Biomechanics is the study of the forces that act on and within living organisms and the effect

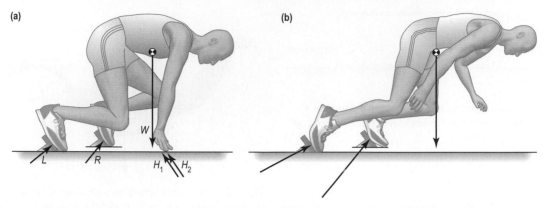

Fig. 1.3   The forces acting on a sprinter in the set position (a) and just after the start (b). H_1 and H_2 = forces acting on the hands; W = weight of the sprinter; L = force exerted on the left foot; R = force exerted on the right foot

Fig. 1.4   Subdisciplines of mechanics

Focus of study	Subdisciplines	
Mechanical properties of material	Mechanics of materials	
Mechanics of liquids and gases	Fluid mechanics	
Mechanics of bodies under the action of balanced forces	Statics	
Mechanics of bodies under the action of unbalanced forces	Dynamics	{ Kinetics { Kinematics

of the forces on the size, shape, structure and movement of the organisms (Watkins 2001). Human movement is brought about by the musculoskeletal system (skeleton, joints, skeletal muscles) under the control of the nervous system. The muscles pull on the bones in order to control the movements of the joints and, in doing so, control the movement of the body as a whole. By coordination of the various muscle groups, the forces generated by the muscles are transmitted by the bones and joints to enable the body to apply forces to the external environment (usually by the hands and feet) in order to maintain an upright posture, transport the body (such as walking, running and swimming) and manipulate objects (ranging from fine dexterity such as threading a needle to gross whole body movement such as throwing a ball). Biomechanics of sport and exercise is the study of the relationship between the external forces (due to body weight and physical contact with the environment) and internal forces (active forces generated by muscles and passive forces

exerted on connective tissues) that act on and within the body and the effect of these forces on the size, shape, structure and movement of the body.

FORMS OF MOTION

There are two fundamental forms of motion, linear motion and angular motion. Linear motion, which is also referred to as translation, occurs when all parts of a body move the same distance in the same direction in the same time (Watkins 2000). In all types of self-propelled human movement, such as walking, running and swimming, the orientation of the body segments to each other continually changes and, therefore, pure linear motion seldom occurs in human movement. The human body may experience pure linear motion for brief periods in activities such as skating (Fig. 1.5) and ski jumping (Fig. 1.6). When the linear movement is in a

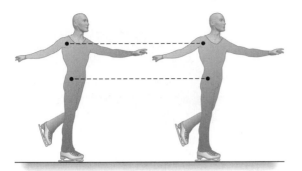

Fig. 1.5   Rectilinear motion in skating

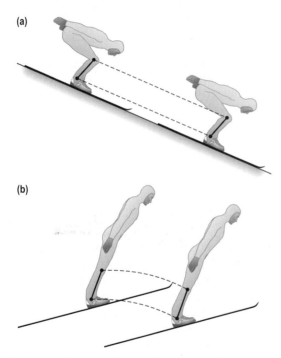

Fig. 1.6   Linear motion: a ski jumper is likely to experience rectilinear motion on the runway (a) and curvilinear motion during flight (b)

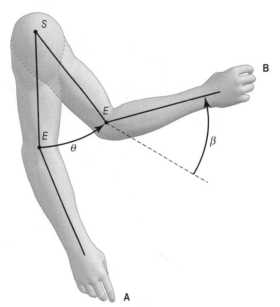

Fig. 1.7   Angular motion: as the arm swings from position (a) to position (b) the upper arm rotates through an angle θ about the transverse (side-to-side) axis S through the shoulder joint and the lower arm and hand rotate through an angle β about the transverse axis E through the elbow joint

straight line, the motion is called rectilinear motion (Figs 1.5, 1.6a). When the linear movement follows a curved path, the motion is referred to as curvilinear motion (Fig. 1.6b).

Angular motion, also referred to as rotation, occurs when a body or part of a body, such as an arm or a leg, moves in a circle or part of a circle about a particular line in space, referred to as the axis of rotation, such that all parts of the body move through the same angle in the same direction in the same time. The axis of rotation may be stationary or it may experience linear motion (Fig. 1.7). Figure 1.8 shows a gymnast rotating about a horizontal bar. Provided that the orientation of the body segments to each other does not change, the gymnast as a whole and each of the body segments will experience angular motion about the bar. Most whole body human movements are combinations of linear and angular motion. For example, in walking, the movement of the head and trunk is fairly linear but the movements of the arms and legs involve simultaneous linear and angular motion as the body as a whole moves forward (Fig. 1.9). Similarly, in cycling, the movement of the trunk, head and arms is fairly linear but the movements of the legs involve simultaneous linear and angular motion (Fig. 1.10). The movement of a multisegmented body, such as the human body, which involves simultaneous linear and angular

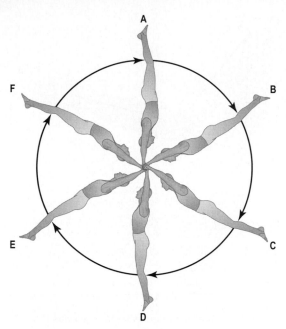

Fig. 1.8 A gymnast rotating about a high bar

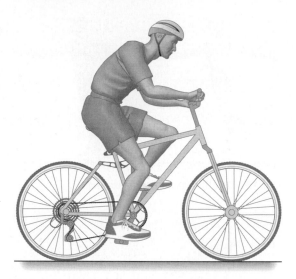

Fig. 1.10 General motion: in cycling, the movement of the trunk, head and arms is fairly linear but the movements of the legs involve simultaneous linear and angular motion

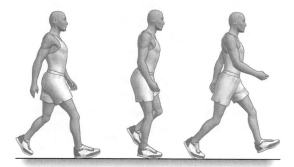

Fig. 1.9 General motion: in walking, the movement of the head and trunk is fairly linear but the movements of the arms and legs involve simultaneous linear and angular motion

motion of the segments, is usually referred to as general motion.

> There are two fundamental forms of motion, linear motion and angular motion. Most whole body human movements are combinations of linear and angular motion.

UNITS OF MEASUREMENT

Commerce and scientific communication are dependent on the correct use and interpretation of units of measurement. With the advent of the industrial revolution in the 18th century and the progressive increase in international trade that resulted from it, the need for uniformity in measurement became increasingly evident. At that time, one of the most widely used systems of units was the British imperial system, but lack of clarity and consistency with regard to definitions and symbols for many variables resulted in resistance to the use of this system internationally (Rowlett 2004). The metric system of measurements originated in France around 1790. The name of the system is derived from the base unit for length, the metre, which was defined as one 10-millionth of the distance from the equator to the North Pole. In contrast to the British imperial system, each unit in the metric system has a unique definition and a unique symbol. Largely

Table 1.1 Mechanical units and (symbols) of measurement

Quantity	British imperial system	SI system
Distance	foot (ft)	metre (m)
Time	second (s)	second (s)
Speed	feet per second (ft/s)	metres per second (m/s)
Acceleration	feet per second per second (ft/s^2)	metres per second per second (m/s^2)
Mass	pound (lb)	kilogram (kg)
Linear momentum	pounds feet per second (lb.ft/s)	kilogram metres per second (kg.m/s)
Force	poundal (pdl)	newton (N)
	1 pdl = 1 lb × 1 ft/s^2	1 N = 1 kg × 1 m/s^2
Weight*	pound force (lbf)	kilogram force (kgf)
	1 lbf = 1 lb × 32.2 ft/s^2 = 32.2 pdl	1 kgf = 1 kg × 9.81 m/s^2 = 9.81 N
Pressure	pounds force per square inch (lbf/in^2)	pascal (Pa) (Pa = N/m^2)
Angular distance	radian (rad)	radian (rad)
Angular speed	radians per second (rad/s)	radians per second (rad/s)
Angular acceleration	radians per second per second (rad/s^2)	radians per second per second (rad/s^2)
Moment of inertia	pound foot squared (lb.ft^2)	kilogram metres squared (kg.m^2)
Angular momentum	pound foot squared per second (lb.ft^2/s)	kilogram metres squared per second (kg.m^2/s)
Turning moment	poundal foot (pdl.ft)	newton metre (N.m)
Energy and work	foot poundal (ft.pdl)	joule (J) (J = N.m)
Power	horsepower (hp) 1 hp = 550 ft lb/s[†]	watt (W) (W = J/s)

*Pound force (lbf) and pound weight (lbwt) are different names for the same unit, i.e. the weight of a mass of 1 lb; kilogram force (kgf), kilopond (kp) and kilogram weight (kgwt) are different names for the same unit, i.e. the weight of a mass of 1 kg.
[†]The horsepower symbol is usually written as ft lb/s, but the 'lb' is actually 'lbf' (pound force). Consequently, the correct symbol for horsepower is ft lbf/s (foot pounds force per second). Fortunately, the horsepower is rarely used in biomechanics.

for this reason, the metric system progressively gained ground internationally. The metric system was officially adopted in the Netherlands and Luxembourg in 1820 and in France in 1837. In 1875, many of the industrialized countries signed the Treaty of the Metre, which established the International Bureau of Weights and Measures (BIPM for *Bureau International des Poids et Mésures*) and a single system of units, the International System of Units, to include all physical and chemical, metric and non-metric units. The system is usually referred to as the SI system after its French language name *Système International d'Unites*. The SI system is now the most widely used system of units, especially in science and international commerce. The system is maintained and updated by the BIPM as new units are proposed and accepted. The system now consists of a large number of units but all the units are derived from a set of base units. The base units for mechanical variables in the SI system are the metre (length), the kilogram (mass) and the second (time). These three units give rise to a subsection of the SI system called the metre–kilogram–second (m–kg–s) system. The corresponding subsection of the British imperial system is the foot–pound–second (ft–lb–s) system. These two subsystems are shown in Table 1.1. Apart from in a few examples, the m–kg–s system is used throughout this book.

> The International System of Units (SI system) includes all physical and chemical, metric and non-metric units. It is the most widely used system of units, especially in science and international commerce.

Table 1.2 Equivalences between SI and British imperial system units

Mass
1 lb = 0.4536 kg
1 kg = 2.2046 lb
1 ton = 2240 lb = 1016.05 kg

Length
1 in = 25.4 mm (mm = millimetre: 1 m = 1000 mm)
1 in = 2.54 cm (cm = centimetre: 1 m = 100 cm)
1 in = 0.0254 m
1 ft = 0.3048 m
1 yd = 0.914 4 m
1 mile = 1609.34 m
1 mile = 1.609 34 km (km = kilometre: 1 km = 1000 m)
1 cm = 0.3937 in
1 cm = 0.0328 ft
1 m = 39.37 in
1 m = 3.2808 ft
1 m = 1.0936 yd
1 m = 6.2137×10^{-4} miles = 0.000 621 37 miles
1 km = 0.621 37 miles

Time
1 s = 0.0167 min
1 s = 2.7778×10^{-4} h (hours) = 0.000 277 78 h
1 min = 60 s
1 h = 60 min
1 h = 3600 s

Force
1 kgf = 9.81 N
1 N = 0.1019 kgf
1 kgf = 2.2046 lbf
1 lbf = 0.4536 kgf
1 lbf = 4.4498 N
1 N = 0.2247 lbf
1 tonf (ton force) = 2240 lbf
1 tonf = 1016 kgf
1 tonf = 9964 N

Speed
1 m/s = 3.2808 ft/s
1 m/s = 2.2369 mph (miles per hour)
1 m/s = 3.6 km/h

1 km/h = 0.277 78 m/s
1 ft/s = 0.3048 m/s
1 ft/s = 0.6818 mph
1 mph = 0.4470 m/s
1 mph = 1.609 34 km/h
1 km/h = 0.6214 mph

Area
1 m^2 = 10.7639 ft^2
1 m^2 = 1550 in^2
1 m^2 = 1.1960 yd^2
1 yd^2 = 0.8361 m^2
1 ft^2 = 0.0929 m^2
1 in^2 = 0.000 645 16 m^2 = $6.4516 \times 10^{-4} m^2$
Surface area of a sphere = $4\pi.r^2$ where r = radius of the sphere

Volume
1 yd^3 (cubic yard) = 0.764 555 m^3 (cubic metre)
1 ft^3 (cubic foot) = 0.028 316 m^3
1 in^3 (cubic inch) = 16.387 cm^3
1 m^3 = 35.3144 ft^3
1 m^3 = 1.307 95 yd^3
1 cm^3 = 0.061 023 7 in^3
1 l (litre) = $10^3 cm^3$ = 1000 ml (millilitres)
1 m^3 = $10^6 cm^3$ = 10^3 l
1 l = $10^{-3} m^3$
Volume of a sphere = $4\pi.r^3/3$ where r = radius of the sphere
Volume of an ellipsoid = $4\pi.a.b^2/3$ where a = length radius and b = width radius

Pressure
1 Pa = 0.000 144 988 lbf/in^2 = $1.449 88 \times 10^{-4} lbf/in^2$
1 lbf/in^2 = 6897.15 Pa
1 atm (atmosphere) = 101 325 Pa = 14.69 lbf/in^2

Density
Water (at sea level) = 1000 kg/m^3
Air (at sea level) = 1.25 kg/m^3

Viscosity
Water (at 20°C) = 0.1002 P = 0.010 02 Pl
Air (at 20°C) = 0.0018 P = 0.000 18 Pl

UNIT SYMBOLS IN THE SI SYSTEM

Units in the SI system are represented by symbols, which are derived according to mathematical rules, rather than abbreviations that follow grammatical rules (Rowlett 2004). The mathematical rules include:

- A symbol is not followed by a full stop (period), except at the end of a sentence

- The letter 's' is not added to a symbol to indicate more than one. For example, 2 kilograms is reported as 2 kg, not 2 kgs
- Superscripts are used to indicate 'squared' or 'cubed'. For example, 4 square metres is written as $4\,m^2$, not 4 sq m
- A raised dot (also referred to as a middle dot, centred dot and half-high dot), a decimal point or a space is used to indicate multiplication of one SI unit by another. For example, the symbol for a newton metre is, $N \cdot m$, N.m or N m, but not Nm. The decimal point format is used in this book
- A forward slash or raised dot with a negative power is used to indicate division of one unit by another. For example, the symbol for metres per second is m/s or $m.s^{-1}$. However, only one slash or raised dot is permitted. For example, the symbol for metres per second per second is m/s^2 or $m.s^{-2}$, not m/s/s. The slash format is used in this book
- A space is placed between the number and the associated symbol. For example, 2.4 kg and 3.25 s are correct, but 2.4kg and 3.25s are incorrect. Percentage and degrees (temperature and angles) are not part of the SI system and are represented by abbreviations rather than symbols. However, they are frequently used in science literature. These variables are reported without a space between the number and the abbreviation, i.e. 7.6%, 5.5°C and 25.4° are all correct
- In numbers with five or more digits on either side of the decimal point, groups of three digits are separated by a space instead of a comma (which is used as a decimal point in some countries) as, for example, 10 000 m or 0.123 46 kg.

CONVERSION OF UNITS

Whereas most countries use the SI system, units from the British imperial system are still widely used in the UK and the USA. These units include, for example, inches (in), feet (ft), yards (yd) and miles (as in miles per hour, mph) for distance, and pound (lb) and ton for mass. Table 1.2 shows some frequently used equivalences between SI and British imperial system units.

To convert units, it is necessary to replace the units to be converted by their numerical equivalent in the units required. For example, the maximum speed of elite male sprinters in a 100 m race is approximately 11.7 m/s. This is equivalent to a speed of 26.17 mph:

Since 1 m/s = 2.2369 mph (Table 1.2)
then 11.7 m/s = 11.7 × 2.2369 mph
           = 26.17 mph

Similarly, the standard road vehicle speed limit in built-up areas in the UK is 30 mph. This is equivalent to a speed of 48.28 km/h:

Since 1 mph = 1.609 34 km/h
then 30 mph = 30 × 1.609 34 km/h
          = 48.28 km/h

REVIEW QUESTIONS

1. Define the following terms: force, contact force, attraction force, resultant force, mechanics, biomechanics, mass, inertia, volume, density, stiffness, strength, kinematics, kinetics.

2. Describe the two ways in which forces tend to affect bodies.

3. Describe the four main subdisciplines of mechanics.

4. Describe the two fundamental forms of motion.

5. List the base units for length, mass and time in the International System of Units.

6. Convert 150 m/s to mph, 10 mph to km/h, 25 km/h to m/s.

References

Rowlett R 2004 How many? A dictionary of units of measurement. Available on line at: http://www.unc.edu/~rowlett/units/sipm.html 14 June 2004

Watkins J 2000 Biomechanics of movement. In: Armstrong N, van Mechelen W (eds) Paediatric exercise science. Oxford University Press, Oxford, p 107–122

Watkins J 2001 Structure and function of the foot. In: Lorimer D L, French G, O'Donnell M, Burrow J G (eds) Neale's disorders of the foot, 6th edn. Churchill Livingstone, Edinburgh, p 1–22

Chapter 2

Linear motion

CHAPTER CONTENTS

The human body, like any other body, will only begin to move or, if it is already moving, change its speed or direction, when the resultant force acting on it becomes greater than zero. Furthermore, the amount of change in speed and/or direction that occurs will depend upon the magnitude and direction of the resultant force, i.e. there is a direct relationship between change of resultant force and change in movement. Isaac Newton (1642–1725) described this relationship in what has come to be known as Newton's laws of motion. In addition to the three laws of motion, Newton's law of gravitation describes the naturally occurring force of attraction that is always present between any two bodies. A body falls to the ground because of the gravitational attraction between the body and the earth, and the planets are maintained in their orbits round the sun by the gravitational attraction between the planets and the sun. The purpose of this chapter is to introduce the fundamental mechanical concepts underlying the study of linear motion, in particular Newton's laws of motion and gravitation.

SPACE AND NEWTONIAN FRAME OF REFERENCE

In mechanics, position and change in position of a body in space is defined in relation to a newtonian frame of reference (after Isaac Newton). In a newtonian frame of reference, the three dimensions of space (forward–backward, side-to-side, up–down) are represented by three orthogonal axes (three lines at right angles to each other) that intersect at a point called the origin (Fig. 2.1). The three axes are usually referred to as the X (forward–backward), Y (vertical) and Z (side-to-side) axes. Each axis has a positive and a negative sense with respect to the origin. Forward is positive and backward is negative on the X axis, upward is positive and downward is negative on the Y axis. Positive Z may be to the left or to the right, giving rise to the so-called left-handed and right-handed axis systems respectively. In the right-handed axis system, as shown in Figure 2.1, positive Z is to the right. If the

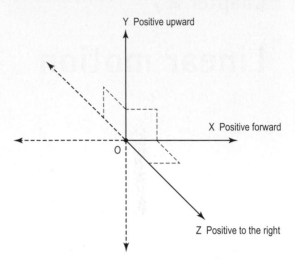

Fig. 2.1   The right-handed axis system: O = origin

thumb and first two fingers of the right hand are held at right angles to each other with the index finger pointing forward (positive X) and the second finger pointing upward (positive Y), then the thumb will point to the right (positive Z); hence the name right-handed axis system. The right-handed axis system is the most widely used system. The right-handed axis system will be used in this book.

In a newtonian frame of reference, the position of a point is defined by the coordinates of the point with respect to the three axes, i.e. the lengths x, y and z along the X, Y and Z axes that correspond to the point. The coordinates of a point are listed in the order x, y and z. For example, the coordinates of the points A, B and C in Figure 2.2 are (0,0,2), (0,3,2) and (4,3,2) respectively. The three axes give rise to three orthogonal planes, XY, YZ, XZ (Fig. 2.3). Analysis of human movement may be concerned with movement along an axis (such as the movement of the body as a whole along the X axis in a 100 m sprint), in a plane (such as the movement of the head in the XY plane in a 100 m sprint) or in three-dimensional space.

> In a newtonian frame of reference, the three dimensions of space are represented by three orthogonal axes that intersect at a point called the origin.

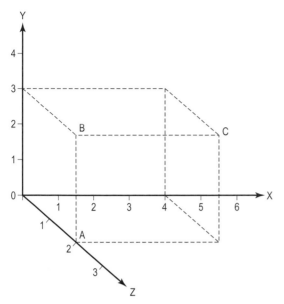

Fig. 2.2   Coordinates of points in the right-handed axis system: A (0,0,2), B(0,3,2), C(4,3,2)

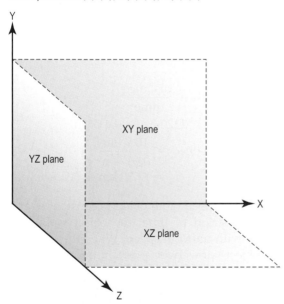

Fig. 2.3   Reference planes in the right-handed axis system

ANATOMICAL FRAME OF REFERENCE

In order to describe the spatial orientation of a particular part of the body in relation to another, it is necessary to use standard terminology

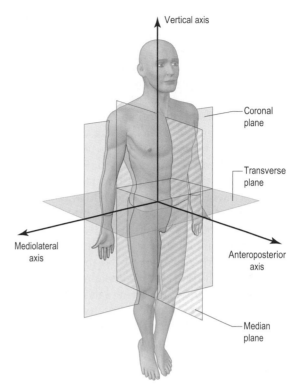

Fig. 2.4   Anatomical frame of reference

with reference to a standard body posture. The generally accepted convention, referred to as the anatomical, relative or cardinal frame of reference, utilizes the right-handed newtonian frame of reference axis system in relation to a standard body posture called the anatomical position. In the anatomical position, the body is upright with the arms by the sides and palms of the hands facing forward. The anatomical frame of reference (Fig. 2.4) describes three principal planes (median, coronal, transverse) and three principal axes (anteroposterior, vertical, mediolateral).

The median plane is a vertical plane that divides the body down the middle into more-or-less symmetrical left and right portions. The median plane is also frequently referred to as the sagittal plane; the terms sagittal, paramedian and parasagittal (para = beside or against) are also sometimes used to refer to any plane parallel to the median plane. In this book the term sagittal is used to refer to any plane parallel to the median plane. The mediolateral axis is perpendicular to the median plane. The terms lateral and medial are used to describe the position of structures with respect to the mediolateral axis. Lateral means further away from the median plane and medial means closer to the median plane. For example, in the anatomical position, the fingers of each hand are medial to the thumbs (and the thumbs are lateral to the fingers). Lateral and medial are also used to describe the direction of forces acting on the body in a mediolateral direction. For example, a laterally directed force acting on the right foot tends to move the body to the right and a medially directed force acting on the right foot tends to move the body to the left.

The coronal plane (or frontal plane) is a vertical plane perpendicular to the median plane that divides the body into anterior and posterior portions. The anteroposterior axis is perpendicular to the coronal plane. The terms anterior (in front of) and posterior (behind) are used to describe the position of structures with respect to the anteroposterior axis. For example, in the anatomical position, the toes of each foot are anterior to the heels (and the heels are posterior to the toes). The terms ventral and dorsal are synonymous with anterior and posterior respectively.

The transverse plane is a horizontal plane, perpendicular to both the median and coronal planes, that divides the body into upper and lower portions. The vertical axis is perpendicular to the transverse plane. The terms superior (above) and inferior (below) are used to describe the position of structures with respect to the vertical axis. For example, in the anatomical position, the head is superior to the shoulders (and the shoulders inferior to the head).

There are some spatial terms that apply to some segments, but not to others. For example, the terms proximal and distal are normally only used in reference to the limb segments (upper arm, forearm, hand, thigh, shank, foot). Superior parts or features of the segments (with respect to the anatomical position) are referred to as proximal, whereas inferior parts or features are referred to as distal. For example, the proximal end of the right upper arm articulates with the trunk to form the right shoulder joint. Similarly, the distal end of the right upper arm

articulates with the proximal end of the right forearm to form the right elbow joint.

> The anatomical frame of reference describes three principal planes (median, coronal, transverse) and three principal axes (anteroposterior, vertical, mediolateral).

DISTANCE AND SPEED

The length of the line between two points in three-dimensional space is referred to as the distance between the points. Similarly, the length of the path followed by a body as it moves from one position to another in three-dimensional space is referred to as the distance travelled by the body. Speed is defined as rate of change of position, i.e. the distance travelled in moving from one position to another divided by the length of time taken to change position. For example, if a cross country runner completes the race distance of 10.7 km (6.65 miles) in 37 min 2.5 s, his average speed during the run is given by:

$$\text{average speed} = \frac{\text{distance}}{\text{time}}$$

37 min 2.5 s = 2222.5 s = 0.6174 h

$$\text{i.e. average speed} = \frac{10.7\,\text{km}}{0.6174\,\text{h}}$$
$$= 17.33\,\text{km/h}\ (10.77\,\text{mph})$$

When the speed of an object is constant over a certain period of time, the object is said to move with uniform speed. When the speed of an object varies over a certain period of time, the object is moving with non-uniform speed.

Analysis of the speed of human movement is important in all sports where time is the determinant of performance, such as track athletics and swimming. Knowledge of the average speed and the variation in speed of an athlete during a race is likely to have implications for the training of the athlete. For example, an endurance athlete aiming to run 5000 m in 13 min would need to achieve an average speed of 6.41 m/s, i.e.

$$\text{average speed} = \frac{5000\,\text{m}}{780\,\text{s}} = 6.41\,\text{m/s}$$

However, average lap time would probably be more useful to the athlete and coach. Since there are 12.5 laps (1 lap = 400 m) in a 5000 m race, an average speed of 6.41 m/s corresponds to an average lap time of 62.4 s/lap, i.e.

$$\text{average lap time} = \frac{780\,\text{s}}{12.5\,\text{laps}} = 62.4\,\text{s/lap}$$

> Analysis of the speed of human movement is important in all sports where time is the determinant of performance, such as track athletics and swimming.

AVERAGE SPEED IN A MARATHON RACE

Table 2.1 shows the 5 km split times and average speeds in the 5 km splits of the winner (Paula Radcliffe, UK) of the 2005 women's London marathon. The average speed of the runner over the whole race was 5.11 m/s (11.43 mph), i.e.

distance = 26 miles 385 yd = 42.195 km
time = 2 h 17 min 42 s = 8262 s

$$\text{average speed} = \frac{42\,195\,\text{m}}{8262\,\text{s}} = 5.11\,\text{m/s}$$

The distance–time data (columns 1 and 2 of Table 2.1) are plotted in the distance–time graph in Figure 2.5. The graph is close to linear, indicating little variation in speed throughout the race. This is reflected in the 5 km split times, which range between 15 min 47 s and 16 min 40 s and the corresponding average speed in the 5 km splits, which ranges between 5.00 m/s and 5.28 m/s. The average speed over the final 2.195 km of the race was 5.03 m/s. The average speed–time data are plotted in the average speed–time graph in Figure 2.5. Since the speed data are average speeds, each data point is plotted at the midpoint of the corresponding time interval.

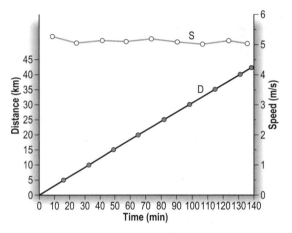

Fig. 2.5 Distance–time graph (D) and average speed–time graph (S) of the winner of the 2005 women's London marathon: see data in Table 2.1

Table 2.1 Race time, time after each 5 km, 5 km split times and average speed in the 5 km splits of the winner of the 2005 women's London marathon

Distance (km)	Time (min:s)	5 km split time* (min:s)	Average speed in each 5 km split* (m/s)
5	15:47	15:47	5.28
10	32:17	16:30	5.05
15	48:34	16:17	5.12
20	65:55	16:21	5.10
25	81:03	16:08	5.17
30	97:27	16:24	5.08
35	114:07	16:40	5.00
40	130:26	16:19	5.11
42.195	137:42	7:16	5.03

* The time for the final 2.195 km of the race was 7 min 16 s, resulting in an average speed of 5.03 m/s.

EFFECT OF RUNNING WIDE IN MIDDLE–DISTANCE TRACK EVENTS

A runner's energy reserves are fixed at the start of a race and, consequently, in order to maximize performance, correct pace judgement is essential. Ideally, the runner would be completely exhausted, i.e. have used all his/her available energy reserves as s/he crosses the finish line. The runner's fixed energy reserves will determine the maximum average speed that s/he can maintain during the race. The runner's maximum average speed will also depend upon the distance covered, i.e. the longer the distance the lower the average speed that can be maintained. Whereas the race distance is ostensibly fixed, the distance covered by the runner is not, i.e. it is likely, if only as a result of overtaking, that a runner will run further than the race distance. For example, if a runner completes one lap of a 400 m track on the inside of the second lane, s/he will run 7.04 m further than if s/he had run on the inside of the first lane (Jones & Whipp 2002).

In the finals of the men's 800 m and 5000 m at the Sydney 2000 Olympic Games, the pre-race favourite in each race was beaten into second place. Jones & Whipp (2002) investigated the possible effect of actual distance covered on the performances of the first- and second-placed runners in each race. Using slow-motion video playback, the actual distances covered by the runners were calculated. The results are shown in Tables 2.2 and 2.3.

The 800 m race was won in 1 min 45.08 s by Schumann (Germany), who ran close to the kerb throughout the race and covered a total distance of 802 m at an average speed of 7.63 m/s. Kipketer (Denmark) finished in second place in a time of 1 min 45.14 s. In contrast to Schumann, Kipketer ran in lanes 2 and 3 throughout the race and covered a total distance of 813 m at an average speed of 7.73 m/s. Schumann won the race even though his average speed during the race was 0.1 m/s slower than Kipketer, but he ran 11 m less than Kipketer. Based on their average velocities, Schumann and Kipketer should have been able to cover the actual race distance of 800 m in times of 1 min 44.84 s and 1 min 43.49 s respectively. This suggests that

Table 2.2   Distance covered, race time, average speed and time to cover race distance at average speed of the gold and silver medal winners in the men's 800 m at the Sydney 2000 Olympic Games

	Schumann (Germany)	Kipketer (Denmark)	Schumann relative to Kipketer
Position in race	1	2	
Distance run (m)	802	813	−11
Race time (min:s)	1:45.08	1:45.14	−0.06
Average speed (m/s)	7.63	7.73	−0.10
Time to cover 800 m at average speed (min:s)	1:44.84	1.43.49	+1.35

Table 2.3   Distance covered, race time, average speed and time to cover race distance at average speed of the gold and silver medal winners in the men's 5000 m at the Sydney 2000 Olympic Games

	Wolde (Ethiopia)	Saidi–Sief (Algeria)	Wolde relative to Saidi–Sief
Position in race	1	2	
Distance run (m)	5022	5028	−6
Race time (min:s)	13:35.49	13:36.20	−0.71
Average speed (m/s)	6.158	6.160	−0.002
Time to cover 5000 m at average speed (min:s)	13:31.95	13.31.69	+0.26

Kipketer might have been able to win the race if his race tactics had been more closely related to his energy reserves.

The situation in the 5000 m race was similar to that in the 800 m race. The race was won by Wolde (Ethiopia) in 13 min 35.49 s at an average speed of 6.158 m/s. Saidi-Sief (Algeria) finished in second place in 13 min 36.2 s at an average speed of 6.160 m/s. Whereas Wolde ran close to the kerb whenever possible, Saidi-Sief tended to run on the outside shoulder of the leader. Wolde won the race even though his average speed during the race was 0.002 m/s slower than Saidi-Sief, but he ran 6 m less than Saidi-Sief.

Based on their average velocities, Wolde and Saidi-Sief should have been able to cover the actual race distance of 5000 m in times of 13 min 31.95 s and 13 min 31.69 s respectively. This suggests that Saidi-Sief might have been able to win the race if his race tactics had been more closely related to his energy reserves. Jones & Whipp (2002) concluded that performance in middle-distance running events is dependent not only on energy reserves but also on race tactics in terms of total distance covered.

LINEAR KINEMATIC ANALYSIS OF A 100 M SPRINT

Whereas an analysis of performance based on average speed is likely to be useful to athlete and coach in middle and long-distance running events, average speed is of limited value in the short sprints of 100 m and 200 m. In these events, the aim of the sprinter is to achieve maximum speed as soon as possible and then maintain it to the end of the race. Consequently, analysis of the variation in speed during the race rather than average speed is likely to provide the most useful performance indicators. These include:

- Time taken to achieve maximum speed
- Maximum speed
- Length of time that maximum speed is maintained
- Difference between maximum speed and speed at the finish.

In order to produce a speed–time graph, it is first of all necessary to obtain distance–time data. The most frequently used method of recording sprint performance for the purpose of obtaining distance–time data is video.

VIDEO RECORDINGS FOR MOVEMENT ANALYSIS

A video recording consists of a series of discrete images of the subject separated by a fixed time interval. The time interval between images is determined by the frame rate setting of the camera, i.e. the number of images (frames) recorded per second. In the SI system of units, frequency (the rate at which a periodic event or cycle of events occurs) is measured in hertz (Hz), i.e. the number of times that the event occurs per second ($1 Hz = 1/s$). The minimum frame rate available on most standard digital video cameras is 25 Hz. The human eye cannot detect discrete changes in the environment that occur more frequently than approximately 15 Hz. Consequently, to the human eye, a video playing at 25 Hz appears to be continuous rather than a series of discrete images. Whereas the frame rate of a digital video camera may be 25 Hz, the way that the images are stored by the camera allows the user to view discrete images at twice the frame rate, i.e. 50 Hz. Many analyses of human movement are based on measurements taken from sequences of discrete images in video recordings.

The type of analysis that can be carried out will depend upon the frame rate (which will determine the number of discrete images of the action under consideration) and the exposure (which will determine the sharpness and brightness of the images). The required frame rate of a recording will be determined by the duration of the action under consideration. For example, whereas 25 Hz is adequate for most types of human locomotion, such as walking and running (Winter 1990), a much higher frame rate is normally needed to adequately record high-speed/short-duration events such as impacts. For example, the contact time between clubhead and ball during a golf drive is approximately 0.0005 s, i.e. half a millisecond (0.5 ms) or 1/2000th of a second (Daish 1972). A frame rate in the region of 10000 Hz would provide only five images of this type of impact:

Number of images = frame rate × contact time
= 10 000 Hz (images/s) ×
0.0005 s
= 5 images

The contact time between a tennis racket and ball during impact is approximately 0.005 s i.e. 5 ms or 1/200th of a second (Daish 1972). A frame rate of 2000 Hz would provide approximately 10 images of this type of impact:

Number of images = frame rate × contact time
= 2000 Hz (images/s) ×
0.005 s
= 10 images

Exposure determines the sharpness (of contours and particular reference points) and brightness of the images. Sharpness is determined by the shutter speed setting of the camera, i.e. the length of time that the image sensor of the camera is exposed to the image. The faster the shutter speed, the sharper the image. A shutter speed of 0.002 s (1/500th of a second) is usually adequate to capture sharp images in fast human movement. However, the faster the shutter speed, the shorter the duration of the exposure. This has to be balanced with the aperture setting of the camera (referred to as the f-stop), which determines the amount of light entering the camera during the exposure to ensure that the images are not too light or too dark.

> Many analyses of human movement are based on measurements taken from sequences of discrete images in video recordings. The type of analysis that can be carried out will depend upon the frame rate and the exposure.

DISTANCE–TIME AND SPEED–TIME DATA FROM VIDEO ANALYSIS

Video was used to record the performance of a 19-year-old male junior international sprinter as he sprinted 100 m with maximum effort on a straight, level track (frame rate = 25 Hz; shutter speed = 0.002 s; aperture = f8). Figure 2.6 shows

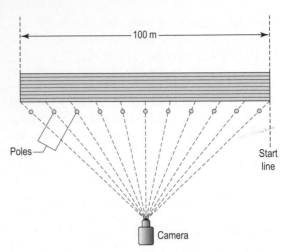

Fig. 2.6 Layout of the video camera, track and sighting poles for recording a 100 m sprint for the purpose of obtaining distance–time data

the layout of the camera and track. The camera was placed close to the centre of the infield area, in line with the 50 m mark on the track.

Prior to videotaping the sprint, the inside lane, i.e. the lane nearest to the camera, was marked at 10 m intervals from the start line. The sprinter was then asked to stand at the 10 m mark while a white wooden pole was placed in the infield area approximately 1 m away from the track on a line between the camera lens and the sprinter. This procedure was repeated at each of the other nine 10 m marks, the last one being the finish line. The sprinter was then videotaped as he ran 100 m flat out under normal race start conditions. By viewing the video frame by frame (50 Hz) from the start of the run, the time taken by the sprinter to run the first 10 m, the first 20 m, the first 30 m, etc. up to 100 m was estimated by counting the frames and multiplying the number of frames by the frame rate, i.e. 0.02 s (1/50th of a second). The results are presented in the second column of Table 2.4. Column 3 of Table 2.4 shows the time for each successive 10 m of the sprint. Based on this data, the average speed of the sprinter in each successive 10 m is shown in column 4 of Table 2.4. For example,

$$\text{average speed over the first 10 m} = \frac{10\,\text{m}}{1.92\,\text{s}}$$
$$= 5.21\,\text{m/s}$$

Table 2.4 Cumulative distance, cumulative time, time for each successive 10 m and average speed during each successive 10 m in a 100 m sprint by a male junior international athlete

Distance (m)	Cumulative time (s)	Time for 10 m (s)	Average speed for 10 m (m/s)
10	1.92	1.92	5.21
20	3.10	1.18	8.47
30	4.16	1.06	9.43
40	5.06	0.90	11.11
50	6.08	1.02	9.80
60	7.00	0.92	10.87
70	8.02	1.02	9.80
80	9.04	1.02	9.80
90	10.02	0.98	10.20
100	11.12	1.10	9.09

Elite performance in the 100 m sprint is characterized by a rapid increase in speed just after the start followed by a more gradual increase in speed up to maximum speed, which is then maintained till the end of the race (Wagner 1998, Murase et al 1976). The average speed–time data in column 4 of Table 2.4 does not indicate a smooth change in speed; indeed the data indicate marked fluctuations in speed during the last 60 m, involving two phases of increasing speed alternating with three phases of decreasing speed. This almost certainly reflects error in the distance–time data from which the average speed–time data was obtained. Timing errors could be related to the variation in body position of the sprinter at each 10 m marker and the restriction of the frame rate, which both create difficulties in trying to locate the same point on the body, such as the pelvic region, at each marker post. More accurate distance–time data can be obtained from a 'line of best fit' distance–time graph. The line of best fit is a line drawn through the distance–time data that more accurately reflects the normal changes in speed during a 100 m sprint, i.e. a progressive smooth change in speed (absence of marked fluctuations in speed) involving an increase in speed up to maximum speed followed by maintenance of maximum speed or slight decrease in speed toward the end of the race. Figure 2.7 shows the distance–time data (columns 1 and 2 of Table 2.4 plotted on square-centimetre graph paper) and the corresponding

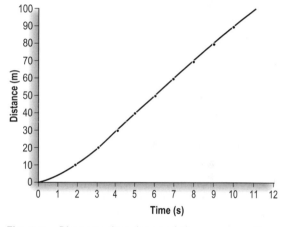

Fig. 2.7 Distance–time data and the corresponding line of best fit distance–time graph

line of best fit distance–time graph. Some of the distance–time data points lie on the line of best fit graph but others do not. Very small errors in distance–time data will result in much larger errors in speed–time data derived from it.

To obtain more accurate distance–time data from the line of best fit distance–time graph, parallel lines perpendicular to the distance axis are drawn to intersect the distance axis at intervals of 1 s (Fig. 2.8). The points of intersection with the distance axis indicate the cumulative distance after successive intervals of 1 s (column 2 of Table 2.5). The distance covered in each 1 s interval (column 3 of Table 2.5) and, therefore, the average speed in each 1 s interval (column 4 of Table 2.5) can then be calculated. Unlike the average speed–time data obtained directly from the original distance–time data (column 4 of Table 2.4), the average speed–time data obtained from the line of best fit distance–time graph (column 4 of Table 2.5) indicate that the speed of the sprinter increased fairly smoothly to a maximum value and then gradually decreased. This is typical of maximal effort sprinting over 100 m.

The average speed–time data obtained from the line of best fit distance–time graph (column 4 of Table 2.5) are plotted in Figure 2.9 together with the line of best fit average speed–time graph. Since the average speed–time data represent average speeds, each data point is plotted at the midpoint of the corresponding time interval. The line of best fit distance–time graph is also shown in Figure 2.9. Note the shallow S shape of the distance–time graph (look along the graph at eye level). The dotted vertical line

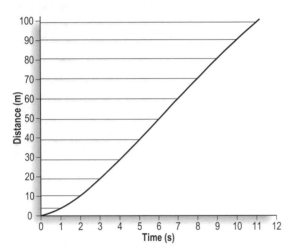

Fig. 2.8 Method of determination of distance–time data from the line of best fit distance–time graph

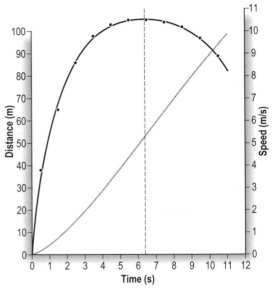

Fig. 2.9 Line of best fit distance–time and speed–time graphs together with average speed–time data points obtained from the line of best fit distance–time graph

Table 2.5 Cumulative time, cumulative distance, distance covered in each one second interval and average velocity in each one second interval in a 100 m sprint by a male junior international athlete

Time (s)	Cumulative distance (m)	Distance travelled in each second (m)	Average speed in each second (m/s)
1	3.8	3.8	3.8
2	10.3	6.5	6.5
3	18.9	8.6	8.6
4	28.7	9.8	9.8
5	39.0	10.3	10.3
6	49.5	10.5	10.5
7	60.0	10.5	10.5
8	70.4	10.4	10.4
9	80.6	10.2	10.2
10	90.3	9.7	9.7
11	99.2	8.9	8.9

distinguishes the two main phases of the run. The first phase is characterized by a progressive increase in the slope of the distance–time graph, corresponding to a progressive increase in speed to maximum speed of about 10.5 m/s (0–6.4 s, 0–53 m). The second phase is characterized by a progressive decrease in the slope of the distance–time graph corresponding to a steady decrease in speed to a finishing speed of approximately 8.2 m/s (6.4–11.12 s, 53–100 m). The average speed–time data in column 4 of Table 2.5 indicate a brief period of constant maximum speed (5.5–6.5 s), but this is not evident in the line of best fit average speed–time graph.

In order to show that the distance–time and speed–time graphs in Figure 2.9 were truly representative of the sprinter's performance, it would be necessary to repeat the process on a number of trials, not just the one described here. However, assuming that the graphs in Figure 2.9 were representative, it would be useful to compare the speed–time graph with that of a senior elite sprinter in order to highlight areas for improvement. Figure 2.10 shows the junior international sprinter's speed–time graph (as in Figure 2.9) in relation to that of Carl Lewis (USA) in the final of the 100 m at the 1987 World

Athletics Championships in Rome (Wagner 1998). Lewis finished second in a time of 9.93 s. Table 2.6 shows a comparison of the performances of the two sprinters. Whereas Lewis took longer to achieve maximum speed (7.5 s, 6.4 s), he was far superior to the junior athlete in relation to maximum speed (11.7 m/s, 10.5 m/s), length of time that maximum speed was maintained (2.4 s, 0 s) and finishing speed (11.7 m/s, 8.2 m/s).

ACCELERATION

Acceleration is defined as rate of change of speed, i.e. change in speed divided by the length of time in which the change in speed occurred

$$a = \frac{v - u}{t_2 - t_1}$$

where a = acceleration, u = speed at time t_1 and v = speed at some later time t_2.

When the speed of a body increases during a particular period of time, the acceleration is positive. When the speed of a body decreases during a particular period of time, the acceleration is negative. Negative acceleration is usually referred to as deceleration.

The speed–time graph of the junior international sprinter shown in Figure 2.10 shows that his speed increased from zero at the start to a maximum speed of about 10.5 m/s in about 6.0 s. Consequently, his acceleration during this period is given by:

$$a = \frac{v - u}{t_2 - t_1} = \frac{10.5 \, \text{m/s} - 0 \, \text{m/s}}{6.0 \, \text{s} - 0 \, \text{s}}$$
$$= 1.75 \, \text{m/s}^2 \text{ (metres per second per second)}$$

i.e. his speed increased at an average of 1.75 m/s for each second between the start and 6.0 s into the run. Figure 2.10 also shows that his speed decreased from a maximum speed of 10.5 m/s at about 6.5 s to about 8.2 m/s at the end of the run, which was completed in 11.12 s, i.e.

$$a = \frac{v - u}{t_2 - t_1} = \frac{8.2 \, \text{m/s} - 10.5 \, \text{m/s}}{11.12 \, \text{s} - 6.5 \, \text{s}}$$
$$= \frac{-2.3 \, \text{m/s}}{4.62 \, \text{s}} = -0.50 \, \text{m/s}^2$$

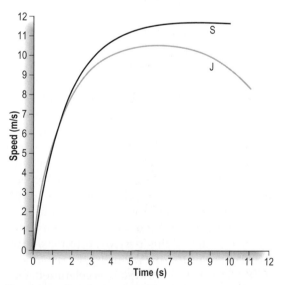

Fig. 2.10 Speed–time graphs for a male junior international sprinter (J) and a male senior (S) elite sprinter in the 100 m sprint

Table 2.6   Comparison of performance of a male junior international (time = 11.12 s) with that of a senior elite sprinter (Carl Lewis, USA, final of the 1987 World Athletics Championships in Rome; time = 9.93 s) in the 100 m sprint

	Junior international	Senior elite
Time taken to achieve maximum speed (s)	6.4	7.5
Maximum speed (m/s)	10.5	11.7
Length of time that maximum speed was maintained (s)	0	2.4
Finishing speed (m/s)	8.2	11.7
Difference between maximum speed and speed at the finish (m/s)	−2.3	0

Table 2.7   Cumulative time, cumulative speed, change in speed in each one second interval and average acceleration in each one second interval in a 100 m sprint by a male junior international athlete

Time (s)	Cumulative speed (m/s)	Change in speed in each second (s)	Average acceleration in each second (m/s^2)
1	5.35	5.35	5.35
2	7.80	2.45	2.45
3	9.25	1.45	1.45
4	10.00	0.75	0.75
5	10.38	0.38	0.38
6	10.50	0.12	0.12
7	10.50	0	0
8	10.30	−0.20	−0.20
9	9.90	−0.40	−0.40
10	9.30	−0.60	−0.60
11	8.25	−1.05	−1.05

The negative sign indicates that the sprinter was decelerating during the period under consideration, i.e. his speed decreased at an average of 0.50 m/s for each second during the period 6.5 s to the end of the run.

Using the same method used to obtain distance–time data from the line of best fit distance–time graph, the speed of the junior international sprinter after each second of the run was obtained from the line of best fit speed–time graph in Figure 2.9. This data is shown in column 2 of Table 2.7. Column 3 of Table 2.7 shows the change in speed during each second of the run and the corresponding average acceleration of the sprinter in each one

second interval is shown in column 4 of Table 2.7. The average acceleration–time data (plotted at the midpoints of the corresponding time intervals) and line of best fit acceleration–time graph are shown in Figure 2.11 together with the corresponding distance–time and speed–time graphs. The acceleration–time graph shows that the sprinter's acceleration was positive for about 6.4 s, i.e. his speed increased progressively during this period up to maximum speed of about 10.5 m/s. During the remainder of the sprint, the sprinter's acceleration was negative, resulting in a steady decrease in speed. Whereas it was not possible to estimate the acceleration of the sprinter just after the

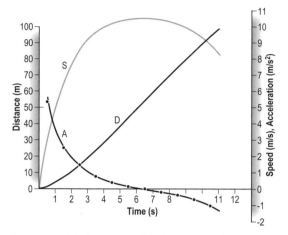

Fig. 2.11   Distance–time (D), speed–time (S) and acceleration–time (A) graphs of a male junior international sprinter in a 100 m sprint

start, data reported by Baumann (1976) indicates that, 0.2 s after the start, acceleration would be approximately 13 m/s² for this standard of sprinter (100 m time of 10.9–11.4 s). This is consistent with the acceleration–time data in Figure 2.11.

Practical worksheet 1 involves the collection of distance–time data over a 15 m sprint, which is then used to produce the corresponding distance–time, speed–time and acceleration–time graphs.

VECTOR AND SCALAR QUANTITIES

All quantities in the physical and life sciences can be categorized as either scalar or vector quantities. Quantities that can be completely specified by their magnitude (size) are called scalar quantities. These include volume, area, time, temperature, mass, distance and speed. Quantities that require specification in both magnitude and direction are called vector quantities. These include displacement (distance in a given direction), velocity (speed in a given direction), acceleration and force. A vector quantity can be represented by a straight line with an arrow head. The length of the line, with respect to an appropriate scale, corresponds to the magnitude of the quantity and the orientation of the line and arrow head, with respect to an appropriate reference axis (usually horizontal or vertical) indicates the direction.

> All quantities in the physical and life sciences can be categorized as either scalar or vector quantities. Quantities that can be completely specified by their magnitude (size) are called scalar quantities. Quantities that require specification in both magnitude and direction are called vector quantities.

DISPLACEMENT VECTORS

If a man runs 3 miles from a point A to a point B and then walks 2 miles from point B to a point C, it is clear that he has travelled a total distance of 5 miles. However, it is not possible to determine the position of C with respect to A since no information is given concerning the directions in which he ran and walked. However, if we are given the directions as well as the distances, we are then dealing with vector quantities, i.e. displacements and can, therefore, determine the position of C in relation to A. For example, if we are told that the man ran 3 miles due north from A to B and then walked 2 miles due east from B to C, the position of C in relation to A can be determined by considering the displacement vectors *AB* and *BC*. The bold italics indicates a vector. The displacements *AB* and *BC* are shown in Figure 2.12a. The position of C in relation to A is specified by the vector *AC*, which is the vector sum of *AB* and *BC*, i.e. *AC* = *AB* + *BC*. The distance between A and C can be determined by measuring the line AC and converting this to miles using the distance scale. The direction of C in relation to A is specified by the angle θ. *AC* is referred to as the resultant vector of *AB* and *BC*, and *AB* and *BC* are referred to as component vectors. *AC* (3.6 miles N 33° E) is the resultant displacement of the man from the point A. Vector addition is clearly not the same as arithmetic (scalar) addition.

If the man walked 2 miles due south from C to a point D, the position of D in relation to A would be specified by the vector *AD* (Fig. 2.12b).

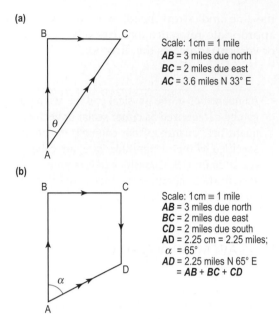

(a)

Scale: 1 cm ≡ 1 mile
AB = 3 miles due north
BC = 2 miles due east
AC = 3.6 miles N 33° E

(b)

Scale: 1 cm ≡ 1 mile
AB = 3 miles due north
BC = 2 miles due east
CD = 2 miles due south
AD = 2.25 cm = 2.25 miles;
α = 65°
AD = 2.25 miles N 65° E
= **AB** + **BC** + **CD**

Fig. 2.12   Resultant of displacement vectors

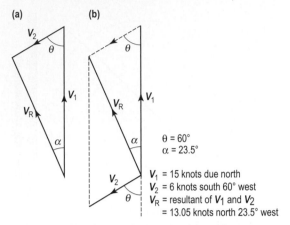

$\theta = 60°$
$\alpha = 23.5°$

V_1 = 15 knots due north
V_2 = 6 knots south 60° west
V_R = resultant of V_1 and V_2
= 13.05 knots north 23.5° west

Fig. 2.13   Resultant velocity of a ship without a keel. (a) Vector chain method. (b) Parallelogram of vectors method. Scale: 1 cm ≡ 5 knots

In this case, the resultant vector **AD** is the resultant of the three vectors **AB**, **BC** and **CD**. This example illustrates the fact that, irrespective of the number of component displacement vectors used to describe the movement of a body, the net result of all the component vectors can be specified by a single resultant displacement vector. This general principle applies to all vector quantities.

The method used in Figure 2.12 to determine the resultant of the component vectors is called the vector chain method, i.e. the component vectors are linked together in a chain (in any order) and the resultant vector runs from the starting point of the first component vector to the end point of the last component vector.

VELOCITY VECTORS

In addition to the vector chain method of determining the resultant of a number of component vectors, there is another method, the parallelogram of vectors, that is useful when there are only two component vectors but somewhat laborious when there are three or more component vectors. In this method two component

vectors extend from the same point to form adjacent sides of a parallelogram. The resultant of the two component vectors is given by the diagonal of the completed parallelogram. For example, if a ship without a keel starts to sail due north in a wind blowing S 60° W, the resultant velocity of the ship is specified by the resultant of the velocity V_1 of the ship resulting from the drive of the engines and the velocity V_2 of the ship resulting from the wind. The vector chain and parallelogram of vectors methods of determining the resultant velocity of the ship are shown in Figure 2.13. If V_1 = 15 knots due north and V_2 = 6 knots S 60° W, the resultant velocity of the ship V_R = 13.05 knots N 23.5° W.

When using the parallelogram of vectors method to determine the resultant of three or more component vectors, the first step is to find the resultant R_1 of any two component vectors. The resultant of R_1 and another component vector is then found and the process is repeated until the resultant of all the component vectors is found.

In the above example of the ship without a keel, the component velocities were constant. However, component velocities are frequently variable, resulting in variable resultant velocities. Consider a rugby player attempting a penalty kick at goal. If there is no cross-wind, the kicker has only to kick the ball in the direction

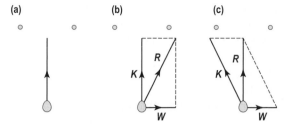

(a)   **(b)**   **(c)**

Fig. 2.14   Effect of a cross-wind on the direction of a rugby ball following a place kick. K = velocity due to the kick; W = velocity due to the wind; R = resultant of K and W

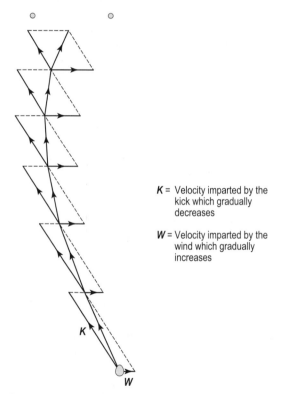

K = Velocity imparted by the kick which gradually decreases

W = Velocity imparted by the wind which gradually increases

Fig. 2.15   Effect of a cross-wind and air resistance on the direction of a rugby ball following a place kick

Even then, the ball does not travel in a straight line but along a curve, as shown in Figure 2.15. Assuming that the wind continues to blow throughout the period of ball flight, the speed of the ball imparted by the wind will gradually increase during the flight. However, the speed of the ball imparted by the kick will gradually decrease during the flight due to air resistance. Consequently, the direction of the ball will continually change (Fig. 2.15). In this example, it is assumed that the kick does not impart spin to the ball. The mechanics of a spinning ball are considered in Chapter 5.

CENTRE OF GRAVITY

The human body consists of a number of segments linked by joints. Each segment contributes to the body's total weight (Fig. 2.16a). Movement of the body segments relative to each other alters the weight distribution of the body. However, in any particular body posture the body behaves (in terms of the effect of body weight on the movement of the body) as if the total weight of the body is concentrated at a single point called the centre of gravity (also referred to as centre of mass) (Fig. 2.16b). Body weight acts vertically downward from the centre of gravity along a line called the line of action of body weight. The concept of centre of gravity applies to all bodies, animate and inanimate.

> The centre of gravity of an object is the point at which the whole weight of the object can be considered to act.

of the middle of the posts (Fig. 2.14a). However, if there is a cross-wind, the movement of the ball will be determined by the velocity K imparted by the kick and the velocity W imparted by the wind. If the kicker does not take account of the wind, the ball will not travel in the direction of the middle of the posts (Fig. 2.14b). A good kicker will take account of the wind such that the combined effect of the kick and the wind will direct the ball between the posts (Fig. 2.14c).

The position of an object's centre of gravity depends on the distribution of the weight of the object. For a regular-shaped object (of uniform density) such as a cube, oblong or sphere, the centre of gravity is located at the object's geometric centre (Fig. 2.17).

For an irregular-shaped object the centre of gravity may be inside or outside the object. For example, consider a triangle-shaped card with sides 15 cm, 20 cm and 25 cm in length, with

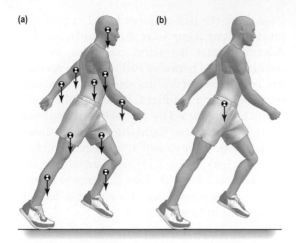

Fig. 2.16 (a) Centres of gravity of body segments and lines of action of the weights of the segments. (b) Centre of gravity of the whole body and line of action of body weight

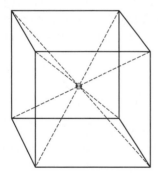

Fig. 2.17 The centre of gravity of a regular-shaped object of uniform density, such as a cube, is located at the geometric centre of the object

vertices A, B and C. Figure 2.18a shows the card suspended from a freely movable pin joint close to vertex A. The line of action of the weight of the card coincides with the vertical line through the point of suspension. By suspending a plumb line in front of the card from the same pin joint, the line of action of the weight of the card can be determined. Figure 2.18b and c show this process repeated from points of suspension close to vertices B and C respectively. In Figure 2.18d the lines of action of the weight of the card in positions 2 and 3 are shown superimposed on the line of action in position 1. The lines of action of the weight of the card in the three positions intersect at a single point, the centre of gravity of the card. In this example, the card's centre of gravity lies inside the body of the card.

Figure 2.19 shows the same process carried out with an L-shaped card with arms of length 15 cm and 20 cm and of width 4 cm. In this case the centre of gravity of the card is found to lie outside the body of the card (Fig. 2.19d).

The human body is an irregular shape. When standing upright, the centre of gravity of an adult is located inside the body close to the level of the navel (56.4 ± 2.8% of stature for females and 57.1 ± 2.3% of stature for males) and midway between the front and back of the body (Fig. 2.20a; Watkins 2000). Moving the arms forward to a horizontal position will move the centre of gravity slightly forward and upward (Fig. 2.20b). Moving the arms from this position to overhead (Fig. 2.20c) will move the

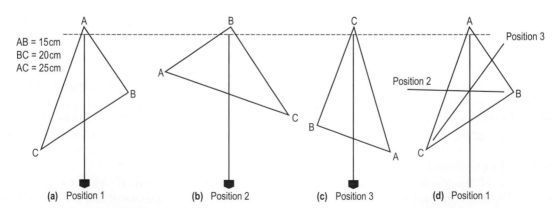

Fig. 2.18 Suspension method of locating the centre of gravity of an irregular-shaped object: a triangular piece of card

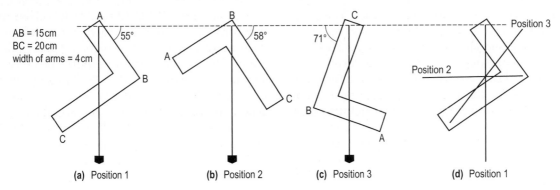

Fig. 2.19   Suspension method of locating the centre of gravity of an irregular-shaped object: an L-shaped piece of card

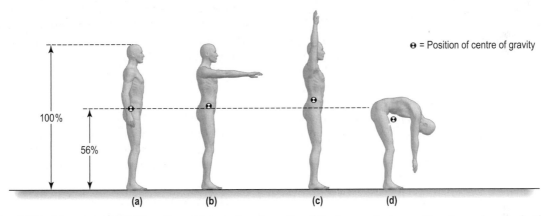

Fig. 2.20   Movement of the location of the centre of gravity of the human body resulting from changes in the mass distribution of the body

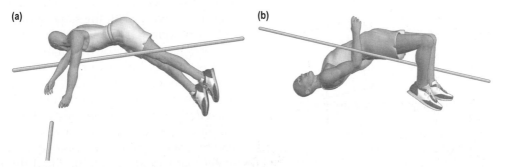

Fig. 2.21   During bar clearance in pole vault (a) and high jump (b) the centre of gravity of the body may lie outside the body

centre of gravity slightly backward and upward. Since the combined weight of both arms comprises about 11% of body weight, any movement of the arms results in a fairly slight change in the position of the centre of gravity. However, movement of the trunk, which comprises approximately 50% of body weight, will result in a relatively large change in the position of the centre of gravity. For example, full flexion of the trunk will result in the centre of gravity being located outside the body (Fig. 2.20d). This position is similar to the position adopted by a pole vaulter when clearing the bar (Fig. 2.21a). The body's centre of gravity may also be located outside the body during postures involving full extension of the trunk, as in clearing the bar using the Fosbury flop technique in high jumping (Fig. 2.21b). Movements involving continuous change in the orientation of body segments to each other, such as walking and running, result in continuous change in the position of the body's centre of gravity.

STABILITY

Figure 2.22 shows a regular cube-shaped block of wood resting on a horizontal surface. The centre of gravity of the block of wood is located at its geometric centre and the line of action of the weight of the wood intersects the base of support ABCD on which it is resting. If the block of wood is tilted over on any of the edges of the

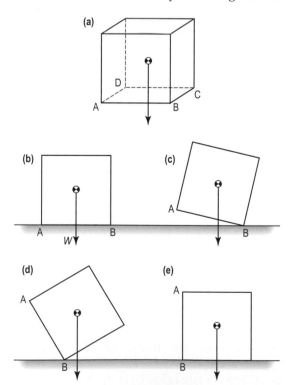

Fig. 2.22 The line of action of the weight of a cube in relation to its base of support

base of support, AB, BC, CD or AD, it will return to its original position provided that, at release, the line of action of its weight intersects the plane of the original base of support ABCD. This situation is shown in Figure 2.22c with respect to the edge BC. However, if, at release, the line of action of its weight does not intersect the original base of support, the block of wood will fall on to one of its other faces, as shown in Figure 2.22d and e. With respect to a particular base of support, an object is stable when the line of action of its weight intersects the plane of the base of support and unstable when it does not. Consequently, the block of wood in Figure 2.22 is stable with respect to the base of support ABCD in the positions shown in Figure 2.22b and c, and unstable with respect to the base of support ABCD in the position shown in Figure 2.22d.

> With respect to a particular base of support, an object is stable when the line of action of its weight intersects the plane of the base of support and unstable when it does not.

The stability of an object with respect to its base of support depends on the size of the base of support and the height of the object's centre of gravity above the base of support. Figure 2.23 shows two blocks of wood, 10 cm and 20 cm long respectively, with the same square cross-section of 4 cm × 4 cm. When the two pieces of wood rest on any of their larger faces the heights of their centres of gravity above the base of support are the same, i.e. 2 cm. With respect to the X axis (CD in the longer block of wood and RS in the shorter block of wood) the stability of the longer block of wood is greater than that of the shorter block of wood since the longer one would need to be tilted through a larger angle (79°) than the shorter one (68°) before it became unstable (Fig. 2.23c and d). However, with respect to the Y axis (AD in the longer block of wood and PS in the shorter block of wood) the stability of the two blocks is the same; each block would need to be tilted through an angle of 45° before it became unstable (Fig. 2.23e).

Clearly, for a given height of centre of gravity, the broader the base of support with respect to a particular axis of tilt, the greater the object's stability. In Figure 2.24a the longer block of wood is shown standing on one of its ends, and in Figure 2.24c the shorter block is shown standing on one of its ends. In this situation the dimensions of the base of support of each block are the same, but the centre of gravity of the taller block is 10 cm above its base and that of the shorter block is 5 cm above its base. When both blocks are tilted on one edge, the taller block becomes unstable after being tilted through a much smaller angle (11°) than the shorter block (22°). Consequently, in this situation the taller block is less stable than the shorter block.

It follows from the above examples that for any particular object the lower the ratio of the height of the centre of gravity to the length of the base of support (with respect to each possible tilt axis), the greater the stability of the object. This principle is used, for example, in the design of vehicles in order to minimize their risk of overturning during normal use.

With regard to human movement, the terms stability and balance are often used synonymously. Maintaining stability of the human body is a fairly complex, albeit largely unconscious, process (Roberts 1995). In upright standing the line of action of body weight intersects the base of support formed by the area beneath and

between the feet (Fig. 2.25a and b). The size of the base of support can be increased by moving the feet further apart. For example, moving one foot in front of the other increases anteroposterior stability, and moving one foot laterally increases side-to-side stability (Fig. 2.25c and d). Combining these movements with a degree of flexion of the hips, knees and ankles, as in certain movements in wrestling and boxing, reduces the height of the centre of gravity and thereby further increases stability.

Movement of the body from one base of support to another, such as in moving from standing to sitting, illustrates the unconscious way in which the balance systems of the body automatically redistribute body weight to maintain stability. Figure 2.26 shows a person moving from a standing position to sitting on a chair. The person moves his feet close to the front of the chair and then lowers his body by flexing his knees and bending his trunk forward while maintaining the same base of support, i.e. the area beneath and between his feet (Fig. 2.26a and b). He may or may not take hold of the sides of the chair as his thighs approach the seat of the chair. If he does take hold of the chair, his base of support immediately increases to include the area bounded by the legs of the chair as well as that beneath and between his feet, but the line of action of his body weight will still be over the area between his feet (Fig. 2.26c). When his thighs come close to the seat of the chair he begins to transfer his weight from over his feet to over the seat by gently rocking the trunk backward (Fig. 2.26d). These movements are reversed when moving from a sitting to a standing position.

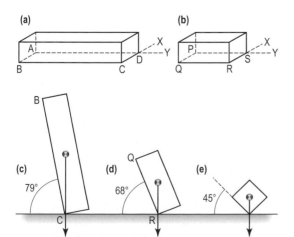

Fig. 2.23   The effect of the length of the base of support on stability

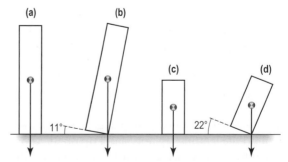

Fig. 2.24   The effect of the height of the centre of gravity above the base of support on stability

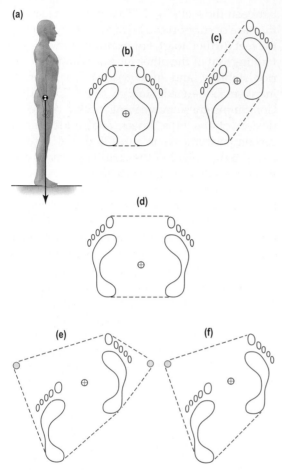

Fig. 2.25 The line of action of body weight in relation to the base of support. (a, b) Standing upright. (c) Standing upright with the right foot in front of the left foot. (d) Standing upright with feet apart, side-by-side. (e) Standing with the aid of crutches or two walking sticks. (f) Standing with the aid of a walking stick in the left hand. The symbol ⊕ denotes the point of intersection of the line of body weight with the base of support

Figure 2.27 shows a person stepping on to a chair. He initiates the movement by putting one foot on the chair. In order to step up with the other foot he must move his centre of gravity forward so that the line of action of his weight passes within a new base of support provided by the foot of the leading leg. He can then extend the leading leg and stand up on the chair. Therefore, in walking up a flight of stairs, the centre of gravity is continually shifted forward over the leading foot.

When bending forward from an upright position, a person's buttocks move backward in relation to his feet so that the line of action of his weight remains over his base of support (Fig. 2.28a and b). This can easily be demonstrated by asking someone to bend forward while standing with his/her back and heels against a wall. Since the buttocks are prevented from moving backward, the line of action of the person's weight soon passes in front of his/her base of support and s/he will fall forward unless s/he takes a step forward (Fig. 2.28c and d).

In general, the lower the centre of gravity and the larger the area of the base of support, the greater stability is likely to be. For example, by moving from a standing to a sitting position the body's centre of gravity is lowered and the area of the base of support is increased (Fig. 2.29a, b and c). The recumbent position is one of the most stable positions of the human body, since the area of the base of support is large and the centre of gravity is at its lowest (Fig. 2.29d). Spreading the arms and legs on the floor would further increase stability. As the area of the base of support increases, the degree of muscular effort needed to maintain stability tends to decrease. For example, it is usually easier, in terms of muscular effort, to maintain stability when standing on both feet than when standing on one foot. Similarly, it is usually less tiring to sit than to stand, and less tiring to lie down than to sit. A person recovering from a leg injury may use crutches or a walking stick in order to relieve the load on the injured limb. The use of crutches also increases the area of the base of support and makes it easier for the user to maintain stability (Fig. 2.25e and f).

Adequate stability is vital for good performance in all sports. For example, in boxing, in order to apply a rapid powerful forward jab (Fig. 2.30) the boxer needs to ensure that he has adequate stability so that he can apply a large force without losing his balance as a result of the equal and opposite force exerted on his fist. This is achieved by putting one foot in front of the other, which considerably increases his stability in the direction of the punch. Similarly, a

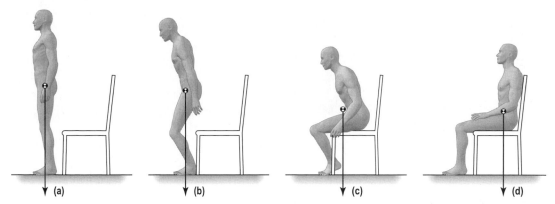

Fig. 2.26 The line of action of body weight in relation to the base of support when moving from standing to sitting

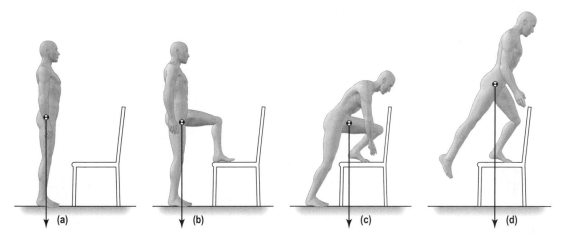

Fig. 2.27 The line of action of body weight in relation to the base of support when stepping on to a chair

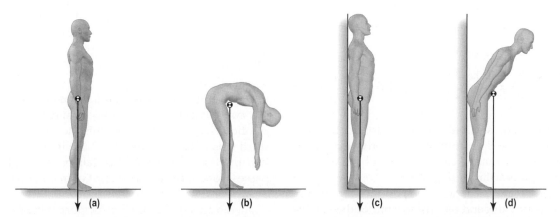

Fig. 2.28 The line of action of body weight in relation to the base of support when (a) standing, (b) bending forward, (c) standing against a wall and (d) bending forward from a standing position against a wall

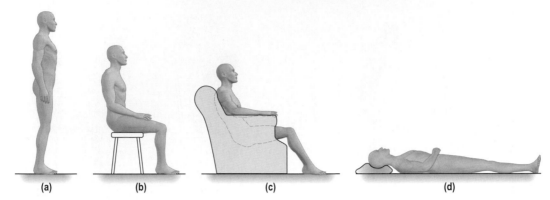

Fig. 2.29   (a) Standing, (b, c) sitting and (d) lying postures

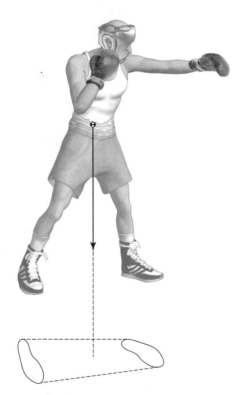

Fig. 2.30   The line of action of the weight of a boxer in relation to his base of support when making a punch

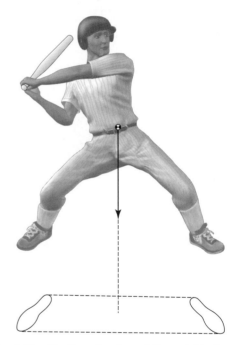

Fig. 2.31   The line of action of the weight of a baseball player in relation to his base of support when hitting the ball

baseball or soft ball player will tend to place one foot well in front of the other when hitting the ball so that he can hit the ball hard without losing his balance (Fig. 2.31).

In certain situations in sport, good performance may depend on unstable rather than stable postures. For example, in the set position of a sprint start the sprinter tends to move his/her centre of gravity as far forward as possible without overbalancing in order to obtain the best position from which to drive his/her body forward when the gun goes (Fig. 2.32). In this position the line of action of his/her body weight passes close to the anterior limit of his/her base of support.

As the area of the base of support decreases, the degree of tolerance in the movement of the line of action of body weight also decreases if

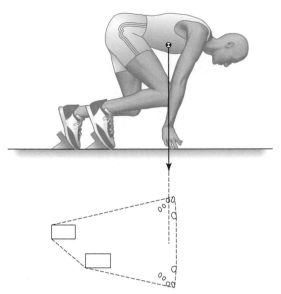

Fig. 2.32   The line of action of the weight of a sprinter in the set position in relation to his base of support

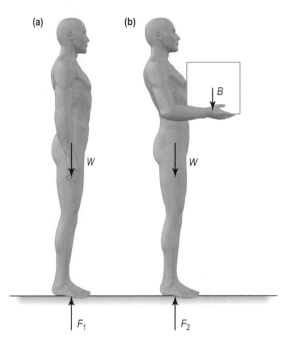

Fig. 2.33   Compression load on the body in upright postures. W = body weight; B = weight of object; F_1, F_2 = ground reaction forces

stability is to be maintained. When the base of support becomes a knife-edge or something similar, such as a tightrope or very narrow beam, the amount of tolerance in the movement of the centre of gravity is zero in any direction other than along the line of support. Consequently, when an object is in a balanced position on a knife-edge support the centre of gravity of the object is located in the vertical plane through the line of support. By balancing an object in a number of different positions and noting the orientation of the vertical support plane to the object in each position, it may be possible to determine the position of the centre of gravity of the object, which will be located at the point of intersection of the support planes. This method could be used with the triangle-shaped piece of card in Figure 2.18.

MUSCULOSKELETAL SYSTEM FUNCTION

Posture refers to the orientation of body segments to each other and is usually applied to static or quasi-static positions such as sitting and standing. When standing upright there are two forces acting on the body, body weight and the ground reaction force (Fig. 2.33a). The ground reaction force is the force exerted by the ground on the body. When standing upright the ground reaction force is equal in magnitude but opposite in direction to body weight. The combined effect of body weight and the ground reaction force is a compression load that tends to collapse the body in a heap on the ground. This compression load increases with any additional weight carried by the body (Fig. 2.33b). To prevent the body from collapsing while simultaneously bringing about desired movements, the movements of the various joints need to be carefully controlled by coordinated activity between the various muscle groups. For example, when standing upright the joints of the neck, trunk and legs must be stabilized by the muscles that control them, otherwise the body would collapse. Consequently, the weight of the whole body is transmitted to the floor by the feet but the weights of the individual body segments above the feet (head, arms, trunk and legs) are transmitted indirectly to the floor by the skeletal chain formed by the bones and joints of the neck, trunk and legs.

Transmitting body weight to the ground while maintaining an upright body posture illustrates the essential feature of musculoskeletal function, i.e. the generation (by the muscles) and transmission (by the bones and joints) of forces. In biomechanical analysis of human movement, the forces generated and transmitted by the musculoskeletal system are referred to as internal forces, and forces that act on the body from external sources, such as body weight, ground reaction force, water resistance and air resistance, are referred to as external forces. The musculoskeletal system generates and transmits internal forces to counteract the effects of gravity and create the ground reaction forces (and propulsion forces in water) necessary to maintain upright posture, transport the body and manipulate objects, often simultaneously (Watkins 1999).

> Transmitting body weight to the ground while maintaining an upright body posture illustrates the essential feature of musculoskeletal function, i.e. the generation and transmission of forces.

LOAD, STRAIN AND STRESS

A load is any force or combination of forces applied to an object (Watkins 1999). There are three types of load: tension, compression and shear (Fig. 2.34). Loads tend to deform the objects on which they act. Tension is a pulling (stretching) load that tends to make an object longer and thinner along the line of the force (Fig. 2.34a and b). Compression is a pushing or pressing load that tends to make an object shorter and thicker along the line of the force (Fig. 2.34a and c). A shear load comprises two equal (in magnitude), opposite (in direction), parallel forces that tend to displace one part of an object with respect to an adjacent part along a plane parallel to and between the lines of force (Fig. 2.34a and d). The cutting load produced by scissors and garden shears is a shear

load, while the cutting load produced by a knife is a compression load. It is also a shear load that forces one object to slide on another (Fig. 2.34e). The sliding or tendency to slide is resisted by a force called friction, which is exerted between and parallel to the two contacting surfaces.

The three types of load frequently occur in combination, especially in bending and torsion (Fig. 2.34 f and g). An object subjected to bending experiences tension on one side and compression on the other. An object subjected to torsion simultaneously experiences tension, compression and shear.

In mechanics, the deformation of an object that occurs in response to a load is referred to as strain. For example, when a muscle contracts it exerts a tension load on the tendons at each end of the muscle and, consequently, the tendons experience tension strain, i.e. they are very slightly stretched. Similarly, an object subjected to a compression load experiences compression strain and an object subjected to a

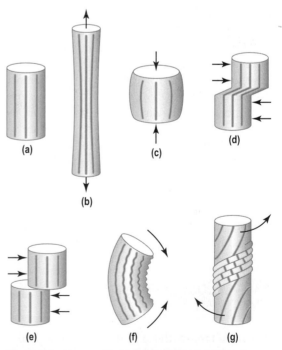

Fig. 2.34   Types of load. (a) Unloaded. (b) Tension. (c) Compression. (d) Shear. (e) Shear producing friction. (f) Bending. (g) Torsion

shear load experiences shear strain. Strain denotes deformation of the intermolecular bonds that comprise the structure of an object. When an object experiences strain, the intermolecular bonds exert forces that tend to restore the original (unloaded) size and shape of the object. The forces exerted by the intermolecular bonds of an object under strain are referred to as stress. Stress is the resistance of the intermolecular bonds to the strain caused by the load.

The stress on an object resulting from a particular load is distributed throughout the whole of the material sustaining the load. However, the level of stress in different regions of the material varies depending upon the amount of material sustaining the load in the different regions: the more material sustaining the load, the lower the stress. Consequently, stress is measured in terms of the average load on the plane of material sustaining the load at the point of interest.

> A load is any force or combination of forces applied to an object. Strain is the deformation of an object that occurs in response to a load. Stress is the resistance of the intermolecular bonds to the strain caused by the load.

TENSION STRESS

Figure 2.35a shows a person standing upright with the line of action of body weight slightly in front of the ankle joints. In this posture stability is maintained by isometric (static) contraction of the ankle plantar flexors, as shown in the simple two-segment model in Figure 2.35b. If the force exerted by the ankle plantar flexors is 350 N (in each leg) and the cross-sectional area of the Achilles tendon at P in Figure 2.35b, perpendicular to the tension load, is 1.8 cm^2, then the tension stress on the tendon at P is 194.4 N/cm^2, i.e.

$$\text{tension stress at P} = \frac{350\,\text{N}}{1.8\,\text{cm}^2}$$
$$= 194.4\,\text{N/cm}^2$$

(newtons per square centimetre)

In the SI system the unit of stress is the pascal (Pa), which is defined as the stress produced by a force of 1 newton uniformly distributed over an area of 1 square metre ($1\,\text{Pa} = 1\,\text{N/m}^2$). As $1\,\text{N/cm}^2 = 10\,000\,\text{Pa}$, the tension stress on the Achilles tendon is equivalent to $1\,944\,000\,\text{Pa}$ or $1.944\,\text{MPa}$ (MPa = megapascal = $10^6\,\text{Pa}$).

COMPRESSION STRESS

When standing barefoot, as in Figure 2.36a, the ground reaction force exerts a compression load on the contact area of the feet. In an adult the contact area is approximately 260 cm^2 (both feet) (Hennig et al 1994). For a person weighing 687 N (70 kgf), the compression stress on the contact area of the feet (on a level floor, contact area perpendicular to the compression load) is 2.64 N/cm^2, i.e.

$$\text{Compression stress} = \frac{687\,\text{N}}{260\,\text{cm}^2}$$
$$= 2.64\,\text{N/cm}^2 = 26\,400\,\text{Pa}$$
$$= 26.4\,\text{kPa}$$

(kPa = kilopascal = $10^3\,\text{Pa}$)

By raising the heels off the ground the contact area is approximately halved (Fig. 2.36b). Since

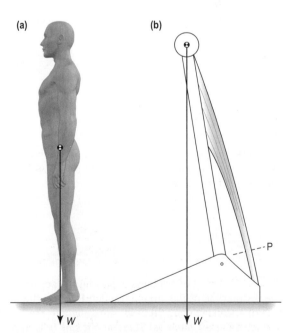

(a)   (b)

↓ W   ↓ W

Fig. 2.35 Tension load on the Achilles tendon

the compression load (body weight) is the same as before, it follows that the compression stress on the reduced contact area is approximately doubled. Compression stress is usually referred to as pressure.

In some sports played on grass pitches, such as soccer and rugby, the players wear studded boots to reduce the risk of slipping. Ideally, the studs should sink fully into the playing surface when weight-bearing; this reduces the risk of slipping and ensures that the ground reaction force is distributed evenly across the whole of the soles of the boots (Fig. 2.37a). However, when playing on a hard surface, the studs may not sink fully into the playing surface such that the ground reaction force will be transmitted directly by the studs and only indirectly by the soles of the boots (Fig. 2.37b). The combined area of the studs is very small compared to the soles of the boots. Consequently, there will be an increase in pressure on those parts of the feet directly above the studs. The actual pressure on any part of each foot will depend upon the flexibility of the soles of the boots; the more flexible the soles, the greater the increase in pressure above the studs. Any kind of propulsive or braking movement (starting, stopping, turning) will increase the pressure even more. As the pressure increases, so does the risk of injury to the feet. There are 26 bones and about 40 joints in each foot. Consequently, most movements of the foot involve a large number of joints (Watkins 2001). Boots with inflexible soles will seriously impair the natural movement of the feet and probably result in blisters, calluses and other disorders.

SHEAR STRESS

Many of the joints, especially those in the lower back and pelvis, are subjected to shear load during normal everyday activities such as standing and walking. For example, in walking, there is a phase when one leg supports the body while the other leg swings forward (Fig. 2.38). In this situation the unsupported side of the body tends to move downward relative to the supported side, subjecting the pubic symphysis joint to shear load. The area of the pubic symphysis in the

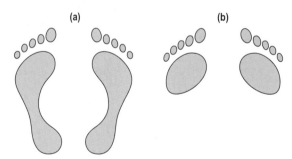

Fig. 2.36 Supporting area of the feet. (a) Normal upright standing posture. (b) Standing upright with the heels off the floor

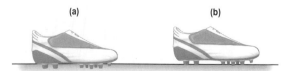

Fig. 2.37 Effect of hardness of playing surface on the distribution of the ground reaction force on the sole of a studded boot. (a) Studs sink fully into the surface on a soft pitch. (b) Studs do not sink fully into the surface on a hard pitch

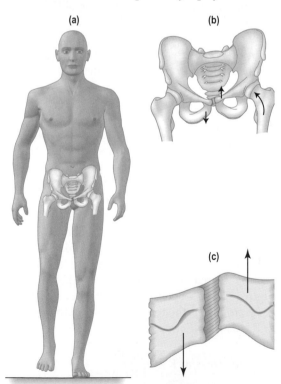

Fig. 2.38 Shear load on the pubic symphysis resulting from single-leg support while walking

plane of the shear load is approximately $2\,\mathrm{cm}^2$. If the shear load at the instant shown in Figure 2.38 is, for example, $20\,\mathrm{N}$, then the shear stress on the joint is $10\,\mathrm{N/cm}^2$, i.e.

$$\text{shear stress} = \frac{20\,\mathrm{N}}{2\,\mathrm{cm}^2}$$
$$= 10\,\mathrm{N/cm}^2 = 100\,000\,\mathrm{Pa}$$
$$= 100\,\mathrm{kPa}$$

FRICTION

When one object moves or tends to move across the surface of another, there will be a force parallel to the surfaces in contact that will oppose the movement or tendency to move. This force is called friction. Consider a block of wood resting on a level table (Fig. 2.39). The only forces acting on the block are the weight of the block W and the force R exerted by the table on the block. Since the block is at rest, R is equal and opposite to W (Fig. 2.39a). If an attempt is made to push the block along the surface of the table by applying a horizontal force P, the frictional force F between the contacting surfaces will begin to operate and oppose the tendency of the block to move (Fig. 2.39b). As P increases, so does F until the block begins to move, i.e. F has a maximum value. This value is directly proportional to the degree of roughness of the two surfaces in contact and the force R. The three variables are related as follows:

$$F = \mu.R \qquad\qquad \text{Eq. 2.1}$$

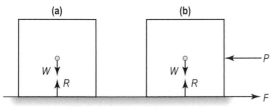

Fig. 2.39   (a) The forces acting on a block of wood resting on a level table. (b) The forces acting on a block of wood resting on a level table but tending to slide horizontally. W = weight of the block; R = normal reaction force; P = horizontal force applied to the side of the block; F = friction

where μ (Greek letter mu) is a measure of the roughness of the two surfaces in contact and is called the coefficient of friction between the two surfaces. The force R is referred to as the normal reaction force and is perpendicular to the plane of contact between the two surfaces.

The magnitude of μ depends upon the types of surface in contact and whether the surfaces are sliding on each other. Surfaces are never perfectly smooth and the minor irregularities of the contacting surfaces interdigitate and resist sliding between the surfaces (Fig. 2.40a). To initiate sliding, the minor irregularities have to be dragged over each other. In doing so, the surfaces tend to separate slightly, which reduces the resistance to sliding, providing that the sliding is maintained (Fig. 2.40b). Consequently, for any two surfaces in contact, μ (and therefore F) will be slightly less when the surfaces are sliding on each other than when the surfaces are not sliding on each other but tending to slide. Therefore, for any two surfaces, there is a coefficient of limiting (static) friction and a coefficient of sliding (dynamic) friction.

When no sliding occurs, the normal reaction force is distributed over those parts of the adjacent surfaces that are in contact; this will include the irregularities and some of the surfaces between the irregularities (Fig. 2.40a). However, during sliding, the normal reaction force is exerted almost entirely by the irregularities (Fig. 2.40b). Consequently, during sliding, the pressure exerted by the irregularities of one surface on the other surface is likely to be considerably increased and result in wear of the surface (similar to the effect of sandpaper on wood). The introduction of a fluid between the surfaces tends to separate not only the surfaces, but also the surface irregularities, resulting in a

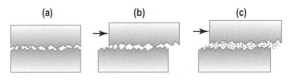

Fig. 2.40   (a) Interdigitation of surface irregularities. (b) Slight separation of surfaces as a result of sliding. (c) Complete separation of surfaces as a result of lubrication

considerable reduction in friction and wear. This is the principle of lubrication (Fig. 2.40c).

In the absence of lubrication, μ is about 0.25–0.50 for wood on wood, 0.15–0.60 for metal on metal, 0.20–0.60 for wood on metal and 0.4–0.9 for wood on rubber (Serway & Jewett 2004). The difference between limiting and sliding friction between different pairs of materials can be easily demonstrated with a spring balance and a block of wood. For example, place a block of wood weighing about 1 kgf on a level wooden table. Apply a horizontal force to the block very gradually with a spring balance and note the maximum force recorded just before the block begins to move. The coefficient of limiting friction μ_L between the block and the table can then be estimated by using Equation 2.1, i.e. $\mu_L = F_1/R$ where F_1 is the maximum force recorded on the spring balance just before the block begins to move and R is the weight of the block. Repeat the experiment and observe the force F_2 required to maintain sliding. The coefficient of sliding friction μ_S between the block and the table can then be estimated from $\mu_S = F_2/R$. Results similar to those shown in the first row of Table 2.8 will be obtained.

Different combinations of materials have different coefficients of friction and this can be demonstrated by varying the support surface in the above experiment. The second, third and fourth rows of Table 2.8 show the results obtained for μ_L and μ_S for the same block of wood and three other materials.

Equation 2.1 shows that the amount of friction, limiting and sliding, between two surfaces is independent of the area of contact when the normal reaction force stays the same. The compression stress on the surfaces will vary with the area of contact but the amount of friction will not change if the normal reaction force remains constant.

The development of adequate friction between the human body and the environment is essential for most actions of daily living, in particular, body transport (friction between the feet and the floor) and manipulation of objects (friction between the fingers and objects). The importance of the need for adequate friction in these types of actions is, perhaps, more obvious in sport, where the quality of performance is likely to depend largely upon the ability of the players to create adequate friction between feet and playing surface and between hands and racket or other implement. In such cases, adequate friction is maintained by using materials that have appropriate coefficients of friction with the playing surface and with the hands. For example, in volleyball, basketball, squash and badminton, the soles of shoes are normally made of materials that will provide adequate friction with the playing surface. It follows that, for most indoor sports, the playing surfaces should not be highly polished, since this will reduce the coefficient of friction and increase the possibility of slipping. However, too much friction is likely to impair performance and result in injury, especially in sports that require rapid changes in speed and/or direction. Ideally, the sole of the shoe should turn as the player turns, but excessive friction may prevent the shoe turning and result in a twisting injury to the ankle or knee. This is also a potential problem

Table 2.8 Coefficient of limiting friction (μ_L) and sliding friction (μ_S) for a number of materials with wood

Support surface	Limiting friction F (kgf)	μ_L	Sliding friction F (kgf)	μ_S
Polished wooden table	0.55	0.50	0.23	0.21
Formica	0.33	0.30	0.18	0.16
Resin floor tile	0.80	0.70	0.38	0.34
Plain rubber mat	0.90	0.80	0.45	0.41

F = horizontal force.

in sports played on grass pitches where the players use studded boots. In these situations, the horizontal forces produced between boots and playing surface are largely shear forces on the studs rather than friction. However, if the studs are too long and sink fully into the pitch, the sole of the boot may not turn as the player turns, which will increase the risk of injury.

There are many non-sporting situations in which it is important to ensure adequate friction in order to reduce the risk of injury. For example, an injured or aged person may rely heavily on walking sticks or crutches for support. It is very important that the sticks or crutches do not slip on the floor. Rubber has a high coefficient of friction with most materials; consequently, rubber tips are usually fitted to the ends of the walking sticks and crutches to reduce the risk of slipping.

In some activities, skilful performance depends upon reducing friction between shoes and floor. For example, in ballroom dancing, good technique is largely dependent on the ability to slide and turn the feet on the floor with as little resistance as possible. Consequently, not only is the floor highly polished, but so are the soles of the dancer's shoes. Similarly, elite skiers wax the underside of their skis in order to reduce the amount of friction between the skis and the snow.

Whereas the development of adequate friction between the human body and the environment is essential for daily living, friction between the different body tissues inside the body must be reduced as much as possible in order to minimize the risk of injury or wear. The human body is made up of a number of different tissues that lie adjacent to each other. Even the slightest movement involves a certain amount of sliding of the various tissues on each other. Unless the adjacent surfaces are adequately lubricated, frictional forces will operate when sliding occurs. Whenever friction develops, a certain amount of heat is generated. Too much heat will injure or wear body tissues. In machines, parts that slide on each other are usually highly polished and friction is reduced even more by lubricating the sliding surfaces with oil or grease. Similar mechanisms exist within the human body. All the freely movable joints of the body are lined by synovial membrane, which produces synovial fluid (Fig. 2.41). The latter is a transparent viscous fluid, resembling the white of an egg, that lubricates and nourishes the articular surfaces (articular cartilage) of the joints. The articular surfaces are normally extremely smooth so that in association with the synovial fluid $\mu_L \simeq 0.01$ and $\mu_S \simeq 0.003$ (Serway & Jewett 2004). Consequently, the amount of friction developed in healthy joints during normal movements is usually extremely small. Joint injury, disease and degeneration due to ageing may reduce the quality of lubrication in synovial joints, resulting in excessive wear and, eventually, painful joints.

Adequate lubrication in synovial joints is particularly important in the major weight-bearing joints of the body, i.e. the hips, knees and ankles. The articular surfaces of these joints are under considerable pressure even when the person is just standing upright and any kind of propulsive movement of the legs will increase the pressure even more. The greater the pressure, the greater the friction between the articular surfaces. Therefore, it is extremely important that any kind of injury to these joints is treated promptly in order to restore normal lubrication as soon as possible. Wearing of articular surfaces is similar to the wearing of brake pads in the wheels of a motor vehicle. When braking occurs, an enormous amount of friction and, therefore, heat is generated between brake pad and wheel. Consequently, the brake pads eventually wear out and have to be replaced. In a

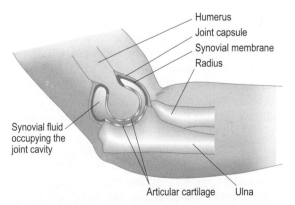

Fig. 2.41   Vertical section through the elbow joint

healthy joint, any wear is usually repaired by normal metabolic processes. However, progressive joint degeneration will occur when the rate of wear outpaces the rate of repair.

As well as in joints, synovial membranes are located in other parts of the body where different tissues slide over each other. For example, most of the tendons of muscles that cross the wrists and ankles pass over, through or around bones and ligaments. To reduce friction between the tendons and adjacent structures the tendons are enclosed within synovial sheaths (Fig. 2.42). A synovial sheath consists of a closed flattened sac made up of synovial membrane containing a capillary film of synovial fluid. The synovial sheath forms a protective sleeve around the tendon. Unaccustomed overuse of the associated muscles is likely to result in tenosynovitis, a condition characterized by inflammation of the synovial sheaths. Squash and badminton players are particularly prone to this type of injury to the flexor and extensor tendons of the wrist. A synovial bursa is a closed sac comprising synovial membrane containing synovial fluid that is interposed between different tissues that slide on each other. Bursae are located most frequently between the deeper layers of the skin and underlying bone (subcutaneous bursa), between tendons and bone (subtendinous bursa) and between individual muscles (submuscular bursa). For example, there is a large subcutaneous bursa between the skin and the patella (the prepatellar bursa; Fig. 2.43). Unaccustomed pressure on a bursa is likely to result in bursitis, i.e. a condition characterized by inflammation of the bursa.

A blister on the skin is a form of bursa that occurs in response to unaccustomed friction. A blister is a short-term safety mechanism that protects the deep layers of the skin from sustained and/or excessive friction resulting from relatively infrequent experiences such as stiff shoes rubbing against the feet or the handle of a screwdriver rubbing against the hand. The body responds to this friction by producing a layer of fluid between the superficial and deep layers of the skin, thereby protecting the deep layers from further damage. In the long term, the body will respond to a sustained increase in friction on a particular part of the skin by thickening the superficial layer of the skin. For example, in comparison with other parts of the body, the skin on the heel and ball of each foot is subjected to fairly sustained pressure and/or frictional force. Not surprisingly, the skin on the heel and ball of each foot is usually much thicker than in other places, except, perhaps, for the palmar surfaces of the hands of manual workers.

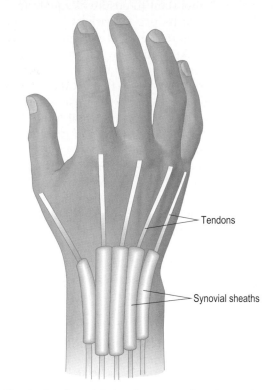

Fig. 2.42 Synovial sheaths surrounding the tendons of the wrist and finger extensors

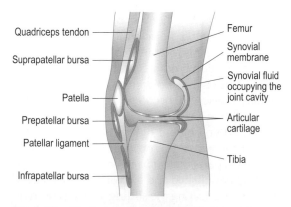

Fig. 2.43 Vertical section through the knee joint

Whereas the development of adequate friction between the human body and the environment is essential for daily living, friction between the different body tissues inside the body must be reduced as much as possible in order to minimize the risk of injury or wear.

FORCE VECTORS AND RESULTANT FORCE

When standing upright, there are three forces acting on the human body, body weight W, the ground reaction force L on the left foot and the ground reaction force R on the right foot (Fig. 2.44). The point of application of W in Figure 2.44 and subsequent figures is the centre of gravity of the body. In Figure 2.44, the resultant ground reaction force (resultant of L and R) is equal in magnitude but opposite in direction to W, i.e. the resultant force acting on the body is zero. In Figure 2.45a the force F_1 is the resultant ground

reaction force (resultant of the ground reaction forces acting on the left and right feet). Additional load on the body, such as holding an object as in Figure 2.45b, simply increases the total downward load on the body and results in a corresponding increase in the magnitude of the ground reaction force. Figure 2.46 shows the forces acting on a man sitting on a chair. In this case, there are three upward forces counteracting body weight, the force exerted by the chair and the ground reaction forces on the feet. In the examples in Figures 2.44–2.46, all the forces are vertical forces and, consequently, the upward and downward force vectors are presented in parallel in the vector diagrams.

Figure 2.47 shows a sprinter in the set position of a sprint start, i.e. when the body is at rest and the resultant force acting on the body is zero. In this situation there are five forces acting on the body, body weight W, the forces L and R at the hands and the forces P and Q at the feet.

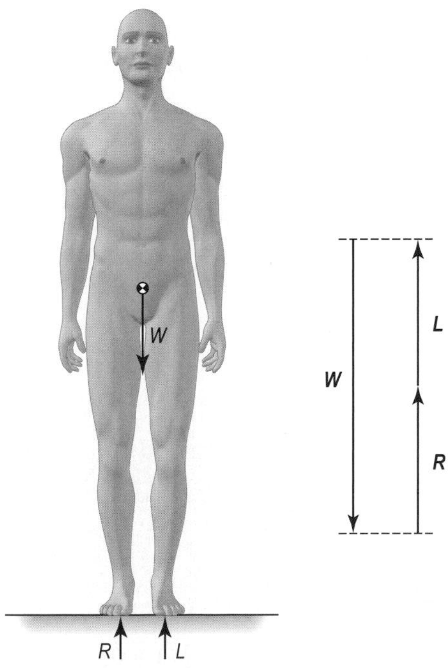

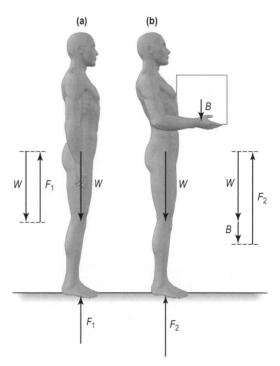

Fig. 2.44   The forces acting on the human body when standing upright and the corresponding vector chain. W = body weight; L = force on the left foot; R = force on the right foot

Fig. 2.45   The forces acting on the human body (a) when standing upright and (b) standing upright with additional load, with the corresponding vector chains. W = body weight; B = weight of object; F_1, F_2 = ground reaction forces

The force vectors are shown in Figure 2.47a and the corresponding vector chain is shown in Figure 2.47b. Since the resultant force acting on the sprinter is zero, the vector chain is a closed loop; in other words, irrespective of the order of the force vectors in the chain, the end of the last vector coincides with the start of the first vector. Figure 2.48a shows the sprinter just after the start as he accelerates forward under the action

of the resultant force acting on his body, i.e. the resultant of his body weight and the forces acting on his feet. Figure 2.48b shows the corresponding vector chain and resultant force.

TRIGONOMETRY OF A RIGHT–ANGLED TRIANGLE

Whereas the vector chain and parallelogram of vectors methods of determining the resultant of a number of component vectors are very useful, it is often more practical to use trigonometry, especially when there are a large number of vectors. Trigonometry is the branch of mathematics that deals with the relationships between the lengths of the sides and the sizes of the angles in a triangle. Figure 2.49 shows a right-angled triangle in which one angle (between sides a and b) is 90°. The angles between sides a and c, and sides b and c, are α and θ respectively.

In a right-angled triangle the two angles less than 90° (α and θ in Figure 2.49) can be specified by the ratio between the lengths of any two sides of the triangle. The three most common ratios are sine, cosine and tangent, and they are defined in relation to the particular angle under

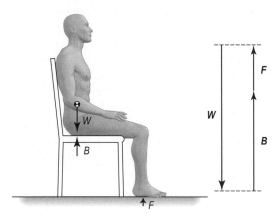

Fig. 2.46 The forces acting on a man sitting on a chair and the corresponding vector chain. W = body weight; F = combined upward force exerted on both feet; B = upward force exerted by the chair

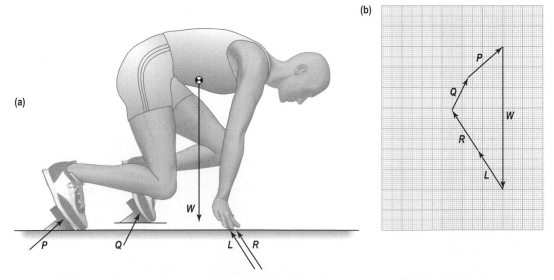

Fig. 2.47 (a) The forces acting on a sprinter in the set position of a sprint start. (b) The corresponding vector chain. W = body weight; P = force on the right foot; Q = force on the left foot; L = force on the left hand; R = force on the right hand. Scale: 1 cm = 10 kgf. W = 70 kgf; P = 21.5 kgf at 40.6° to the horizontal; Q = 18.5 kgf at 63.1° to the horizontal; L = 23.3 kgf at 58.0° to the horizontal; R = 23.3 kgf at 58.0° to the horizontal

consideration. For example, in relation to angle θ in Figure 2.49, side a is referred to as the opposite side, side b is referred to as the adjacent side and side c is the hypotenuse, the side of the triangle opposite the right angle.

The sine of θ is defined as the ratio of the opposite side to the hypotenuse, i.e.

$$\text{sine } \theta = \frac{\text{opposite side}}{\text{hypotenuse}} = \frac{a}{c}$$

The cosine of θ is defined as the ratio of the adjacent side to the hypotenuse, i.e.

$$\text{cosine } \theta = \frac{\text{adjacent side}}{\text{hypotenuse}} = \frac{b}{c}$$

The tangent of θ is defined as the ratio of the opposite side to the adjacent side, i.e.

$$\text{tangent } \theta = \frac{\text{opposite side}}{\text{adjacent side}} = \frac{a}{b}$$

Most electronic calculators provide a range of trigonometric ratios including sine (sin), cosine (cos) and tangent (tan). Alternatively, tables of sine, cosine and tangent (for angles between 0° and 90°) can be obtained in publications such as Castle (1969). The lengths of sides and sizes of angles in right-angled triangles can be calculated using sine, cosine and tangent functions provided that two sides, or one side and one other angle, are known. With reference to Figure 2.49, for example, if $c = 10\,\text{cm}$ and $\theta = 30°$, the lengths of sides a and b and the size of angle α can be determined as follows.

1. Calculation of the length of side a

$$\frac{a}{c} = \sin \theta$$
$$a = c.\sin \theta \text{ (i.e. } c \text{ multiplied by } \sin \theta)$$
$$a = c.\sin 30°$$

From sine tables, sin 30° = 0.5 (i.e. the ratio of the length of side a to the length of side c is 0.5). Since $c = 10\,\text{cm}$ and sin 30° = 0.5, it follows that

$$a = 10\,\text{cm} \times 0.5$$
$$a = 5\,\text{cm}$$

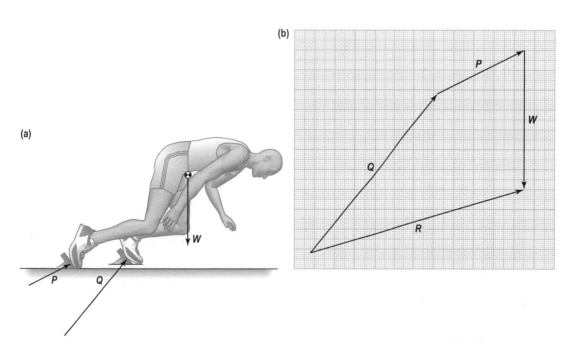

Fig. 2.48   (a) The forces acting on a sprinter just after the start of a race and (b) the corresponding vector chain. W = body weight; P = force on the right foot; Q = force on the left foot. Scale: 1 cm = 10 kgf. W = 70 kgf; P = 48 kgf at 28° to the horizontal; Q = 102 kgf at 51° to the horizontal; R = 11.1 cm = 111 kgf at 16.5° to the horizontal

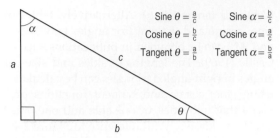

$$\text{Sine } \theta = \tfrac{a}{c} \qquad \text{Sine } \alpha = \tfrac{b}{c}$$
$$\text{Cosine } \theta = \tfrac{b}{c} \qquad \text{Cosine } \alpha = \tfrac{a}{c}$$
$$\text{Tangent } \theta = \tfrac{a}{b} \qquad \text{Tangent } \alpha = \tfrac{b}{a}$$

Fig. 2.49 Definition of sine, cosine and tangent in a right-angled triangle

2. Calculation of the length of side b

$$\frac{b}{c} = \cos \theta$$
$$b = c.\cos \theta \text{ (i.e. } c \text{ multiplied by } \cos \theta)$$
$$b = c.\cos 30°$$

From cosine tables, $\cos 30° = 0.866$ (i.e. the ratio of the length of side b to the length of side c is 0.866). Since $c = 10$ cm and $\cos 30° = 0.866$, it follows that

$$b = 10 \text{ cm} \times 0.866$$
$$b = 8.66 \text{ cm}$$

3. Calculation of angle α
    Angle α can be determined in a number of ways:

    i. The sum of the three angles in any triangle (with or without a right angle) is 180°. Since the sum of θ and the right-angle is 120°, it follows that $\alpha = 180° - 120° = 60°$
    ii. The lengths of all three sides of the triangle are known: $a = 5$ cm, $b = 8.66$ cm and $c = 10$ cm. Consequently, α can be determined by calculating the sine, cosine, or tangent of the angle:

$$\sin \alpha = \frac{b}{c} = \frac{8.66 \text{ cm}}{10 \text{ cm}} = 0.866. \ \alpha = 60°$$

$$\cos \alpha = \frac{a}{c} = \frac{5 \text{ cm}}{10 \text{ cm}} = 0.5. \ \alpha = 60°$$

$$\tan \alpha = \frac{b}{a} = \frac{8.66 \text{ cm}}{5 \text{ cm}} \ 1.732. \ \alpha = 60°$$

Pythagoras' theorem

Pythagoras, a Greek mathematician (572–497 BC), showed that in a right-angled triangle the square of the hypotenuse is equal to the sum of the squares of the other two sides. Therefore, with respect to Figure 2.49,

$$c^2 = a^2 + b^2$$
$$c = \sqrt{(a^2 + b^2)}$$

This can be demonstrated with the data from the above example, where $a = 5$ cm, $b = 8.66$ cm and $c = 10$ cm: $a^2 = 25$, $b^2 = 75$ and $c^2 = 100$.

Resolution of a vector into component vectors

Just as the resultant of any number of component vectors can be determined, any single vector can be replaced by any number of component vectors that have the same effect as the single vector. The process of replacing a vector by two or more component vectors is referred to as the resolution of a vector. In analysing human movement, displacement, velocity and force vectors are frequently resolved into vertical and horizontal components using trigonometry. The example of the sprinter in Figure 2.48 will be used to illustrate how the resolution of forces by trigonometry is used to determine the resultant force acting on the sprinter. There are three steps in the process.

1. Resolve all the forces into their vertical and horizontal components
Figure 2.50a shows the forces acting on the sprinter, body weight W, the force P on the right foot and the force Q on the left foot. In Figure 2.50b, P and Q have been replaced by their vertical (PV and QV) and horizontal (PH and QH) components. Figure 2.51 shows the calculation of PV and PH. Figure 2.52 shows the calculation of QV and QH.

2. Calculate the vertical component RV and horizontal component RH of the resultant force R acting on the sprinter

$$RV = PV + QV - W$$

$$RV = 22.5 + 79.3 - 70 \text{ kgf} = 31.8 \text{ kgf}$$

$$RH = PH + QH$$

$$RH = 42.4 + 64.2 \text{ kgf} = 106.6 \text{ kgf}$$

(a)

(b)

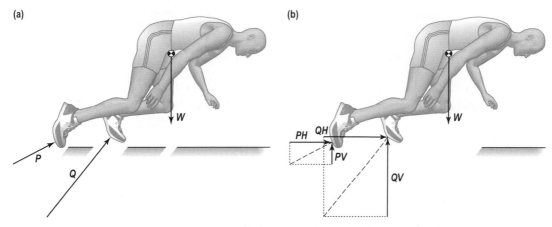

Fig. 2.50   (a) The forces acting on a sprinter just after the start of a race and (b) the vertical and horizontal components of the forces. W = 70 kgf; P = 48 kgf at 28° to the horizontal; Q = 102 kgf at 51° to the horizontal

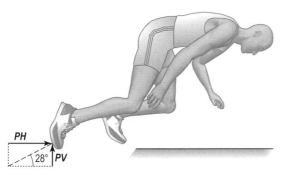

Fig. 2.51   Calculation of the vertical and horizontal components of the force acting on the right foot of a sprinter just after the start of a race. PV = vertical component of P; PH = horizontal component of P; PV/P = sin 28°; $PV = P \times$ sin 28° = 48 kgf × 0.4695 = 22.5 kgf; PH/P = cos 28°; $PH = P \times$ cos 28° = 48 kgf × 0.8829 = 42.4 kgf

3. Calculate R and the angle θ of R with respect to the horizontal

R, RV and RH are shown in Figure 2.53. From Pythagoras' theorem,

$$R^2 = RV^2 + RH^2$$
$$R^2 = 12\ 374.8$$
$$R = 111.2 \text{ kgf}$$
$$\tan \theta = \frac{RV}{RH} = 0.2983$$
$$\theta = 16.6°$$

As expected, R and θ are the same as in the vector chain solution in Figure 2.48.

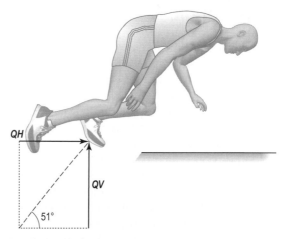

Fig. 2.52   Calculation of the vertical and horizontal components of the force acting on the left foot of a sprinter just after the start of a race. QV = vertical component of Q; QH = horizontal component of Q. QV/Q = sin 51°; $QV = Q \times$ sin 51° = 102 kgf × 0.7771 = 79.3 kgf; QH/Q = cos 51°; $QH = Q \times$ cos 51° = 102 kgf × 0.6293 = 64.2 kgf

Any single vector can be replaced by any number of component vectors that have the same effect as the single vector. The process of replacing a vector by two or more component vectors is referred to as the resolution of a vector.

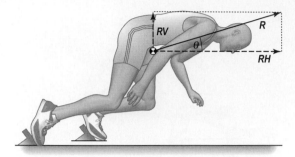

Fig. 2.53 Resultant force acting on a sprinter just after the start of a race. R = resultant force; RV = vertical component of R; RH = horizontal component of R; $R^2 = RV^2 + RH^2$; $R^2 = 12\,374.8$; $R = 111.2$ kgf; $\tan \theta = RV/RH = 0.2983$; $\theta = 16.6°$

CYCLE LENGTH, CYCLE RATE AND SPEED OF MOVEMENT IN HUMAN LOCOMOTION

Human locomotion refers to all forms of self-propelled transportation of the human body with or without the use of equipment. Human locomotion occurs mainly on land, such as walking, running and cycling, and in water, such as swimming, canoeing and rowing. All forms of human locomotion involve cycles of movement of the body in which each cycle of movement moves the body a certain distance. The distance achieved in each cycle of movement, referred to as cycle length, and the number of cycles per unit of time, referred to as the cycle rate, determine the speed of movement. For example, when cycle length is measured in m/cycle and cycle rate in Hz, speed is in m/s, i.e.

speed (m/s) = cycle length (m/cycles)
$\times$ cycle rate (Hz)

STRIDE PARAMETERS AND STRIDE CYCLE IN WALKING AND RUNNING

In walking and running, cycle length and cycle rate are usually referred to as stride length and stride rate respectively. Each cycle of movement from heel-strike to heel-strike of the same foot moves the body forward one stride (Fig. 2.54a). One stride consists of two consecutive steps. The

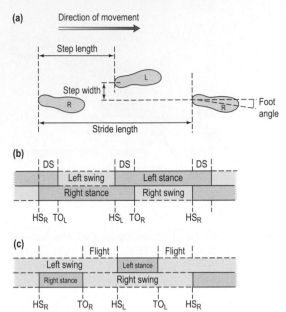

Fig. 2.54 (a) Stride parameters and (b, c) stride cycle in walking (b) and running (c). HS_L = heel-strike left; HS_R = heel-strike right; TO_L = toe-off left; TO_R = toe-off right; DS = double support

stride cycle refers to the movement of the body during a single stride. In walking, the stride cycle of the right leg begins with right heel-strike (contact of the ground with the right heel or, more often, the posterolateral part of the heel) which initiates the stance phase of the right leg, i.e. the period of the stride cycle when the right leg is in contact with the ground. The first part of the stance phase is a period of double support, i.e. when both feet are in contact with the ground (Fig. 2.54b). This period of double support lasts for approximately 10% of the cycle, at which point the left foot leaves the ground (referred to as toe-off) and the left leg swings forward. During the swing phase of the left leg the right leg supports the body on its own; this period lasts for approximately 40% of the cycle and is referred to as the single-support phase of the right leg. At the end of the swing phase of the left leg the left foot contacts the ground and another period of double support ensues. At approximately 60% of the cycle the right foot leaves the ground to begin its swing phase while the left leg experiences a period of single support. The cycle is completed by heel-strike of the right foot. As

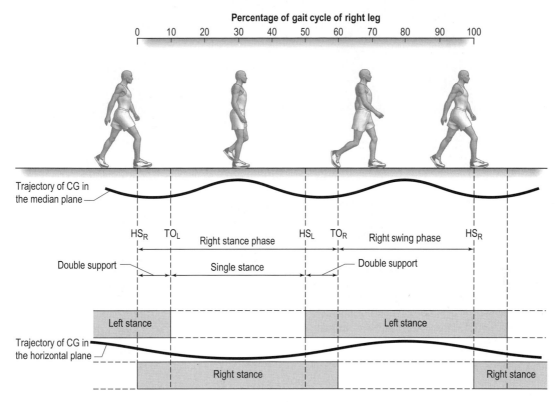

Fig. 2.55   The stride cycle in walking. CG = centre of gravity; HS_L = heel-strike left; HS_R = heel-strike right; TO_L = toe-off left; TO_R = toe-off right

the speed of walking increases, the duration of the periods of double support decrease until there is a sudden change from walking to running. The change is characterized by the absence of periods of double support and the presence of flight phases (when both feet are off the ground) between the single support phases of each leg (Fig. 2.54b & c).

TRAJECTORY OF THE CENTRE OF GRAVITY IN WALKING

During walking, the movement of the body as a whole is reflected in the movement of the whole-body centre of gravity, which tends to follow a fairly smooth up–down, side-to-side trajectory. When viewed from the side, as shown in the upper part of Figure 2.55, the centre of gravity moves up and down twice during each stride with the low points of the trajectory occurring close to the midpoints of the double-support

phases and the high points of the trajectory occurring close to the midpoints of the single-support phases. When viewed from overhead, as shown in the lower part of Figure 2.55, the trajectory of the centre of gravity follows the support phases, moving right during the period from the midpoint of single support of the left leg to the midpoint of single support of the right leg and moving left during the period from the midpoint of single support of the right leg to the midpoint of single support of the left leg. The ranges of up–down and side-to-side movement of the centre of gravity during each stride at normal walking speed (1–1.5 m/s) are approximately 46 mm and 44 mm respectively (Dagg 1977).

GROUND REACTION FORCE IN WALKING

The trajectory of the centre of gravity reflects the magnitude and direction of the ground

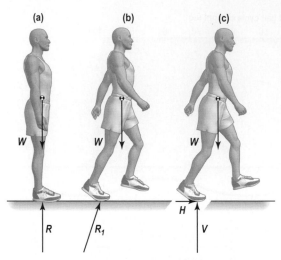

Fig. 2.56 The ground reaction force in standing and walking. (a) Standing upright. (b, c) Push-off in walking. W = body weight; R = ground reaction force while standing; R_1 = ground reaction during push-off; H = horizontal component of R_1; V = vertical component of R_1

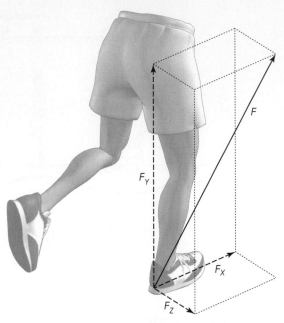

Fig. 2.57 Anteroposterior (F_X), vertical (F_Y) and mediolateral (F_Z) components of the ground reaction force F

reaction force. When standing upright the ground reaction force is equal in magnitude but opposite in direction to body weight, i.e. the resultant force acting on the body is zero (Fig. 2.56a). To start walking or running (or move horizontally by any other type of movement such as jumping or hopping) the body must push or pull against something to provide the necessary resultant force to move it in the required direction. In walking and running, forward movement is achieved by pushing obliquely downward and backward against the ground. Provided that the foot does not slip, the leg thrust results in a ground reaction force directed obliquely upward and forward, which moves the body forward while maintaining an upright posture (Fig. 2.56b). To understand the effect of the ground reaction force it is useful to resolve it into its vertical and horizontal components (Fig. 2.56c). The vertical component counteracts body weight, i.e. the resultant vertical force acting on the body remains close to zero, and the horizontal component (resultant horizontal force) results in forward movement.

Components of the ground reaction force

Figure 2.57 shows the anteroposterior (X), vertical (Y) and mediolateral (Z) components of the ground reaction force. When walking straight forward, the mediolateral component is normally very small, resulting in little side-to-side movement of the body. Figure 2.58 shows the X, Y and Z components of the ground reaction force (force–time curves) exerted on each leg during one stride of the right leg (heel-strike of the right foot to the next heel-strike of the right foot). The movement of the centre of gravity during walking (as in any movement) is determined by the resultant force acting on the body. During a period of single support the resultant force acting on the body is determined by body weight and the ground reaction force exerted on the grounded foot. During a period of double support the resultant force acting on the body is determined by body weight and the ground reaction forces exerted on both feet.

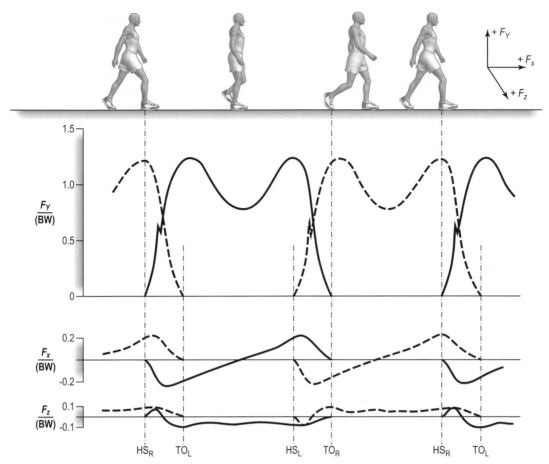

Fig. 2.58   Anteroposterior (F_X), vertical (F_Y) and mediolateral (F_Z) components of the ground reaction force during the walking stride cycle of the right leg. BW = body weight; HS_L = heel-strike left; HS_R = heel-strike right; TO_L = toe-off left; TO_R = toe-off right; solid line = right leg; dotted line = left leg

The vertical component of the ground reaction force exerted on each leg is characteristically dominated by two smooth peaks, with the rise and fall of each peak taking up about half of the stance phase (Fig. 2.58). The rise and fall of the first peak roughly corresponds to the period from heel-strike to heel-off and the rise and fall of the second peak roughly corresponds to the period from heel-off to toe-off.

Like the vertical component, the anteroposterior component is normally characteristically dominated by two smooth peaks whose rise and fall correspond to the rise and fall of the two peaks of the vertical component. The resultant anteroposterior component of force acts backward from the midpoint of double support to heel-off (a braking force), indicating deceleration of the centre of gravity, i.e. the forward speed of the body is decreased. In the heel-off to toe-off period the resultant anteroposterior component acts forward, indicating forward acceleration of the centre of gravity, i.e. the forward speed of the body is increased.

The resultant mediolateral component of force acts medially during single stance and changes direction during double support, i.e. from medial on right foot to medial on left foot during the left heel-strike to right toe-off period (Fig. 2.58).

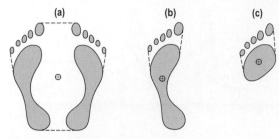

Fig. 2.59 Location of the centre of pressure when (a) standing upright on both feet, (b) standing on the left foot and (c) standing on the left foot with the heel off the floor

In addition to the characteristic smooth phases of the vertical, anteroposterior and mediolateral components of the ground reaction force, all three components are often characterized by a single spike or multiple transient spikes soon after heel-strike that reflect the impact of the heel with the ground (see F_Y in Figure 2.58). Shock-absorbing footwear will reduce or eliminate these transient spikes (Czerniecki 1988).

Centre of pressure

The ground reaction force is distributed across the whole of the area of contact between the feet and the floor. Figure 2.59a shows the contact area when standing barefoot on both feet; the contact area is much smaller than the area of the base of support. Figure 2.59b shows the contact area when standing on one foot and Figure 2.59c shows the contact area when standing on one foot with the heel raised off the ground. In Figures 2.59b and c the contact area is very similar to the base of support. Whereas the ground reaction force is distributed across the whole of the contact area, the effect of the ground reaction force on the movement of the body is as if the ground reaction force acted at a single point, which is referred to as the centre of pressure (just as the whole weight of the body appears to act at the whole body centre of gravity in terms of the effect of body weight on the movement of the body). With respect to Figures 2.59a, b and c, the centre of pressure is at the point of intersection of the line of action of body weight with the base of support.

Path of centre of pressure in walking

As indicated in Figure 2.58 the magnitude and direction of the ground reaction force change continuously during the gait cycle. Figure 2.60a shows the change in the resultant (F_{XY}) of the anteroposterior (F_X) and vertical (F_Y) components. Because of the dominance of F_Y, the change in F_{XY} from heel-strike to toe-off reflects the double-peaked F_Y component in Figure 2.58. F_Y always acts upward, so the progressive change in direction of F_{XY} from upward and backward at heel-strike through more or less vertical at heel-off to upward and forward at toe-off is due to the change in the direction of F_X from backward (heel-strike to heel-off) to forward (heel-off to toe-off) (Fig. 2.58).

During stance, the foot essentially rolls forward from heel to toe such that the contact area between foot and ground and, consequently, the centre of pressure of the ground reaction force on each foot change continuously, as shown in Figure 2.60b to f.

> The effect of the ground reaction force on the movement of the body is as if the ground reaction force acted at a single point, which is referred to as the centre of pressure.

EFFECT OF SPEED OF WALKING AND RUNNING ON STRIDE LENGTH AND STRIDE RATE

Figure 2.61 shows the relationships between stride length (SL), stride rate (SR) and speed (S) of walking and running for a male student (Hay 2002). The SL–S and SR–S graphs are based on data obtained from five walking trials and 10 running trials. In the walking trials, the student was requested to walk at a constant speed in each trial but at a slightly faster pace in each successive trial. All trials were recorded on video at 60 Hz and the SL and SR in each trial (during a period of constant speed) were obtained by frame-by-frame playback using appropriate distance reference markers. A similar procedure was used in the running trials. SL and SR data were obtained for five speeds of

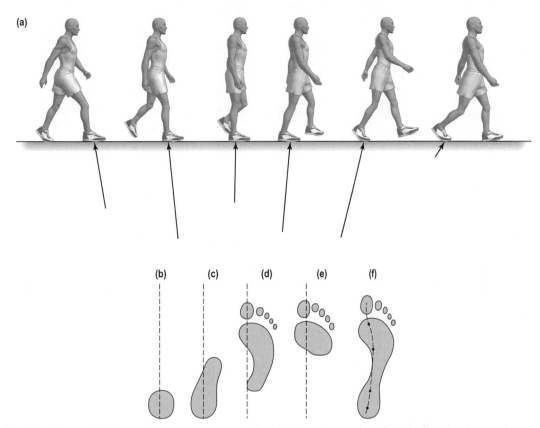

Fig. 2.60 Movement of the centre of pressure along the plantar surface of the foot during the stance phase of the right foot. (a) Change in the magnitude and direction of F_{XY}. (b–e) Plantar contact area (b) just after HS_R, (c) at the middle of double support, (d) at HO_R and (e) at HS_L. (f) Path of the centre of pressure and location of the centre of pressure at the points corresponding to (b), (c), (d) and (e) respectively

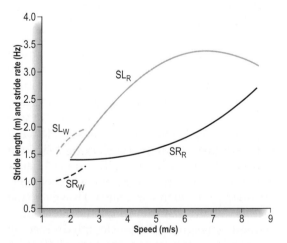

Fig. 2.61 Stride length–speed and stride rate–speed graphs for a male student, walking and running.
SL_W = stride length walking; SR_W = stride rate walking;
SL_R = stride length running; SR_R = stride rate running

walking over the range 1.5–2.6 m/s (moderate to fast pace) and 10 speeds of running over the range 2.1–8.2 m/s (very slow to fast pace). The SL–S and SR–S graphs are the lines of best fit, reflecting the smooth change in SL and SR that normally occurs with increasing speed of walking and running for a given individual. Most people will naturally change from walking to running at about 2.3 m/s because it is more economic in terms of energy expenditure to do so (Alexander 1992). This change in form of locomotion is reflected in the distinct SL–S and SR–S graphs for walking to running. However, the shapes of the SL–S and SR–S graphs for walking and running are very similar. In particular, the SL–S graphs are concave downward and the SR–S graphs are concave upward. In addition, SL makes the greatest contribution to

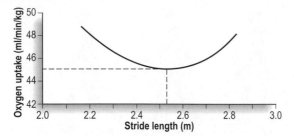

Fig. 2.62 The relationship between stride length and oxygen uptake (energy expenditure) for a distance runner running on a treadmill at 3.83 m/s at different stride length–stride rate combinations. The most economical combination was a stride length of 2.53 m and stride rate of 1.51 Hz

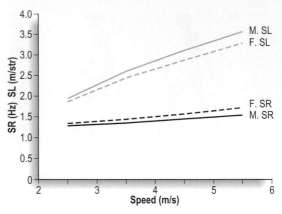

Fig. 2.63 Average stride length and average stride rate for groups of male and female recreational runners running at 2.5 m/s, 3.5 m/s, 4.5 m/s and 5.5 m/s on a treadmill

increase in speed in the lower half of the speed range and SR makes the greatest contribution to increase in speed in the upper half of the speed range. Hay (2002) demonstrated that these relationships hold true for most forms of human locomotion, including walking, running, hopping, wheelchair racing, swimming, canoeing and kayaking.

OPTIMAL STRIDE LENGTH

Running economy, i.e. the rate of energy expenditure (oxygen uptake) for a given submaximal running speed, depends upon a number of biomechanical and physiological variables, but the interaction between the variables appears to be very complex (Williams & Cavanagh 1987, Kyrolainen et al 2001). In any given situation, the stride length–stride rate combination adopted by a runner will depend upon the runner's personal anthropometric, anatomical and physiological characteristics and the environmental demands on the runner. For example, if the runner develops an injury, he is likely to alter his stride length and stride rate in order to minimize pain. Similarly, if the terrain is uneven or slippery, it is likely that the runner will adopt a stride length–stride rate combination that reduces the risk of falling. However, when there are no particular constraints, most runners naturally tend to adopt a stride length–stride rate combination that is optimal in terms of energy expenditure (Cavanagh & Williams 1982, Heinert et al 1988). Figure 2.62 shows the relationship between oxygen uptake (energy expenditure) and stride length for a male distance runner running on a treadmill at 3.83 m/s (7 min/mile) at different stride length–stride rate combinations, including his preferred combination. The graph indicates that the most economical stride length would be approximately 2.53 m, corresponding to a stride rate of 1.51 Hz. This was very close to the runner's preferred combination. Running at stride lengths longer or shorter than the optimal resulted in an increase in energy expenditure.

A number of researchers have investigated the relationship between stride length, height and leg length (Cavanagh et al 1977, Elliot & Blanksby 1979). Figure 2.63 shows the average stride length and average stride rate for 10 male and 10 female well practised recreational runners running at 2.5 m/s, 3.5 m/s, 4.5 m/s and 5.5 m/s (Elliot & Blanksby 1979). The average heights and leg lengths of the males and females were 178.1 cm, 89.5 cm, 166.0 cm and 83.1 cm respectively. At each speed, the females had a shorter average stride length and a higher average stride rate than the males. However, the average relative stride length (stride length divided by height and stride length divided by leg length) at each speed was very similar for both groups (Fig. 2.64). This may reflect a subconscious optimization of personal and environmental constraints, common to males and females,

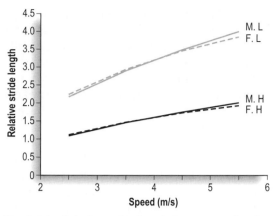

Fig. 2.64 Relative stride length for groups of male and female recreational runners running at 2.5 m/s, 3.5 m/s, 4.5 m/s and 5.5 m/s on a treadmill. H = stride length divided by height; L = stride length divided by leg length

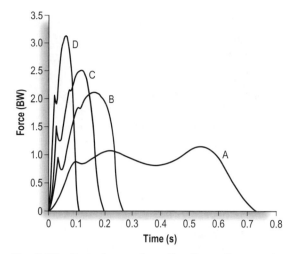

Fig. 2.65 Typical ground reaction force–time graphs (vertical component) for physically active adults walking at 1.0 m/s (A) and running at 3.0 m/s (B), 6.0 m/s (C) and 9.0 m/s (D). BW = body weight (Based on data in Alexander 1992 and Weyland et al 2000)

that results in an optimum stride length–stride rate combination for constant speed running, especially in well practised runners.

Practical worksheet 2 involves the collection of stride length, stride rate and relative stride length data for subjects running on a treadmill over a speed range of 1.5–3.5 m/s, which is then used to produce the corresponding stride length–speed, stride rate–speed and relative stride length–speed graphs.

GROUND REACTION FORCE IN RUNNING

The stride rate–speed and stride length–speed graphs in Figure 2.61 are based on the performance of a single male student as reported by Hay 2002. However, the relationships between stride rate, stride length and speed shown in the graphs are typical of males and females at all levels of performance (Hay 2002). Figure 2.61 shows that stride rate progressively increases throughout the upper half of the speed range. In contrast, stride length increases slightly and then decreases by about the same amount as maximum speed is achieved. Consequently, stride rate and, therefore, step rate, is largely responsible for increase in speed in the upper half of the speed range. Increase in step rate (steps per

second) depends upon step time (seconds per step), i.e. the shorter the step time, the higher the step rate. Step time for each leg is the sum of contact time (the time that the foot is in contact with the ground) and flight time (the time from toe-off of the foot to touchdown of the other foot). The decrease in step time (and increase in step rate) that occurs with increase in sprinting speed in the upper half of the speed range is due to a progressive decrease in contact time with little or no change in flight time (Weyland et al 2000). In order to reduce contact time and maintain the same flight time, the average magnitude of the resultant upward force acting on the sprinter during contact time must increase. Consequently, the average magnitude of the vertical component F_Y of the ground reaction force must increase. In general, the faster the sprinting speed, the greater the average magnitude of F_Y. This is reflected in Figure 2.65, which shows typical ground reaction force–time graphs (vertical component) for physically active adults walking at 1.0 m/s and running at 3.0 m/s, 6.0 m/s and 9.0 m/s; the shorter the contact time, the higher the peak and average F_Y (Weyland et al 2000). The world's fastest 100 m male sprinters have contact times of approximately 80 ms during the

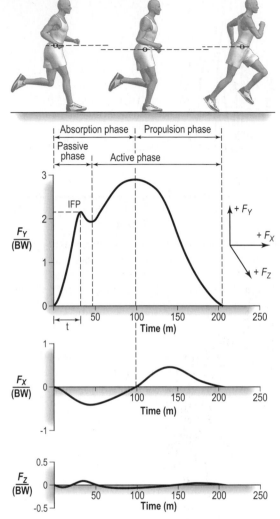

Fig. 2.66 The anteroposterior (F_X), vertical (F_Y) and mediolateral (F_Z) components of the ground reaction force acting on the right foot of a well practised rearfoot striker while running at about 4.5 m/s. BW = body weight; IFP = impact force peak; t = time to impact force peak

peak velocity phase (11.6–11.8 m/s; Moravec et al 1988) and produce ground reaction forces (vertical component) in excess of three times body weight on one leg (Mero & Komi 1986). Consequently, world class sprinting requires great strength of the leg extensor muscles.

Figure 2.66 shows the anteroposterior, vertical and mediolateral components of the ground

reaction force acting on the right foot of a well practised rearfoot striker (contacts the ground with the posterolateral part of the shoe) while running at about 4.5 m/s. Contact time is 205 ms. The graphs are typical of well practised middle- and long-distance rearfoot strikers over the middle- to long-distance speed range (Cavanagh & Lafortune 1980).

The anteroposterior component F_X is responsible for changes in forward velocity. The anteroposterior component exhibits two distinct phases with each phase taking up about half of contact time. In the first phase (48% of contact time) F_X is negative with a single smooth peak of 0.41 body weight (BW) after 45 ms (22% of contact). Consequently, forward velocity decreases during this negative phase. In the second part of contact (52% of contact time) F_X is positive with a single smooth peak of 0.47 BW after 142 ms (69% of contact). Consequently, forward velocity increases during this positive phase. The negative phase is referred to as the absorption (braking) phase and the positive phase is referred to as the propulsion (acceleration) phase. In constant speed running at 4.5 m/s, forward velocity decreases about 0.2 m/s in the absorption phase and increases about 0.2 m/s in the propulsion phase.

The vertical component F_Y is responsible for changes in vertical velocity. The downward vertical velocity of the body at foot-strike is reduced to zero during the absorption phase. In the propulsion phase, upward velocity progressively increases. F_Y exhibits two peaks with the first peak of 2.2 BW occurring after 32 ms (16% of contact time). The second peak of 2.9 BW after 93 ms (45% of contact time) indicates maximum vertical compression of the leg (as vertical velocity is reversed) and corresponds closely with the end of the absorption phase. In constant speed running at 4.5 m/s, vertical velocity decreases about 1.6 m/s in the absorption phase and increases about 1.6 m/s in the propulsion phase. The change in vertical velocity of the body during contact time is reflected in the vertical displacement of the centre of gravity (down during absorption, up during propulsion) as shown in the picture sequence in Figure 2.66.

The mediolateral component F_Z is responsible for changes in mediolateral velocity. The mediolateral component is very small (maximum of 0.1 BW) relative to the anteroposterior and vertical components. It is negative for most of contact time, indicating a small medially directed force.

ACTIVE AND PASSIVE LOADING

In most activities of everyday life, the magnitude and direction of the ground reaction force is determined by muscular activity under conscious control. In these circumstances, when the ground reaction force or any other external load (apart from body weight) is completely controlled by conscious muscular activity, the load is called an active load. By definition, active loads are unlikely to be harmful under normal circumstances. In everyday situations the muscles respond to changes in external loading to ensure that the body is not subjected to harmful loads.

However, it takes a finite time for muscles to fully respond (in terms of appropriate changes in the magnitude and direction of muscle forces) to changes in external loading; this time lag is referred to as muscle latency. Muscle latency varies between approximately 30 ms and 75 ms in adults (Nigg et al 1984, Watt & Jones 1971). Consequently, muscles cannot fully respond to changes in external loading that occur in less than the latency period of the muscles. In these circumstances the body is forced to respond passively (by passive deformation) to the external load; this type of load is a passive load. By definition, the body is unable to control passive loads and is vulnerable to injury from high passive loads. The body is subjected to passive loading during the period of muscle latency following foot-strike in walking and running. Approximately 80% of runners and joggers are rearfoot strikers, i.e. they contact the ground initially with the posterolateral aspect of the shoe (Kerr et al 1983). The remaining 20% of runners and joggers contact the ground initially with either the middle of the foot (midfoot strikers) or the front part of the foot (forefoot strikers). The passive phase

of ground contact in walking and running is characterized by a rapid rise in the vertical component of the ground reaction force, resulting in a relatively sharp peak, referred to as the impact force peak, within the first 30–50 ms after impact (Figs 2.58 & 2.66). The force then declines slightly before rising again at the start of the active phase of ground contact.

The slope of the vertical component of the ground reaction force during the passive phase reflects the rate of loading (impact force peak divided by the time to impact force peak); the steeper the slope, the higher the rate of loading. The higher the rate of loading, the higher the strain on the system of materials subjected to the passive load, i.e. the support surface, the shoe (including insole and sock) and the human body, especially the ankle and foot. The higher the strain, the greater the risk of damage/injury. The rate of loading depends upon the stiffness of the system: the greater the stiffness, the higher the rate of loading. Stiffness refers to the resistance of a material to deformation; the greater the resistance, the stiffer the material.

> Muscles cannot fully respond to changes in external loading that occur in less than the latency period of the muscles. In these circumstances the body responds passively and is vulnerable to injury from high passive loads.

EFFECT OF SHOES ON RATE OF LOADING

Figure 2.67 shows the ground reaction force–time graphs (vertical component) for the same male subject running at approximately 4 m/s barefoot (Fig. 2.67a) and in running shoes (Fig. 2.67b). The duration of ground contact time is similar in both conditions, as is the force–time curve in the active phase, but the force–time curve during the passive phase is different. The impact force peak in the barefoot condition is approximately 3 BW compared to approximately 1.9 BW with shoes. However, the most noticeable differences between the two conditions are the time to impact force peak and the

(a)

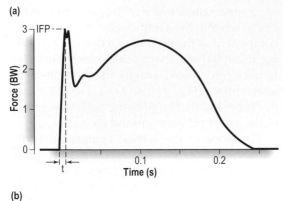

(b)

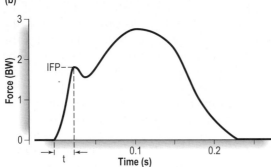

Fig. 2.67   Ground reaction force–time curves (vertical component) for a male rearfoot striker running at approximately 4 m/s (a) barefoot and (b) in running shoes. BW = body weight; IFP = impact force peak; t = time to impact force peak

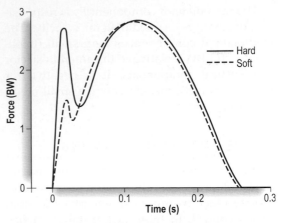

Fig. 2.68   Ground reaction force–time curves (vertical component) for a male rearfoot striker running at 5 m/s in hard- and soft-soled shoes. BW = body weight

rate of loading prior to impact force peak. The time to impact force peak when barefoot is approximately 6 ms compared to 24 ms when wearing shoes. The large difference in time to impact force peak is mainly responsible for the large difference in rate of loading, 500 BW/s (body weights per second) barefoot and 79 BW/s with shoes. The very high rate of loading in the barefoot condition may result in injury.

Figure 2.68 shows the ground reaction force–time graphs (vertical component) for another male subject running at 5 m/s in two types of running shoe, one with a hard (high stiffness) sole and one with a soft (moderate stiffness) sole. The hard-soled shoe results in a higher impact force peak and a higher rate of loading than the softer-soled shoe. Whereas soft-soled shoes reduce the rate of loading more than harder-soled shoes, there is a limit to how soft a shoe can be if it is to be effective in reducing

the rate of loading to an acceptable level. If the shoe material is too soft it can bottom out quickly, such that rate of loading is largely determined by other parts of the system.

EFFECT OF SEGMENTAL ALIGNMENT ON RATE OF LOADING

At foot-strike the alignment of the upper and lower leg and foot in relation to the line of action of the ground reaction force affects the leg's stiffness. The closer the line of action of the ground reaction force to the hip, knee and ankle joints, the more stiffly the leg will tend to respond to foot-strike and, consequently, the higher the rate of loading. This is typical of a rearfoot striker, where the line of action of the ground reaction force passes close to the joint centres of the ankle and knee (Fig. 2.69a).

When the knee is slightly flexed at foot-strike, the leg is more likely to respond like a spring, resulting in flexion of the hip, knee and ankle. This is typical of a forefoot striker, where the line of action of the ground reaction force dorsiflexes the ankle and flexes the knee (Fig. 2.69b). The stiffness of the spring depends considerably on the degree of activation of the muscles controlling the joints. Whereas muscle latency limits the speed with which a muscle can fully respond to a change in external loading, the

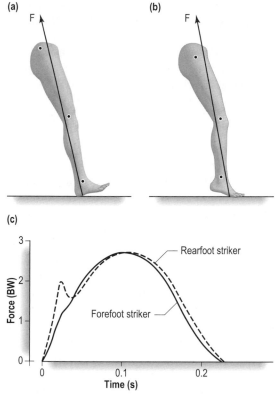

(a)

F

(b)

F

(c)

Force (BW)

3

2

1

0

Rearfoot striker

Forefoot striker

0   0.1   0.2

Time (s)

Fig. 2.69 Effect of the alignment of the upper leg, lower leg and foot at foot-strike on the line of action of the ground reaction force (*F*), impact force peak and rate of loading. (a) Rearfoot striker. (b) Forefoot striker. (c) Ground reaction force–time curves for a rearfoot striker and a forefoot striker

muscles can still influence the rate of loading by setting the rotational stiffness of the joints prior to foot-strike. The greater the degree of tension in the muscles, the greater the degree of rotational stiffness of the joints. A certain amount of rotational stiffness of the joints is necessary to prevent the spring from bottoming out too quickly. In general, the more the leg behaves like a spring at foot-strike, the lower the rate of loading. Striking the ground with the midfoot or forefoot is generally effective in preventing a high rate of loading following foot-strike, such that most midfoot and forefoot strikers do not exhibit a discernible impact force peak (Cavanagh et al 1984) (Fig. 2.69c).

Practical worksheet 3 involves recording the anteroposterior and vertical components of the ground reaction force and carrying out a force–time analysis of the vertical component.

LINEAR MOMENTUM

In terms of linear motion (angular motion is considered in Ch. 3), the inertia of a body at rest, i.e. its reluctance to move, depends entirely on its mass: the larger the mass, the greater the inertia, the greater the force that is needed to move it. The inertia of a moving body, i.e. the reluctance of the body to change its speed and/or direction of movement, depends upon its mass and linear velocity. The product of a body's mass and linear velocity is referred to as the linear momentum of the body. A cricket ball of mass 0.156 kg moving with a linear velocity of 40 m/s (about 90 mph) has a linear momentum of 6.27 kg.m/s, i.e.

linear momentum of ball
= 0.156 kg × 40 m/s
= 6.27 kg.m/s (kilogram metres per second)

Anyone who has ever been hit by a rapidly moving cricket ball or hockey ball will appreciate that the ball exhibits a great reluctance to change its speed and direction, which is reflected in the force exerted by the ball on impact.

In sports, the mass of a player during a game is fairly constant, if the loss of mass due to the exercise is discounted. Consequently the linear momentum of a player will vary directly with his/her linear velocity; the greater the linear velocity, the greater the linear momentum, the greater the force that will be needed to change his/her speed and direction. In rugby, a well-used ploy is to set up a situation in which the ball can be passed to a player who is moving rapidly forward close to the opposition goal line. The greater the linear momentum of the player when he receives the ball, the more difficult it will be for the opposition to stop him going over the goal line. For example, a player of mass 70 kg moving with a linear velocity of 5 m/s has a linear momentum of 350 kg.m/s, i.e.

linear momentum of player = 70 kg × 5 m/s
= 350 kg.m/s

In order to stop the player dead in his tracks, the defending team would have to tackle him with a linear momentum of the same magnitude but opposite in direction. This would be difficult to achieve because of the difference in speed of movement of the attacking player and the tacklers.

Further reference to velocity and momentum in this chapter, unless specified, will refer to linear velocity and linear momentum. Angular velocity and angular momentum are covered in Chapter 3.

NEWTON'S LAWS OF MOTION AND GRAVITATION

Irrespective of the number of forces acting on a body, the resultant force acting on a body at rest is zero. A body at rest will only begin to move when the resultant force acting on it becomes greater than zero. Similarly, the resultant force acting on a body that is moving with uniform linear velocity, i.e. in a straight line with constant speed, is also zero. It will only change direction, accelerate or decelerate when the resultant force acting on it becomes greater than zero. Furthermore, the amount of change in speed and/or direction that occurs will depend upon the magnitude and direction of the resultant force, i.e. there is a direct relationship between change of resultant force and change in movement. Isaac Newton described this relationship in what have come to be known as Newton's laws of motion. There are three laws of motion, sometimes referred to as the law of inertia (first law), the law of momentum (second law) and the law of interaction (third law). In addition to the three laws of motion, Newton's law of gravitation (law of attraction) describes the naturally occurring force of attraction that is always present between any two bodies. A body falls to the ground because of the gravitational attraction between the body and the earth and the planets are maintained in their orbits round the sun by the gravitational attraction between the planets and the sun.

NEWTON'S FIRST LAW OF MOTION

The first law of motion incorporates the fundamental principle that a change in resultant force is necessary to bring about a change in movement. The law may be expressed as follows:

The resultant force acting on a body at rest or moving with uniform linear velocity is zero and the body will remain at rest or continue to move with uniform linear velocity unless the resultant force acting on it becomes greater than zero.

For example, at the start of a soccer match, a player kicks the ball (changes the resultant force acting on the ball) in order to get the ball moving. Similarly, the speed of a passenger travelling on a bus will be the same as that of the bus. If the speed of the bus is suddenly reduced by braking or a collision, the passenger, unless suitably restrained, will be thrown forward (because of the change in resultant force arising from the sudden braking force at her feet) as she will tend to move forward with the speed that she possessed before the bus braked. Seat belts are usually worn by passengers in motor vehicles in order to reduce the risk of injury due to sudden changes in speed.

Not all forces produce or bring about a change in movement. Whether a particular force has any effect on the movement of a body depends upon the size of the force in relation to the inertia of the body. For example, in order to lift a barbell, the lifter must exert an upward force that is greater than the weight of the barbell, otherwise the barbell will not move.

NEWTON'S LAW OF GRAVITATION: GRAVITY AND WEIGHT

It is alleged that Newton was sitting under an apple tree one day when he saw an apple fall from the tree and that this observation led to the formulation of Newton's law of gravitation. The truth of the allegation cannot be confirmed but the phenomenon of natural force of attraction between bodies is a fundamental characteristic of the physical world. The law of gravitation may be expressed as follows:

Every body attracts every other body with a force that varies directly with the product of the masses of the two bodies and inversely with the square of the distance between them.

Thus, the force of attraction F between two objects of masses m_1 and m_2 at a distance d apart is given by,

$$F = \frac{G.m_1.m_2}{d^2}$$ Eq. 2.2

where G is a constant referred to as the gravitational constant and d is the distance between the centres of mass of the two bodies. In very simple terms, the law of gravitation means that the force of attraction between any two bodies will be greater the larger the masses of the bodies and the closer they are together. It is, perhaps, hard to appreciate that a force of attraction exists between any two bodies. However, the force of attraction between bodies is normally minute and has no effect on the movement of the bodies. For example, the force of attraction between two men, each of mass 70 kg, standing 0.5 m apart is approximately 1 10-millionth of a kilogram force (10^{-7} kgf). This force of attraction becomes even smaller the further apart the men move.

There is, however, one body that results in a significant force of attraction between itself and other bodies, i.e. the earth. In relation to the law of gravitation, the earth is simply a massive body (radius 6.37×10^3 km, Elert 2000) with a huge mass (5.98×10^{24} kg, Elert 2000). Even though the distance between the centre of the earth (assumed to be the centre of mass of the earth) and any body on the surface of the earth (or in space close to the surface of the earth) is extremely large, the force of attraction between the earth and any other body is much larger than that which exists between any two bodies on or close to the earth's surface. This is due to the huge mass of the earth. The force of attraction between the earth and any other body is not large enough to have any effect on the movement of the earth but it is certainly large enough to pull any body towards the earth. For example, consider two light bulbs hanging from separate flexes a few feet apart on the same ceiling. By the law of gravitation there will be a force of attraction exerted between each light bulb and the earth, such that each light bulb and flex hangs vertically. There will also be a force of attraction exerted between the two light bulbs. However, the magnitude of this force is insignificant and the light bulbs continue to hang vertically rather than angled toward each other.

The force of attraction between the earth and any body is referred to as the weight of the body. This is the force of attraction that keeps us in contact with the earth or brings us back to the surface of the earth very quickly should we momentarily leave it as, for example, when jumping off the ground. By the law of gravitation, the weight W of an object b may be expressed as,

$$W = \frac{G.m_b.m_e}{d_e^2}$$ Eq. 2.3

where G = gravitational constant = $6.673 \times 10^{-11}.m^3.kg^{-1}.s^{-2}$ (Elert 2000)
m_b = mass of the object
m_e = mass of the earth = 5.98×10^{24} kg
d_e = radius of the earth = 6.37×10^3 km.

Since G and m_e are constants, the term $G.m_e/d_e^2$ is constant for any point on the earth's surface, i.e.

$$W = m_b.g$$ Eq. 2.4

where

$$g = \frac{G.m_e}{d_e^2}$$ Eq. 2.5

g, not to be confused with G, is referred to as gravity. The earth is not a perfect sphere, d being slightly greater at the equator than at the poles. Since g varies inversely with the square of d, g is slightly greater at the poles than at the equator. It follows that the weight of an object will be slightly greater at the poles than at the equator. The law of gravitation applies to all bodies, including all the planets. Since the masses and radii of the planets differ from each other, it follows that the weight of an object on a particular planet (the force of attraction between the object and a particular planet) will be different from its weight on every other planet. For example, the mass of the moon ($0.073\,483 \times 10^{24}$ kg, Elert 2000) is approximately 1/81 of that of the earth and the radius of the moon (1.74×10^3 km, Elert 2000) is approximately 7/25 of that of the earth. Consequently, the weight of the object b on the moon can be expressed as,

$$W_n = \frac{G.m_b.m_n}{d_n^2} \qquad \text{Eq. 2.6}$$

where

W_n = weight of the object on the moon
G = gravitational constant
m_b = mass of the object
m_n = mass of the moon = $0.073\,483 \times 10^{24}$ kg
d_n = radius of the moon = 1.74×10^3 km.

Since $m_n = 0.0123m_e$ and $d_n = 0.2731d_e$, substitution for m_n and d_n in Equation 2.6 results in,

$$W_n = \frac{0.0123G.m_b.m_e}{0.0746d_e^2} = \frac{0.1649G.m_b.m_e}{d_e^2}$$

$$\simeq \frac{G.m_b.m_e}{6d_e^2} \qquad \text{Eq. 2.7}$$

Since

$$W_e = \frac{G.m_b.m_e}{d_e^2} \qquad \text{Eq. 2.8}$$

where W_e = weight of the object on earth, it follows from Equations 2.7 and 2.8 that

$$W_n \simeq \frac{W_e}{6}$$

i.e. the weight of the object on the moon is approximately one-sixth of its weight on earth.

Since the mass of the object is constant, it follows that the moon's gravity is approximately one-sixth of the earth's gravity. This can be clearly demonstrated by manipulating Equation 2.7, i.e.

$$W_n \simeq m_b . \frac{G.m_e}{6d_e^2} = m_b . g_n$$

where

$$g_n = \text{the moon's gravity} = \frac{G.m_e}{6d_e^2} \qquad \text{Eq. 2.9}$$

From Equations 2.5 and 2.9, it follows that $g_n = g/6$, where g is the earth's gravity.

The reduced gravity on the moon has two main effects on the movement of astronauts on the surface of the moon. Firstly, the strength of a particular astronaut on the moon would be the same as on earth, but his weight on the moon would be approximately one-sixth of his weight on earth. Therefore, he would be able to project himself off the surface of the moon far more easily than he could on earth. Secondly, the astronaut would be attracted back to the surface of the moon by a force of approximately one-sixth of the attraction force on earth. Consequently, he would appear to float down to the surface of the moon rather than falling rapidly, as on earth.

NEWTON'S SECOND LAW OF MOTION: THE IMPULSE OF A FORCE

From Newton's first law of motion, the resultant force acting on a body must be greater than zero in order to alter the motion of the body. A change in the velocity of a body will result in a simultaneous change in the momentum of the body (momentum = mass × velocity). When the resultant force acting on a body is greater than zero, the change in momentum, increase or decrease, experienced by the body depends upon the magnitude and direction of the resultant force and the length of time that the resultant force acts on the body. It was this realization that led Newton to formulate his second law of motion. The law may be expressed as follows:

When a force (resultant force greater than zero) acts on a body, the change in momentum experienced by the body takes place in the direction of the force and is directly proportional to the magnitude of the force and the length of time that the force acts.

The law can be expressed algebraically as follows:

$$F.t \propto m.v - m.u \qquad \text{Eq. 2.10}$$

where

F = magnitude of the resultant force
t = duration of force application
m = mass of the object
u = velocity of the object at the start of force application
v = velocity of the object at the end of force application.

The term $F.t$ (the product of the force F and duration of force application t) is referred to as the impulse of the force. The term $m.v - m.u$ is the change in momentum experienced by the object as a result of the impulse of the force. When v is greater than u, i.e. an increase in momentum, F is an accelerating force. When v is less than u, i.e. a decrease in momentum, F is a decelerating or braking force.

From Equation 2.10,

$$F \propto \frac{m.v - m.u}{t} \qquad \text{Eq. 2.11}$$

The right side of the equation indicates rate of change of momentum. The second law is often expressed in terms of Equation 2.11, i.e.

When a force (resultant force greater than zero) acts on a body, the rate of change of momentum experienced by the body is directly proportional to the magnitude of the force and takes place in the direction of the force.

From Equation 2.11,

$$F \propto \frac{m(v - u)}{t} \qquad \text{Eq. 2.12}$$

Since $a = (v - u)/t$, where a = the average acceleration of the body during time t, it follows from Equation 2.12 that

$$F \propto m.a \qquad \text{Eq. 2.13}$$

The second law is often expressed in terms of Equation 2.13, i.e.

When a force (resultant force greater than zero) acts on a body, the acceleration experienced by the body is directly proportional to the magnitude of the force and takes place in the direction of the force.

Since mass is constant, it is clear from Equation 2.13 that there is a direct relationship between F and a, i.e. the constant of proportionality between F and a is 1. Consequently,

$$F = m.a \qquad \text{Eq. 2.14}$$

Newton's second law of motion is often expressed as Equation 2.14, but the impulse–momentum expression is more widely used in the context of sport, i.e.

$$F.t = m.v - m.u \qquad \text{Eq. 2.15}$$

Newton's second law of motion is sometimes referred to as the impulse–momentum relationship or impulse–momentum principle. It has wide application in sport, since performance in many sports is concerned with increasing and decreasing speed of movement (and, therefore, changes in momentum) of the human body or associated implements such as bats and balls. The principle has directly or indirectly led to the development or modification of some sports techniques. For example, in the shot put, the velocity of the shot as it leaves the thrower's hand is determined by the impulse of the force exerted on it by the thrower. The force exerted by the thrower depends largely on his/her strength; in general, the stronger the thrower, the greater the amount of force that s/he will be able to apply to the shot. The length of time that the thrower can apply force to the shot depends upon his/her technique, i.e. the movement pattern (the way the body segments move in relation to each other) during the whole putting action.

Originally, shot put technique consisted largely of a standing put (Fig. 2.70e–g). In a standing put the thrower stands sideways to the intended direction of the shot with the left foot (for a right-handed thrower) against the stop board and the right foot close to the centre of the 2.135 m (7 ft) diameter shot put circle. The thrower then rotates the trunk and flexes the right leg to obtain a position (Fig. 2.70e) from which a powerful thrusting action can be made (Fig. 2.70e–g). Development of the technique resulted from attempts to utilize the rear part of the circle in order to apply force to the shot for a longer period of time (and over a greater distance, see Ch. 4) and, thereby, increase the impulse applied to the shot. The greater the impulse, the greater the release velocity of the shot and, other things being equal such as the height and angle of release, the greater the distance achieved. At the 1952 Olympic Games in Helsinki the winner of the men's shot put (Parry O'Brien, USA) demonstrated a new technique, which is still the most popular. In the O'Brien or glide technique, as it is called, the thrower takes up a starting position in the rear of the circle, facing in the opposite direction

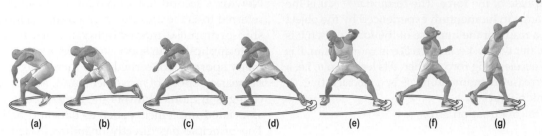

Fig. 2.70   Glide (O'Brien) shot put technique

to that of the intended direction of the shot, with the toe of the right foot (for a right-handed thrower) against the inner side of the circle. The thrower then flexes his/her hips and knees such that the shot may actually be outside the circle (Fig. 2.70a). From this position the movement across the circle is initiated by an explosive extension of the left leg closely followed by and in association with extension of the right leg (Fig. 2.70b). The purpose of this movement is to generate velocity of the shot in the direction of the put. Prior to landing with the left foot close to the stop-board, the thrower flexes the right knee and moves the right foot underneath his/her body such that it lands about half way across the circle (Fig. 2.70c–d). At this stage the thrower is close to a position from which the final thrusting movement, basically a standing put, can be made (Fig. 2.70d–g). The advantage of the O'Brien technique is that, as a result of the impulse of the force applied to the shot during the movement across the circle, the shot will already be moving in the direction of the put before the final putting action is initiated. Consequently, the total impulse applied to the shot during the complete sequence of movements will be greater than that applied in a standing put, resulting in a greater release velocity.

The technique of discus throwing originally consisted of a standing throw, i.e. half a turn that was made from the front of the 2.5 m (8 ft 2½ in) diameter discus circle (Fig. 2.71f–i). The most popular technique now involves one and three-quarter turns from a starting position in the back of the circle with the thrower facing the opposite direction to that of the throw. The thrower starts the turning movement from a position with the shoulders turned as far as possible to the right (for a right-handed thrower; Fig. 2.71a). The thrower then turns to his/her left and performs a fast rotating-stepping movement across the circle into a position from which the final slinging action can be initiated. The impulse of the force applied to the discus using the one-and-three-quarter turns technique is greater than that in a half turn standing throw and, consequently, results in a greater release velocity. Some shot putters use a one-and-three-quarter turns technique (rotation shot put technique) similar to that used in discus (Fig. 2.72).

> Newton's second law of motion is sometimes referred to as the impulse–momentum relationship or impulse–momentum principle. It has wide application in sport, since performance in many sports is concerned with increasing and decreasing speed of movement of the human body or associated implements such as bats and balls.

UNITS OF FORCE

From Newton's second law of motion, the relationship between the acceleration a experienced by a mass m when acted upon by a resultant force F is given by Equation 2.14, i.e. $F = m.a$. In the SI system, the unit of force is the newton (N). In accordance with Equation 2.14, a newton is defined as the force acting on a mass of 1 kg that accelerates it at $1 \, m/s^2$, i.e.

$$1\,N = 1\,kg \times 1\,m/s^2 \text{ (i.e. } 1\,N = 1\,kg.m/s^2)$$

Eq. 2.16

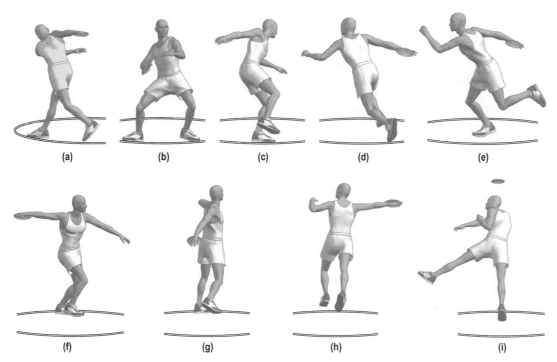

Fig. 2.71 One-and-three-quarter turn discus throw technique

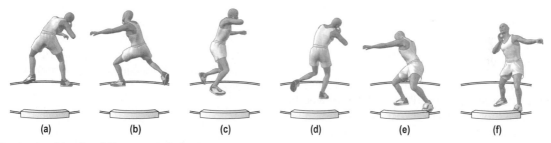

Fig. 2.72 Rotational shot put technique

From Newton's law of gravitation

$$W = m.g \qquad \text{Eq. 2.17}$$

where W = weight of the mass m and g = gravity.

It follows from Equations 2.14 and 2.17 that gravity is an acceleration. The magnitude of gravity varies slightly at different points on the earth's surface (see earlier section on Newton's law of gravitation), with an average value of $9.81 \, \text{m/s}^2$; in other words, in the absence of air resistance an object falling freely close to the earth's surface will accelerate at $9.81 \, \text{m/s}^2$ (and decelerate at $9.81 \, \text{m/s}^2$ if thrown vertically upward). From Equation 2.17, the weight of a mass of 1 kg, referred to as 1 kgf (kilogram force, see Table 1.1) is 9.81 N, i.e.

$$1 \, \text{kgf} = 1 \, \text{kg} \times 9.81 \, \text{m/s}^2 = 9.81 \, \text{N}$$

The kgf is referred to as a gravitational unit of force. Most weighing machines in everyday use, such as kitchen scales and bathroom scales, are graduated in kgf or lbf (pounds force). Thus the weight of a man of mass 70 kg can be expressed as 70 kgf or 686.7 N, i.e.

$$70 \, \text{kgf} = 70 \, \text{kg} \times 9.81 \, \text{m/s}^2 = 686.7 \, \text{N}$$

(a)   (b)

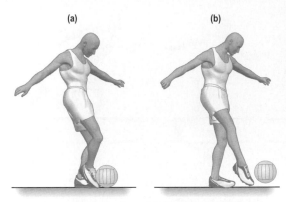

Fig. 2.73   A soccer player kicking a ball. (a) Ball at rest as the foot contacts the ball. (b) The instant of separation of the ball from the player's foot following the kick

In calculations using SI units, the unit of force is the newton and all forces, including weights, must be expressed in newtons. For example, consider the sprinter in Figure 2.53. If the resultant force acting on the sprinter is 111.2 kgf and his mass is 70 kg, it follows from Equation 2.14 that the acceleration a of the sprinter in the direction of the resultant force at the instant shown in the figure is given by

$$a = \frac{F}{m}$$

where $F = 111.2$ kgf and $m = 70$ kg. To complete the calculation, F (equivalent to the weight of a mass of 111.2 kg) must be expressed in newtons, i.e.

$$F = 111.2 \text{ kgf} = 111.2 \text{ kg} \times 9.81 \text{ m/s}^2 = 1090.9 \text{ N}$$

Therefore

$$a = \frac{1090.9 \text{ N}}{70 \text{ kg}} = 15.58 \text{ m/s}^2$$

Similarly, consider the average force exerted on a soccer ball of mass 0.45 kg during a kick. In Figure 2.73a the ball is at rest and in Figure 2.73b the ball has just separated from the player's boot following the kick. If the time of contact between the player's boot and the ball is 0.05 s and the velocity of the ball following the kick is 30 m/s (67.1 mph), the average force F exerted on the ball during the kick can be

determined by using the impulse–momentum form of Newton's second law of motion (Equation 2.15), i.e.

$$F.t = m.v - m.u$$

and

$$F = \frac{m(v - u)}{t}$$

where $t = 0.05$ s, $m = 0.45$ kg, $u = 0$ and $v = 30$ m/s.

Therefore,

$$F = \frac{0.45 \text{ kg } (30 \text{ m/s} - 0 \text{ m/s})}{0.05 \text{ s}}$$

$$F = \frac{13.5 \text{ kg.m/s}}{0.05 \text{ s}} = 270 \text{ N}$$

Since 1 kgf = 9.81 N, then

$$F = \frac{270}{9.81} \text{ kgf} = 27.52 \text{ kgf}$$

The average force exerted on a golf ball during a drive can be calculated in the same way. For example, if F is the average force exerted on the ball, the mass of the ball $m = 0.046$ kg (1.62 ounces), $u = 0$, $v = 70$ m/s (156.6 mph) and t (time of contact between club-head and ball) = 0.0005 s, then

$$F = \frac{m(v - u)}{t}$$

$$F = \frac{0.046 \text{ kg } (70 \text{ m/s} - 0 \text{ m/s})}{0.0005 \text{ s}} = 6440 \text{ N}$$

$$= 656 \text{ kgf}$$

Since 1 tonf = 1016 kgf, then $F = 0.64$ tonf.

FREE BODY DIAGRAM

A diagram showing, in vector form, all the forces acting on a body as if isolated from its surroundings is called a free body diagram. The forces represented may be contact forces such as pulls, pushes, support forces, wind resistance and buoyancy forces, or attraction forces such as weight. The only forces acting on the man in Figure 2.74a are his weight W and the ground

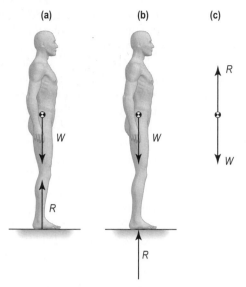

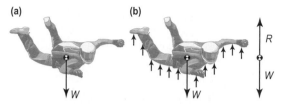

Fig. 2.75 The forces acting on a skydiver. (a) Immediately after jumping from the aeroplane, the skydiver will experience downward acceleration due to gravity. (b) Air resistance will quickly increase to equal body weight in about 5 s. W = weight of skydiver; clothing and parachute; R = air resistance

Fig. 2.74 The forces acting on a man standing upright. W = body weight; R = ground reaction force

reaction force R. In a free body diagram, the point of application of a force may be indicated by either the tail end or the arrow tip of the vector. In Figure 2.74a the point of application of R is indicated by the tail of the vector and in Figure 2.74b the point of application of R is indicated by the arrow tip of the vector. In Figures 2.74a and b the point of application of W is the whole body centre of mass. When only the linear effect of the forces acting on a body are considered (rather than linear and angular), the free body diagram may be simplified by representing the body as a point from which the forces arise, as in Figure 2.74c.

RESULTANT FORCE AND EQUILIBRIUM

When the resultant force acting on an object is zero, the body is described as being in a state of equilibrium. Consequently, Newton's first law of motion can be expressed as follows:

A body will remain in a state of equilibrium (at rest or moving with uniform linear velocity) until the resultant force acting on it becomes greater than zero.

The motion of a skydiver and a person travelling in a lift will be described to illustrate the concept of equilibrium.

Skydiver

When a skydiver jumps out of an aeroplane she will be accelerated toward the earth by the force of her body weight W (weight of skydiver, parachute and clothing; Fig. 2.75a). For the first few seconds of the fall, she will experience uniform downward acceleration, i.e. gravity. However, as her downward velocity increases, so will the air resistance R, i.e. the upward force exerted by the air on the underside of her body. After about 5 seconds, when downward velocity is approximately 50 m/s (112 mph), R will be equal in magnitude but opposite in direction to W (Fig. 2.75b). Consequently, the resultant force on the skydiver will be zero and provided that the orientation and shape of her body does not change, she will continue to fall with uniform velocity of about 50 m/s (Fig. 2.76a and b). The skydiver will therefore be in a state of equilibrium. In order to land safely the skydiver must reduce her downward velocity to about 10 m/s (22 mph). This is achieved by opening the parachute, which suddenly presents a massive area to the air and greatly increases the air resistance. So great is the increase in air resistance that for about 2 seconds the air resistance is greater than the weight of the skydiver, i.e. $R > W$. Therefore, during this short period of time, there will be a resultant upward force acting on the skydiver. Consequently, she will decelerate and her downward velocity will be rapidly reduced to around 10 m/s (Fig. 2.76). As she decelerates, the magnitude of the air resistance quickly decreases to again equal body weight, i.e. $R = W$. Consequently, a new state of

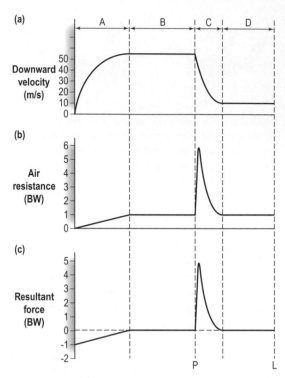

(a)

(b)

(c)

Fig. 2.76 (a) The variation in downward velocity of a skydiver. (b) The corresponding air resistance and (c) resultant force. A, Period of acceleration after jumping out of the aeroplane. Downward velocity increases to a maximum at which point the magnitude of $R = W$. B, Period of free fall in equilibrium. P, Parachute opens. C, Period of deceleration. D, Period of equilibrium prior to landing (L)

this example, the resultant force acting on the skydiver during the period of deceleration is in the opposite direction to the velocity of the skydiver. Consequently, it is necessary to define a positive and a negative direction and give each vector quantity its correct sign in the impulse–momentum equation. It does not matter which direction is regarded as positive as long as all variables are given their correct sign. The positive direction is usually regarded as the direction of the resultant force. In the example of the skydiver, the resultant force during the period of deceleration is upward. Consequently, in the worked example that follows, upward is positive and downward negative, i.e. R is positive because its direction is upward and W, u and v are all negative because their direction is downward. From Newton's second law of motion,

$$F = \frac{m(v - u)}{t}$$

where

$F = R - W$ = average resultant force acting on the skydiver during the period of deceleration

m = mass of the skydiver, clothing and parachute = 70 kg

u = velocity of skydiver before parachute opens = −50 m/s

v = velocity of skydiver at the end of the period of deceleration = −10 m/s

t = 2 s.

$$R - W = 70\,\text{kg}\frac{(-10\,\text{m/s} - (-50\,\text{m/s}))}{2\,\text{s}}$$

$$R - W = 70\,\text{kg}\frac{(-10\,\text{m/s} + 50\,\text{m/s})}{2\,\text{s}}$$

$$R - W = 70\,\text{kg}\frac{(+40\,\text{m/s})}{2\,\text{s}}$$

$$R - W = 1400\,\text{N}$$
$$R = 1400\,\text{N} + W$$
$$R = 1400\,\text{N} + 686.7\,\text{N}$$
$$R = 2086.7\,\text{N} = 3.04\,\text{BW}$$

i.e. the average magnitude of the air resistance acting on the skydiver during the period of deceleration would be in the region of three times the weight (BW) of the skydiver.

equilibrium is established, which continues until the skydiver lands on the ground.

It is possible to estimate the average magnitude of air resistance acting on the skydiver during the period of deceleration by applying Newton's second law of motion. However, it is important to ensure that each of the relevant vector quantities is afforded its correct direction in the impulse–momentum equation. In situations involving accelerating forces, such as the examples concerning the forces on a soccer ball and golf ball described in the earlier section on units of force, force and velocity are in the same direction and it is not necessary to designate a positive and a negative direction. However, in

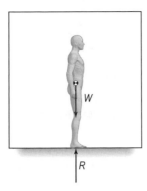

Fig. 2.77 The forces acting on a man standing in a lift. W = the weight of the man; R = ground reaction force

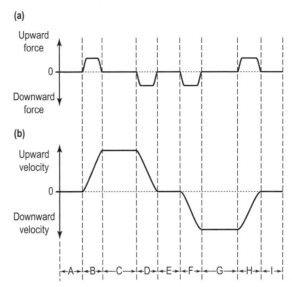

Fig. 2.78 The relationship between the resultant force (a) acting on a man standing in a lift and his velocity (b) as the lift moves up and down. A, Lift at rest, $R = W$, resultant force on the man is zero. B, Lift accelerating upward, $R > W$, resultant upward force on the man and velocity upward increasing. C, Lift moving upward with uniform velocity, $R = W$, resultant force is zero. D, Lift decelerating, $W > R$, resultant downward force, upward velocity decreasing. E, Lift at rest, $R = W$, resultant force is zero. F, Lift accelerating downward, $W > R$, resultant downward force, downward velocity increasing. G, Lift moving downward with uniform velocity, $R = W$, resultant force is zero. H, Lift decelerating downward, $R > W$, resultant upward force, downward velocity decreasing. I, Lift at rest, $R = W$, resultant force is zero

Travelling in a lift

Whether or not the lift is moving, there will be two forces acting on a man standing in a lift, his weight W and the ground reaction force R exerted by the floor of the lift on his feet (Fig. 2.77).

When the lift and, therefore, the man is at rest, $R = W$, i.e. the resultant force acting on the man will be zero. He will be in equilibrium and experience a force at his feet equal to his body weight. As the lift starts to accelerate upward from rest, there will be a resultant upward force acting on the man, i.e. $R > W$. Therefore, during the period of acceleration the man will feel heavier than normal since the force R acting on his feet will be greater than W. At the end of the period of acceleration, i.e. when the lift moves upward with uniform velocity, the force R will again be equal to W and equilibrium will be restored. When the lift starts to decelerate (as the upward velocity of the lift is reduced to zero) there will be a resultant downward force acting on the man, i.e. $W > R$. Therefore, during the period of deceleration, the man will feel lighter than normal since the force R will be less than W. As the lift starts to accelerate downward there will be a resultant downward force acting on the man, i.e. $W > R$, such that he will feel lighter than normal. At the end of the period of acceleration, i.e. when the lift moves downward with uniform velocity, the force R will again be equal to W and equilibrium restored. When the lift starts to decelerate (as the downward velocity of the lift is reduced to zero), there will be a resultant upward force acting on the man, i.e. $R > W$, such that he will feel heavier than normal. Figure 2.78 shows the relationship between the resultant force acting on the man and his velocity as the lift moves upward and downward from rest. You can easily verify these observations by travelling in a lift while standing on a set of bathroom scales.

The amount by which a person feels heavier or lighter during periods of acceleration and deceleration in a lift can be estimated by applying Newton's second law of motion. For example, consider a man of mass 70 kg standing in a lift which accelerates upward from rest at $0.6\,\text{m/s}^2$. During the period of acceleration there will be a resultant upward force acting on the man, i.e. $R > W$. From Newton's second law of motion,

$F = m.a$

where

$F = R - W =$ resultant upward force acting on the man during the period of upward acceleration
$m =$ mass of the man $= 70\,\text{kg}$
$a =$ acceleration of the man $= 0.6\,\text{m/s}^2$

$R - W = 70\,\text{kg} \times 0.6\,\text{m/s}^2$
$R - W = 42\,\text{N}$
$R = 42\,\text{N} + W$
$R = 42\,\text{N} + 686.7\,\text{N}$
$R = 728.7\,\text{N} = 1.06\,\text{BW}$

Therefore, during the period of upward acceleration, the man would feel heavier than normal by about $4.28\,\text{kgf}$ ($42\,\text{N}$). The greater the upward acceleration, the heavier the man would feel. For example, when a rocket lifts off from its launching pad, the acceleration is so great that the upward force exerted on an astronaut inside the rocket is many times the body weight of the astronaut, i.e. the acceleration is many times the acceleration due to gravity but in an upward direction. Consequently, during the period of acceleration, the astronaut will feel many times heavier than normal.

If the lift in the above example accelerated downward at $0.6\,\text{m/s}^2$, there would be a resultant downward force acting on the man, i.e. $W > R$. From Newton's second law of motion,

$F = m.a$

where

$F = W - R =$ resultant downward force acting on the man during the period of downward acceleration
$m =$ mass of the man $= 70\,\text{kg}$
$a =$ acceleration of the man $= 0.6\,\text{m/s}^2$

$W - R = 70\,\text{kg} \times 0.6\,\text{m/s}^2$
$W - R = 42\,\text{N}$
$R = W - 42\,\text{N}$
$R = 686.7\,\text{N} - 42\,\text{N}$
$R = 644.7\,\text{N} = 0.94\,\text{BW}$

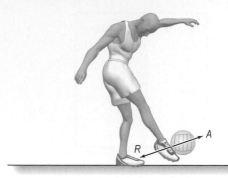

Fig. 2.79   The force A exerted by a soccer player on a ball when kicking the ball and the simultaneous equal and opposite force R exerted by the ball on the kicker's foot

Therefore, during the period of downward acceleration, the man would feel lighter than normal by about $4.28\,\text{kgf}$ ($42\,\text{N}$). The greater the downward acceleration, the lighter the man would feel.

NEWTON'S THIRD LAW OF MOTION

When a soccer player kicks a ball, there is a period of time in which the ball and the player's boot are in contact. During contact, the player exerts a force on the ball and simultaneously experiences a force exerted by the ball on his foot (Fig. 2.79). Furthermore, the greater the force exerted by the player on the ball, the greater the force exerted by the ball on his foot. Similarly, the greater the force exerted by a shot putter on the shot, the greater the force exerted by the shot on the putter's hand (Fig. 2.80). These examples indicate that whenever one body A exerts a force on another body B, then body B will simultaneously exert a force on body A. What is not so evident is that the forces are equal in magnitude and opposite in direction. This phenomenon is the basis of Newton's third law of motion. The law may be expressed as follows:

Whenever one body A exerts a force on another body B, body B simultaneously exerts an equal and opposite force on body A.

Consider the force exerted by and, therefore, on the head of a soccer player when heading a ball (Fig. 2.81). Assume that the ball travels

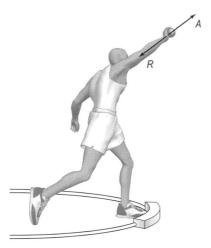

Fig. 2.80 The force *A* exerted by a shot putter on a shot during a putting action and the simultaneous equal and opposite force *R* exerted by the shot on the putter's hand

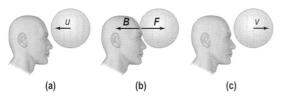

Fig. 2.81 Heading a soccer ball. (a) The direction of the ball just prior to contact with the player's head. (b) The force *F* exerted by the player's head on the ball and the equal and opposite force *B* exerted by the ball on the player's head. (c) The direction of the ball just as it leaves the player's head

horizontally just before and just after contact with the player's head and that the direction of the ball as it contacts the player's head (Fig. 2.81a) is opposite to that at which it leaves the player's head (Fig. 2.81c). From Newton's second law of motion,

$$F = \frac{m(v - u)}{t}$$

where

F = average force exerted on the ball during contact with the player's head

m = mass of the ball = 0.45 kg

u = velocity of the ball as it comes into contact with the player's head = −20 m/s (65.6 mph). u is negative because its direction is opposite to F

v = velocity of the ball as it leaves the player's head = 15 m/s (49.2 mph)

t = contact time between the ball and the player's head = 0.05 s.

$$F = 0.45\,kg\,\frac{(15\,m/s - (-20\,m/s)}{0.05\,s}$$

$$F = 0.45\,kg\,\frac{(15\,m/s + 20\,m/s)}{0.05\,s}$$

$$F = 315\,N = 32.1\,kgf$$

Consequently, the average force acting on the ball and, therefore, on the player's head during contact would be in the region of 32 kgf (about 46% of body weight for a player of mass 70 kg). The values of u, v, m and t used in this example are fairly typical of those that occur during the game (Asken & Schwartz 1998). The average and consequently the peak force acting on the head when heading the ball may be considerably greater than 32 kgf, especially when the ball is travelling very quickly. Considering that some players, particularly those who play in defensive positions, may be required to head the ball many times during a game, it is not surprising that they suffer concussion during or after certain games.

There are many occasions when it is necessary to reduce the magnitude of forces acting on the human body in order to prevent injury. Such occasions occur largely during the performance of two types of movement:

● Stopping a moving object, such as catching a cricket ball, trapping a soccer ball on the chest and riding a punch in boxing
● Stopping the human body, such as landing from a jump and falling in judo, wrestling and skateboarding.

The purpose of these movements is to reduce the momentum of the human body or that of the moving object to zero. In doing so, the deceleration force, as in landing from a jump (the ground reaction force), or the reaction to the deceleration force, as in catching a cricket ball (the force exerted on the hands), will be exerted on the body tissues, i.e. skin, muscles, ligaments, bones. If the moving object slows down very quickly, i.e. if the decelerating force applied to the object is very large, the body tissues may not be able to withstand the force and injury will occur. The underlying mechanical principle involved is still Newton's second law of motion but the technical emphasis in the movement pattern employed is on how to exert sufficient impulse to reduce the momentum of the moving object to zero without injuring the body (momentum–impulse) rather than on trying to increase impulse in order to increase velocity (impulse–momentum). From Newton's second law of motion, the greater the length of time over which the momentum of a moving object is dissipated, the smaller will be the average force required to bring the object to rest and, consequently, the lower the risk of damage to the person or object providing the stopping force. This will be illustrated with respect to catching a cricket ball and landing from a fall.

Catching a cricket ball

When catching the ball, the hands exert a force on the ball, referred to as the action force and the hands simultaneously experience an equal and opposite force, referred to as the reaction force. If the player holds his arms and hands fairly stiff in readiness for the catch, the ball will tend to decelerate rapidly (high action force) on impact with the hands and rebound out of the hands before the fingers have a chance to grasp it. At the same time, the reaction force may injure the hands. However, if the arms and hands are held fairly loosely in readiness for the catch, with the wrists slightly extended and the elbows and fingers slightly flexed, the impact of the ball on the hands will tend to flex the elbows, rather like compressing a spring, so that the hands move with the ball toward the chest (Fig. 2.82). The movement of the hands in the direction of the ball allows the fingers sufficient time to grasp the ball and, since the momentum of the ball is dissipated over a longer period of time, the average size of the action force and, therefore, the reaction force on the hands is considerably reduced. The deceleration period of the ball can be lengthened even further with corresponding further

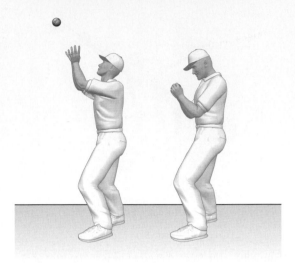

Fig. 2.82 Catching a cricket ball

reduction in the action and reaction forces by moving the trunk in the direction of the ball, i.e. downward and/or backward. A slip fielder may be seen to fall or roll backward in the process of taking a catch. Trapping a soccer ball on the chest is a similar action to catching a ball. As the ball contacts the chest, the trunk is moved backward, thereby dissipating the momentum of the ball over a longer period of time and reducing the force exerted on the ball and chest, with the result that the ball drops at the player's feet rather than bouncing away.

Landing from a jump or fall

Many court sports, including basketball, volleyball, badminton and tennis, involve jumping and landing. Players usually try to land on their feet in order to control the landing and be in a position to move off quickly for the next phase of play. When landing from a vertical jump, the downward momentum of the body has to be dissipated. This is achieved by the player pushing against the floor with his feet, which results in an equal and opposite force exerted by the floor against his feet, i.e. the ground reaction force. A stiff-leg landing will decelerate the body very quickly, but only at the expense of a very large ground reaction force, which may result in injury. Good landing

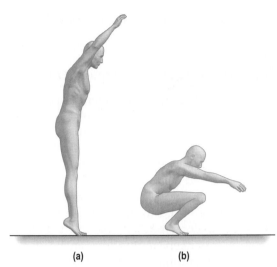

(a)   (b)

Fig. 2.83 Landing from a vertical jump (a) with legs extended at contact with the floor followed by (b) controlled flexion of the hips, knees and ankles

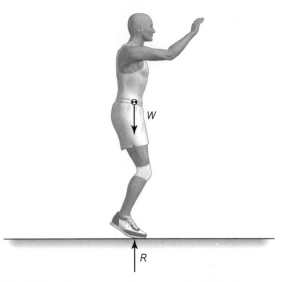

Fig. 2.84 The forces acting on a volleyball player landing from a spike jump. W = body weight; R = ground reaction force

technique involves controlled flexion of the hips, knees and ankles, which significantly increases the period of deceleration and, consequently, reduces the average and peak ground reaction force (Fig. 2.83).

Figure 2.84 shows a volleyball player landing following a spike jump. During the landing period, the body is acted on by two forces, the ground reaction force R and body weight W. If the downward velocity of the player when he contacts the floor is 3.4 m/s (after falling a distance of 0.6 m) and he lands fairly heavily (very little flexion of the hips, knees and ankles), his deceleration will be rapid and he will come to rest very quickly in about 0.1 s. During the period of deceleration there will be a resultant upward force acting on the player, i.e. $R > W$. From Newton's second law of motion,

$$F = \frac{m(v - u)}{t}$$

where

$F = R - W$ = average resultant force acting on the player during the period of deceleration
m = mass of the player = 70 kg
u = velocity of the player on contact with the floor = −3.4 m/s. u is negative because its direction is opposite to that of the resultant force

$v = 0$
$t = 0.1$ s;

i.e.

$$R - W = 70 \text{ kg} \frac{(0 \text{ m/s} - (-3.4 \text{ m/s}))}{0.1 \text{ s}}$$

$$R - W = 2380 \text{ N}$$
$$R = 2380 \text{ N} + W$$
$$R = 2380 \text{ N} + 686.7 \text{ N}$$
$$R = 3066.7 \text{ N} = 4.46 \text{ BW}$$

i.e. the average magnitude of R during the period of deceleration would be in the region of 4.5 times the body weight of the player. Consequently, the peak of R would be much larger than 4.5 BW and could result in injury. If the man landed relatively softly, by flexing his hips, knees and ankles to cushion the impact, the period of deceleration could be increased to approximately 0.3 s, which would considerably reduce the average and peak levels of R, i.e.

$$R - W = 70 \text{ kg} \frac{(0 \text{ m/s} - (-3.4 \text{ m/s}))}{0.3 \text{ s}}$$

$$R - W = 793 \text{ N}$$
$$R = 793 \text{ N} + W$$
$$R = 793 \text{ N} + 686.7 \text{ N}$$
$$R = 1479.7 \text{ N} = 2.15 \text{ BW}$$

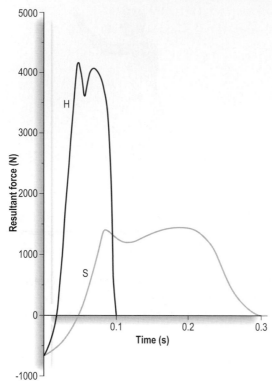

Fig. 2.85 Resultant force–time graphs of a hard (H) and soft (S) landing from a spike jump. Body weight = 686.7 N (70 kgf)

In both of the above examples the momentum of the player on contact with the floor was 238 kg.m/s (70 kg × 3.4 m/s). Consequently, the impulse of F (the average resultant force acting on the player during the period of deceleration) would need to be 238 N.s. In the hard landing this was achieved with an average resultant force $F = 2380$ N over a period of 0.1 s (2380 N × 0.1 s = 238 N.s) and in the soft landing it was achieved with an average resultant force $F = 793$ N over a period of 0.3 s (793 N × 0.3 s = 238 N.s). Figure 2.85 shows the resultant force–time graphs of the two types of landing. In each type of landing, the area between the force–time graph and the time axis represents the impulse of the resultant force. Each graph has a short negative period just after contact with the floor (approximately 16 ms and 47 ms in the hard and soft landings respectively), i.e. before the resultant force begins to decelerate the downward velocity of the player. The sum

of the negative and positive areas of each graph are the same, i.e. 238 N.s.

Protective clothing and equipment

Special clothing and equipment is used in many sports to reduce the risk of injury from impact forces. In sports that involve a lot of jumping and landing, such as basketball and volleyball, the players usually wear fairly thick-soled shoes and thick socks in order to cushion landings. In sports such as gymnastics and judo, mats are used to decrease the forces on the body arising from landing and falling. In athletics, very deep landing areas are needed in order to prevent injury in high jump and pole vault. Helmets are worn to reduce the risk of head injury in a range of sports, including cycling, skateboarding, canoeing, American football, cricket and rock-climbing. Volleyball players and skateboarders wear knee pads and elbow pads. Batsmen and wicket keepers in cricket wear gloves and leg pads. In the days of prize fighting when contestants fought without gloves, the injuries sustained were often very serious. In modern professional boxing the boxers wear gloves of a prescribed weight and structure, which reduces impact forces. In amateur boxing, headguards are compulsory and professional boxers wear headguards in training.

> From Newton's second law of motion, the greater the length of time over which the momentum of a moving object is dissipated, the smaller will be the average force required to bring the object to rest and, consequently, the lower the risk of damage to the person or object providing the stopping force.

The importance of the free body diagram in the solution of mechanical problems

Students sometimes have difficulty understanding the operation of Newton's third law of motion. For example, consider a man pushing a large box across a level floor (Fig. 2.86). From

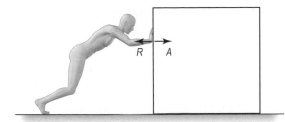

Fig. 2.86 Equal and opposite forces exerted by the man on the box (*A*) and the box on the man (*R*)

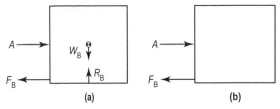

Fig. 2.87 Free body diagram of (a) the forces acting on the box and (b) the horizontal forces acting on the box. W_B = weight of the box; R_B = force exerted by the floor on the box; A = force exerted by the man on the box; F_B = friction force between the box and the floor

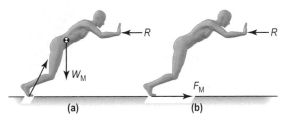

Fig. 2.88 Free body diagram of (a) the forces acting on the man and (b) the horizontal forces acting on the man. W_M = weight of the man; G_R = ground reaction force on the man; R = force exerted by the box on the man; F_M = friction force between the man and the floor

Newton's third law of motion, the force *A* exerted by the man on the box will be equal and opposite to the force *R* exerted by the box on the man. The question often asked is, 'If the force on the box is the same as that on the man's hands, how it is possible to move the box forward?' The misunderstanding arises from not taking into consideration all of the forces acting on the man and on the box. An object at rest will start to move only when the resultant force acting on the object is greater than zero. To determine the resultant force acting on an object it is necessary to consider all the individual forces acting on the object by means of a free body diagram. An understanding of the free body diagram is the key to understanding mechanics. Mechanical problems concerning resultant forces usually involve two or more objects in contact with each other. The first step in solving such a problem should be to draw a complete free body diagram for each object.

Figure 2.87a shows a free body diagram of the forces acting on the box. The only horizontal forces acting on the box, i.e. the only forces that determine whether the box moves horizontally across the floor, are *A* and F_B (Fig. 2.87b). It follows that the box will move forward if the force exerted by the man on the box is greater than the friction between the box and the floor, i.e. if $A > F_B$.

The forces acting on the man pushing the box are shown in Figure 2.88a. The only horizontal forces acting on the man are *R* and F_M (Fig. 2.88b). Consequently, the box will move forward if the frictional force at the man's feet is greater than the resistance of the box, i.e. if $F_M > R$. Since *R* is equal in magnitude to *A*, the box will move forward if $F_M > A$. Since the box will move forward if $F_M > A$ and $A > F_B$, it follows that the box will move forward if $F_M > F_B$, i.e. if the friction between the man's feet and the floor is greater than the friction between the box and the floor.

CONSERVATION OF LINEAR MOMENTUM

When two bodies collide, such as a club-head hitting a golf ball, they exert equal and opposite forces on each other for the same length of time, i.e. the two bodies experience equal and opposite impulses. Since the impulses are equal and opposite, the change in the linear momentum of each body must be equal and opposite. Consequently, the sum of the momentum of the two bodies after the collision will be the same as before the collision, i.e. there will have been a transfer of linear momentum from one body to the other but no loss or gain in the combined momentum of the two bodies. This phenomenon is referred to as conservation of linear momentum. The principle of conservation of linear momentum may be expressed as follows:

> If no external force acts on a system of colliding objects, the total amount of linear momentum in the system remains constant, i.e. the sum of the linear momentum of the colliding objects remains constant.

Algebraically, the principle can be expressed as follows:

$$m_1.u_1 + m_2.u_2 = m_1.v_1 + m_2.v_2 \qquad \text{Eq. 2.18}$$

where

m_1 and m_2 = the masses of the colliding bodies
u_1 = velocity of m_1 before the collision
u_2 = velocity of m_2 before the collision
v_1 = velocity of m_1 after the collision
v_2 = velocity of m_2 after the collision

Practically, it is difficult to demonstrate the principle of the conservation of linear momentum since the weights of the colliding objects will affect their motion in addition to the impulse of the impact force. However, when the contact time is very small and the impact force very large in relation to the weights of the colliding objects, as in driving a golf ball off a tee, conservation of linear momentum of the colliding bodies may be demonstrated experimentally. For example, high-speed film analysis of a golf drive has shown that if a club-head of mass 0.2 kg with a velocity of approximately 50 m/s hits a stationary ball of mass 0.046 kg, the resulting velocity of the ball is approximately 70 m/s (Daish 1972). From Equation 2.18, the linear momentum of the club-head and ball before impact is equal to $m_1.u_1 + m_2.u_2$, where

m_1 = mass of club-head = 0.2 kg
m_2 = mass of the ball = 0.046 kg
u_1 = velocity of m_1 before the collision = 50 m/s
u_2 = velocity of m_2 before the collision = 0

i.e.

$$m_1.u_1 + m_2.u_2 = (0.2\,\text{kg} \times 50\,\text{m/s})$$
$$+ (0.046\,\text{kg} \times 0)$$
$$= 10.0\,\text{kg.m/s}$$

The linear momentum of the club-head and ball after impact is equal to

$$m_1.v_1 + m_2.v_2$$

where

v_1 = velocity of m_1 after the collision
v_2 = velocity of m_2 after the collision = 70 m/s

i.e.

$$m_1.v_1 + m_2.v_2 = (0.2\,\text{kg} \times v_1)$$
$$+ (0.046\,\text{kg} \times 70\,\text{m/s})$$
$$= 0.2\,\text{kg}.v_1 + 3.22\,\text{kg.m/s}$$

In accordance with the principle of the conservation of linear momentum, the total linear momentum after impact is equal to the total linear momentum before impact, i.e.

$$0.2\,\text{kg}.v_1 + 3.22\,\text{kg.m/s} = 10.0\,\text{kg.m/s}$$

$$0.2\,\text{kg}.v_1 = 10.0\,\text{kg.m/s} - 3.22\,\text{kg.m/s}$$
$$= 6.78\,\text{kg.m/s}$$

$$v_1 = \frac{6.78\,\text{kg.m/s}}{0.2\,\text{kg}} = 33.9\,\text{m/s}$$

i.e. the velocity of the club-head after impact is 33.9 m/s, a reduction of 16.1 m/s. Theoretically, the impulse responsible for the reduction in the velocity of the club-head from 50 m/s to 33.9 m/s should be the same as the impulse responsible for increasing the velocity of the ball from zero to 70 m/s. The momentum of the ball after the impact = 3.22 kg.m/s (i.e. 0.046 kg × 70 m/s). Consequently, the impulse exerted on the ball during the impact = 3.22 N.s. It follows that the club-head would have experienced an equal and opposite impulse of 3.22 N.s during the impact, which would have reduced its velocity by

$$\begin{aligned}\text{change in velocity} \atop \text{of club-head} &= \frac{\text{impulse on club-head}}{\text{mass of club-head}} \\ &= \frac{3.22\,\text{N.s}}{0.2\,\text{kg}} = 16.1\,\text{m/s}\end{aligned}$$

The reduction of 16.1 m/s is exactly the same as that obtained by applying the principle of conservation of linear momentum.

UNIFORMLY ACCELERATED MOTION

Acceleration is the rate of change of speed, i.e.

$$a = \frac{v - u}{t_2 - t_1}$$

where

a = average acceleration
u = speed at t_1
v = speed at a later time t_2

i.e.

$$a = \frac{v - u}{t}$$ Eq. 2.19

where $t = t_2 - t_1$.
    From Equation 2.19,

$$v = u + a.t$$ Eq. 2.20

Equation 2.20 shows how the speed v of an object with an initial speed of u changes with time when it experiences uniform (constant) acceleration a. For example, consider the motion of a stone that is dropped from rest from a height of 200 m. Assuming that the effect of air resistance on the stone is negligible, the acceleration of the stone will be constant and the speed of the stone can be calculated using Equation 2.20 where $u = 0$ and a = gravity = 9.81 m/s². Table 2.9 shows the speed of the stone after each second in the first 6 s after release. Figure 2.89 shows the corresponding speed–time graph. As acceleration is constant, the speed–time graph is a straight line.
    In any speed–time graph, the area between the speed–time graph and the time axis is equivalent to the distance travelled by the object during the period of time under consideration. For example, the distance fallen by the stone in the first 3 s after release is represented by the shaded area A in Figure 2.89. The average speed of the stone during this period is equal to $(u + v)/2$ where, $u = 0$ (speed at $t = 0$) and $v = 29.43$ m/s (speed at $t = 3$ s), i.e.

$$\text{average speed} = \frac{0 + 29.43 \, \text{m/s}}{2} = 14.71 \, \text{m/s}$$

Table 2.9   Distance fallen and speed of a stone after each second during the first 6 s after being dropped from rest from a height of 200 m

Time (s)	Speed (m/s)	Distance (m)
0	0	0
1	9.81	4.90
2	19.62	19.62
3	29.43	44.14
4	39.24	78.48
5	49.05	122.62
6	58.86	176.58

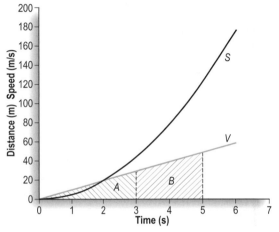

Fig. 2.89   Distance–time (S) and speed–time (V) graphs of a falling stone during the first 6 s after release

Since distance = average speed × time, the distance fallen in the first 3 s after release (s_{0-3}) is 44.14 m (s is the traditional symbol for distance), i.e.

$$s_{0-3} = 14.71 \, \text{m/s} \times 3 \, \text{s} = 44.14 \, \text{m}$$

Similarly, the distance fallen by the stone during the period 3–5 s after release (s_{3-5}) is 78.48 m, i.e.

$$s_{3-5} = \frac{(u + v)}{2} \times 2 \, \text{s}$$

where $u = 29.43$ m/s (speed at $t = 3$ s) and $v = 49.05$ m/s (speed at $t = 5$ s), i.e.

$$s_{3-5} = \frac{(29.43 \, \text{m/s} + 49.05 \, \text{m/s})}{2} \times 2 \, \text{s} = 78.48 \, \text{m}$$

This is represented by the shaded area B in Figure 2.89. The distance fallen during the first 5 s after release is the sum of areas A and B, i.e.

$$s_{0-5} = s_{0-3} + s_{3-5} = 44.14\,\text{m} + 78.48\,\text{m}$$
$$= 122.62\,\text{m}$$

Table 2.9 shows the cumulative distance fallen by the stone after each second in the first 6 s after release. Figure 2.89 shows the corresponding distance–time graph.

For an object moving with uniform acceleration, the distance s travelled by the object is given by,

$$s = \frac{(u + v)}{2}.t \qquad \text{Eq. 2.21}$$

where

u = speed at t_1
v = speed at a later time t_2
$t = t_2 - t_1$

Substituting v from Equation 2.20 in Equation 2.21 gives

$$s = \frac{(u + (u + a.t))}{2}.t$$

$$s = \frac{(2u + a.t)}{2}.t$$

$$s = u.t + \frac{a.t^2}{2} \qquad \text{Eq. 2.22}$$

From Equation 2.21,

$$t = \frac{2s}{(u + v)}$$

Substituting this expression for t in Equation 2.20 gives

$$v = u + \frac{a.2s}{(u + v)}$$

$$v(u + v) = u(u + v) + 2a.s$$

$$v^2 - u^2 = 2a.s \qquad \text{Eq. 2.23}$$

Equations 2.20–2.23 are collectively referred to as the equations of motion for an object

Table 2.10 Equations of motion for an object moving with uniform acceleration

	s	u	v	a	t
$v = u + a.t$		✓	✓	✓	✓
$s = \dfrac{(u + v)}{2}.t$	✓	✓	✓		✓
$s = u.t + \dfrac{a.t^2}{2}$	✓	✓		✓	✓
$v^2 - u^2 = 2a.s$	✓	✓	✓	✓	

moving with uniform acceleration. The equations, summarized in Table 2.10, show the relationships between distance travelled, speed, acceleration and time that describe the motion of the object.

AIR RESISTANCE

In everyday life, including sport, the human body is always surrounded by air or water or a combination of air and water, which presses on the body and affects its movement. The amount of pressure exerted by air or water, usually referred to as air resistance and water resistance, depends upon a number of factors (see below) including the shape and speed of the body and the density of air and water. Whereas water resistance has a considerable effect on movement of the human body, the effect of air resistance is usually negligible. Nevertheless, the constant presence of surrounding air means that the human body is unlikely to experience uniform acceleration, since the resultant force acting on the human body during movement is unlikely to be constant, even for a very short period of time.

In mechanics, air and water are both regarded as fluids, since the factors that determine air resistance and water resistance are the same. Fluid mechanics (the study of the forces that act on bodies moving through fluids and the effects of the forces on the movement of the bodies) is covered in some detail in Chapter 5.

Air resistance and water resistance are examples of drag, i.e. the force exerted by a fluid on a body moving through the fluid that opposes the movement of the body. The magnitude of drag depends upon the coefficient of drag, the density of the fluid, the area of the body presented to the fluid (perpendicular to the direction of movement) and the speed of the body relative to the speed of the fluid. Drag is expressed algebraically as follows:

$$F_D = \frac{C_D.\rho.A.v^2}{2} \qquad \text{Eq. 2.24}$$

where

F_D = drag (N)
C_D = coefficient of drag
ρ = density of fluid (kg/m^3) (ρ = Greek letter rho)
A = area (m^2)
v = relative speed (m/s)

- *Coefficient of drag*: The coefficient of drag is a dimensionless number, i.e. a number without units, that reflects the interaction of the shape, surface texture and speed of movement of the body. Its approximate range is 0–2.3 (Filippone 2005).
- *Density*: The density of air is approximately 1.25 kg/m^3 and the density of water is approximately 1000 kg/m^3 (Cutnell & Johnson 1995). Consequently, for equivalent C_D, A and v, water resistance is about 800 times greater than air resistance.
- *Area*: When standing upright in the anatomical position, the frontal area of an adult male is approximately 0.62 m^2 (Kubaha et al 2003). In running the frontal area of an adult male is approximately 0.45 m^2 (Davies 1980).
- *Relative speed*: In still air (no wind), the speed of the body relative to the air is the same as the speed of the body. For example, if a sprinter is running at 10 m/s through still air, his speed relative to the air is 10 m/s. If the sprinter is running at 10 m/s with a tail wind (in the same direction as the runner) of 1 m/s, the speed of the sprinter relative to the air is 9 m/s (10 m/s − 1 m/s). If the sprinter is running at 10 m/s into a head wind (in the opposite direction to that of the sprinter) of

1 m/s, the speed of the sprinter relative to the air is 11 m/s (10 m/s − (−1 m/s)). Drag increases with the square of the relative speed, i.e. a two-fold increase in relative speed results in a four-fold increase in drag.

All bodies moving through fluids experience drag. Some bodies, because of their shape (such as a discus, javelin and aeroplane wing) or speed of rotation (such as top spin on a tennis ball or side spin on a soccer ball) also experience a force at right angles to the drag force. This force is referred to as hydrodynamic lift. Hydrodynamic lift is covered in some detail in Chapter 5. For the remainder of this section, it is assumed that the motion of the objects described is not affected by hydrodynamic lift.

Table 2.11 shows the estimated drag (based on Eq. 2.24) acting on a male adult when walking at 1.5 m/s, sprinting at 11.7 m/s (maximum speed of an elite male sprinter in a 100 m race) and just after take-off in a long jump (horizontal component of velocity at take-off for an elite male athlete is about 9 m/s). In elite shot putting (male and female), the horizontal component of velocity of the shot at release is about 10 m/s. Table 2.11 shows the estimated drag on a shot just after release by an elite female athlete. Like a shot, balls used in sports are spherical. Table 2.11 shows the estimated drag on a number of different balls (tennis, baseball, cricket, table tennis, squash and golf) moving through air at 10 m/s.

Air resistance slows down or tends to slow down the moving object. Consequently, the effect of air resistance on the movement of an object is reflected in the deceleration that would be produced if the air resistance was the resultant force acting on the object. From Newton's second law (Eq. 2.14), for a given amount of air resistance F, the greater the mass m of the object the smaller the deceleration a produced ($a = F/m$), i.e. the smaller the effect of the air resistance on the movement of the object. This is reflected in the final column of Table 2.11. A direct comparison of the effect of air resistance on the shot and the six types of balls (all spherical and all moving at 10 m/s) can be made by investigating the relationship between the density and deceleration of

Table 2.11   Drag on a male adult when walking, sprinting and at take-off in a long jump, and on a shot and various types of ball

	Mass (g)	Radius (cm)	Coefficient of drag	Density[†] (kg/m³)	Area* (cm²)	Speed (m/s)	Drag (N)	Deceleration (m/s²)
Walking[†§]	85000		0.6	1.25	4500	1.5	0.3797	0
Sprinting[†§¶]	85000		0.6	1.25	4500	11.7	23.1019	0.27
Long jump[†§‖]	85000		0.6	1.25	4500	9	13.6688	0.16
Shot[**††]	4000	5.12	0.45	1.25	82.51	10	0.2321	0.06
Cricket ball[‡‡‡‡]	157	3.58	0.45	1.25	40.29	10	0.1133	0.72
Baseball[‡‡‡‡]	144	4.50	0.45	1.25	63.62	10	0.1789	1.24
Tennis ball[‡‡‡‡]	57	3.25	0.45	1.25	33.18	10	0.0933	1.64
Golf ball[‡‡‡‡]	46	2.20	0.45	1.25	15.20	10	0.0428	0.93
Squash ball[‡‡‡‡]	24	2.03	0.45	1.25	12.97	10	0.0365	1.52
Table tennis ball[‡‡‡‡]	2.7	2.0	0.45	1.25	12.57	10	0.0354	13.11

The data for mass, radius and area are presented in grams, centimetres and square centimetres respectively. For the calculations of drag, the area data have to be converted to square metres (see Eq. 2.24). Similarly, for the calculations of acceleration (drag divided by mass), the mass data have to be converted to kilograms (see Eqs 2.14 and 2.16).

* Area = $\pi.r^2$, where r = radius. [†] Density of air: Cutnell & Johnson 1995. [‡] Coefficient of drag: Linthorne 1994. [§] Area: Davies 1980. [¶] Speed: Wagner 1998. ‖ Speed: Hay et al 1986. ** Mass and radius of shot: International Amateur Athletic Federation 1984. [††] Coefficient of drag: Daish 1972. [‡‡] Mass and radius: http://en.wikipedia.org/

Table 2.12   Mass, radius, volume, density and deceleration of a shot and six types of ball all moving in air at 10 m/s

	Mass (g)	Radius (cm)	Volume* (cm³)	Density (g/cm³)	Deceleration (m/s²)
Shot	4000	5.12	562.2	7.11	0.06
Cricket ball	157	3.58	192.2	0.82	0.72
Baseball	144	4.50	381.7	0.38	1.24
Tennis ball	57	3.25	143.8	0.40	1.64
Golf ball	46	2.20	44.6	1.03	0.93
Squash ball	24	2.03	35.04	0.68	1.52
Table tennis ball	2.7	2.0	33.51	0.08	13.11

* Volume = $4\pi.r^3/3$ where r = radius

the objects (Table 2.12). In general, the greater the density, the smaller the deceleration.

> The magnitude of drag experienced by a body depends upon the coefficient of drag, the density of the fluid, the area of the body presented to the fluid and the speed of the body relative to the speed of the fluid.

As shown in Table 2.11, air resistance on the human body during self-propelled movement is usually very small. At natural walking speed (1.5 m/s), air resistance is extremely small (approximately 0.4 N, resulting in an equivalent deceleration of zero to two decimal places) and certainly imperceptible to the individual. Air resistance is perceptible at maximum sprinting speed (approximately 23 N, resulting in an equivalent deceleration of approximately $0.27\,m/s^2$) but is not likely to have a significant effect on performance (Mureika 2001). In the long jump, air resistance (approximately 14 N, resulting in an equivalent deceleration of approximately $0.16\,m/s^2$) may reduce horizontal distance during the flight phase of the jump by approximately 0.06 m in a 8.79 m jump (see below). Similarly, in shot put, air resistance (approximately 0.23 N, resulting in an equivalent deceleration of approximately $0.06\,m/s^2$) may reduce horizontal distance by approximately 0.11 m in a 19.85 m put (see below). However, the effect of air resistance on the movement of a shot during flight and on human movement during the flight phase of a jumping action is usually small enough to be regarded as negligible. Consequently, during flight, a shot and the human body experience more or less uniform acceleration (gravity) and their movement can be very accurately described by applying the equations of uniformly accelerated motion (Eqs 2.20–2.23).

PROJECTILES

In mechanics, a projectile is an object with no means of self-propulsion that is thrown (e.g. a ball or stone), thrust (e.g. a shot) or in some other way launched into the air. If the effect of air resistance on the movement of a projectile may be regarded as negligible, the only force acting on the projectile during flight is its weight, which acts vertically downward. Consequently, the vertical motion of the projectile will be subject to the uniform acceleration of gravity; in other words, following release, the upward velocity of the projectile will decrease at $9.81\,m/s^2$ until it reaches its maximum height, at which point its vertical velocity will be zero. It will then accelerate downward at $9.81\,m/s^2$ until it hits the ground. In contrast, since there are no horizontal forces acting on the projectile (resultant horizontal force = 0), its horizontal velocity will remain constant during flight. The time of flight and maximum height of the projectile can be determined by considering the vertical motion of the projectile. The horizontal range (horizontal distance from release to landing) can then be

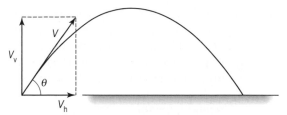

Fig. 2.90 Vertical and horizontal components of release velocity of a projectile. v = release velocity; v_v = vertical component of release velocity; v_h = horizontal component of release velocity. $v_v/v = \sin\theta$, i.e. $v_v = v.\sin\theta$; $v_h/v = \cos\theta$, i.e. $v_h = v.\cos\theta$

determined by considering the horizontal motion of the projectile. The basic equations (based on Eqs 2.20–2.23) will be derived and then applied in a number of real examples.

Step 1: Vertical and horizontal components of velocity of the projectile at release
As shown in Figure 2.90, if a projectile is released with a velocity v and angle of release θ, then the vertical and horizontal components of velocity are $v.\sin\theta$ and $v.\cos\theta$ respectively.

Step 2: Flight time for a projectile that lands at the same level as the release point (as in Figure 2.90)
Consider vertical motion from release to landing.

$$s = u.t + \frac{a.t^2}{2} \qquad \text{(Eq. 2.22),}$$

where

t = flight time
$u = v_0.\sin\theta$ (where v_0 = release velocity)
$a = -g$ (g is negative with respect to u)
s = resultant vertical displacement = 0

The projectile lands at the same level as the release point; in other words, even though the projectile may cover a large distance in rising to its maximum height and then falling back to the ground, its resultant vertical displacement from release to landing is zero, i.e. $s = 0$.

By substitution and rearrangement,

$$0 = v_0.\sin\theta.t - \frac{g.t^2}{2}$$

i.e. flight time $t = \dfrac{2v_0.\sin\theta}{g}$ \qquad Eq. 2.25

From Equation 2.25, it is clear that, for a given release velocity v_0, maximum flight time occurs when $\sin \theta$ has its maximum value, i.e. at 90°. Consequently maximum flight time is achieved by launching the projectile vertically upward.

Step 3: Maximum height
Consider vertical motion from release to maximum height.

$$v^2 - u^2 = 2a.s \qquad \text{(Eq. 2.23),}$$

where

$s = s_m = $ upward vertical distance from release to maximum height
$u = v_0.\sin \theta$ (where $v_0 = $ release velocity)
$v = $ vertical velocity at maximum height $= 0$
$a = -g$

By substitution and rearrangement,

$$0 - (v_0.\sin \theta)^2 = -2g.s_m$$

i.e. maximum height $s_m = \dfrac{v_0^2 . \sin^2 \theta}{2g}$ Eq. 2.26

From Equation 2.26, it is clear that, for a given release velocity v_0, maximum height occurs when $\sin^2 \theta$ has its maximum value, i.e. at 90°. Consequently maximum height is achieved by launching the projectile vertically upward.

Step 4: Range
Consider horizontal motion from release to landing.

$$s = u.t + \dfrac{a.t^2}{2} \qquad \text{(Eq. 2.22),}$$

where

$s = s_r = $ range
$a = 0$
$u = v_0.\cos \theta$ (where $v_0 = $ release velocity)
$t = $ flight time $= (2v_0.\sin \theta)/g$ (Eq. 2.25).

By substitution,

$$s_r = v_0 \cos \theta . \dfrac{2v_0.\sin \theta}{g} - 0$$

i.e. range $s_r = \dfrac{2v_0^2.\cos \theta.\sin \theta}{g}$ Eq. 2.27

(a)
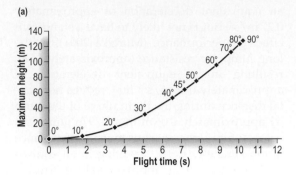

(b)
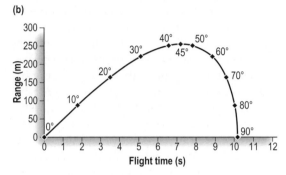

Fig. 2.91   (a) The relationship between flight time, maximum height and angle of release for a projectile (release velocity = 50 m/s) in the absence of air resistance. (b) The relationship between flight time, range and release angle for a projectile (release velocity = 50 m/s) in the absence of air resistance. The data corresponding to the points are shown in Table 2.13

From Equation 2.27, it is clear that, for a given release velocity v_0, maximum range occurs when $\cos \theta.\sin \theta$ has its maximum value, i.e. when $\theta = 45°$. Consequently maximum range is achieved by launching the projectile at 45° to the horizontal.

Equations 2.25, 2.26 and 2.27 only apply to projectiles where the launch point and landing point are on the same level and where air resistance is negligible. However, even with air resistance (but no hydrodynamic lift force), maximum flight time and maximum height are achieved with $\theta = 90°$ and maximum range is achieved with $\theta = 45°$. The relationship between flight time, maximum height and release angle for a projectile (release velocity = 50 m/s) in the absence of air resistance is shown in Figure 2.91a.

Table 2.13 Flight time, maximum height and range for a projectile without air resistance over the release angle range 0–90°

Angle (°)	Flight time (s)	Maximum height (m)	Range (m)
0	0	0	0
10	1.77	3.98	87.16
20	3.49	14.91	163.81
30	5.10	31.86	220.70
40	6.55	52.65	250.97
45	7.21	63.71	254.84
50	7.81	74.77	250.97
60	8.83	95.57	220.70
70	9.58	112.52	163.81
80	10.04	123.58	87.17
90	10.19	127.42	0

Flight time, calculated from Equation 2.25; maximum height, calculated from Equation 2.26; range, calculated from Equation 2.27.

The relationship between flight time, range and release angle for a projectile (release velocity = 50 m/s) in the absence of air resistance is shown in Figure 2.91b. The data corresponding to the points in Figure 2.91 are shown in Table 2.13. It is clear from Figure 2.91a that maximum height increases as release angle increases. Figure 2.91b shows that range increases with increase in release angle between 0° and 45° and then decreases with increase in release angle between 45° and 90°. Figure 2.91b also shows that flight time increases with release angle.

Trajectory of a projectile in the absence of air resistance

Figure 2.92a shows the typical trajectory (horizontal displacement–vertical displacement graph) of a projectile launched from ground level and landing at ground level in the absence of air resistance. In this particular example, the launch velocity of the projectile is 50 m/s and launch angle is 70° to the horizontal. Figure 2.92b shows the corresponding vertical velocity–time and vertical displacement–time graphs and Figure 2.92c shows the corresponding horizontal velocity–time and horizontal displacement–time graphs. Table 2.14 shows the data (at 1 s intervals) used to plot the graphs in Figure 2.92.

1. Flight time
Flight time t is given by Equation 2.25, i.e.

$$t = \frac{2v_0 . \sin \theta}{g}$$

where

v_0 = release velocity = 50 m/s
θ = release angle = 70°
g = 9.81 m/s²

i.e. flight time $t = \dfrac{2 \times 50 \times 0.9397}{9.81} = 9.58 \text{ s}$

2. Maximum height
Maximum height s_m is given by Equation 2.26, i.e.

$$s_m = \frac{v_0^2 . \sin^2 \theta}{2g}$$

where

v_0 = release velocity = 50 m/s
θ = release angle = 70°
g = 9.81 m/s²

i.e. maximum height $s_m = \dfrac{2500 \times 0.883}{19.62}$
$= 112.51 \text{ m}$

(a)

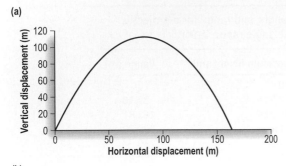

(b)

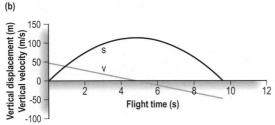

(c)

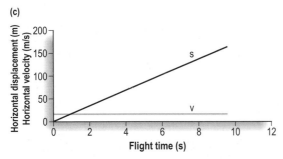

Fig. 2.92 Trajectory of a projectile, in the absence of air resistance, launched from ground level with a launch velocity of 50 m/s, a launch angle of 70° to the horizontal and landing at ground level. (a) Trajectory. (b) Vertical velocity–time (v) and vertical displacement–time (s) graphs. (c) Horizontal velocity–time (v) and horizontal displacement–time (s) graphs. The data used to plot the graphs are shown in Table 2.14

3. Range

Range s_r is given by Equation 2.27, i.e.

$$s_r = \frac{2v_0^2.\cos\theta.\sin\theta}{g}$$

where

v_0 = release velocity = 50 m/s
θ = release angle = 70°
g = 9.81 m/s^2

i.e. range $s_m = \dfrac{5000 \times 0.3421 \times 0.9397}{9.81}$

$\qquad\qquad = 163.84$ m

4. Time to maximum height t_m

Consider vertical motion from release to maximum height.

$$v = u + a.t \qquad\qquad \text{(Eq. 2.20)},$$

where

v = vertical velocity at maximum height = 0
a = -9.81 m/s^2
θ = release angle = 70°
u = vertical component of release velocity v_0
$\quad$ = $v_0.\sin\theta$ = 50 $\times$ 0.9397 = 46.98 m/s

By substitution and rearrangement,

$$0 = 46.98 - 9.81.t_m$$

$$t_m = \frac{46.98}{9.81} = 4.79\text{ s}$$

i.e. time to maximum height $t_m = 4.79$ s

5. Horizontal displacement from release to maximum height s_h

Consider horizontal motion from release to maximum height.

$$s = u.t + \frac{a.t^2}{2} \qquad\qquad \text{(Eq. 2.22)},$$

where

t = time from release to maximum height = 4.79 s
θ = release angle = 70°
a = 0
u = horizontal component of release velocity v_0
$\quad$ = $v_0.\cos\theta$ = 50 $\times$ 0.342 = 17.10 m/s

By substitution,

$$S_h = 17.10 \times 4.79 = 81.92\text{ m}$$

The time to maximum height (4.79 s) is exactly half the flight time (9.58 s) and the horizontal displacement from release to maximum height (81.92 m) is exactly half the range (163.84 m). These results are to be expected, since the release and landing points are on the same level and the acceleration of the projectile is constant. Horizontal acceleration is zero. Therefore, horizontal velocity is constant and horizontal

Table 2.14 Horizontal velocity, horizontal displacement, vertical velocity and vertical displacement of a projectile with release velocity of 50 m/s and release angle of 70° at 1s intervals from release to landing

Time (s)	Horizontal velocity (m/s)	Horizontal displacement (m)	Vertical velocity (m/s)	Vertical displacement (m)
0	17.10	0	46.98	0
1	17.10	17.10	37.17	42.08
2	17.10	34.20	27.36	74.35
3	17.10	51.30	17.55	96.81
4	17.10	68.40	7.74	109.46
5	17.10	85.50	−2.06	112.30
6	17.10	102.61	−11.87	105.33
7	17.10	119.71	−21.68	88.55
8	17.10	136.81	−31.49	61.96
9	17.10	153.91	−41.31	25.56
9.58	17.10	163.81	−46.98	0

Flight time, calculated from Equation 2.22 by consideration of vertical motion; horizontal velocity, constant; horizontal displacement, calculated from Equation 2.22 by consideration of horizontal motion; vertical velocity, calculated from Equation 2.20 by consideration of vertical motion; vertical displacement, calculated from Equation 2.22 by consideration of vertical motion.

displacement increases at a constant rate, which is indicated by the straight line horizontal displacement–time graph (Fig. 2.92c). Vertical acceleration is due to gravity, which results in constant deceleration upward of 9.81 m/s² and constant acceleration downward of 9.81 m/s²; this is reflected in the straight line vertical velocity–time graph (Fig. 2.92b) and the equal and opposite vertical velocity at release and landing (Table 2.14). The results also reflect the main characteristic of the flight of a projectile in the absence of air resistance, i.e. the second half of the trajectory (from maximum height to landing) is a mirror image of the first part of the trajectory (from release to maximum height); see Figure 2.92a. Mathematicians refer to this type of curve as a parabola.

Trajectory of a shot

In shot put, the effect of air resistance on the trajectory of the shot is small enough to be regarded as negligible (Lichtenberg & Wills 1978), i.e. the only force acting on a shot during flight may be considered to be its weight. Therefore, during flight, the horizontal acceleration of the shot may be considered to be zero and the horizontal velocity of the shot may be considered to be constant. Similarly, the vertical acceleration of the shot, i.e. the acceleration due to gravity, may be considered to be constant. Provided that some details of the trajectory of the shot and/or the release conditions of the shot are known, the complete trajectory can be described by applying the equations of uniformly accelerated motion. The actual equations that are used depend upon the variables that need to be quantified. Sometimes only one step (using one equation) is necessary, whereas other calculations may require two or three steps. The guiding principle underlying each calculation is to ensure that the time period under consideration and the direction of motion during the time period are clearly defined at the outset.

The length of a shot put is measured from the inside of a 10 cm high stop board at the front of the circle to the mark in the landing area closest to the circle (Fig. 2.93). Since the shot is normally released from a position outside the circle, referred to as the release distance s_d (horizontal displacement of the centre of the shot from the circle), the measured distance s_0 is the sum of s_d and the flight distance s_r (horizontal distance travelled during flight), i.e. $s_0 = s_d + s_r$. The maximum height of the shot during flight s_m (maximum height above the ground) is the sum

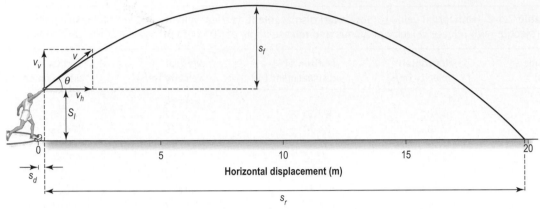

Fig. 2.93 Trajectory of a shot put. s_d = release distance; s_l = release height; s_r = flight distance; s_f = flight height; v = release velocity; v_h = horizontal component of release velocity, v_v = vertical component of release velocity. The data used to plot the trajectory are shown in Table 2.15

of the release height s_l (height of the shot at release) and the flight height s_f (vertical displacement of the shot between release and maximum height), i.e. $s_m = s_l + s_f$.

The women's shot put at the 1999 World Athletics Championships was won by Astrid Kumbernuss (Germany) with a put of 19.85 m. Playback of a video of the put at 25 Hz showed that the flight time was approximately 1.92 s (48 frames × 0.04 s), the release angle was approximately 39° and the release distance was approximately 0.25 m. Using this information, the complete trajectory can be described (Fig. 2.93).

1. Calculate the horizontal component of velocity at release v_h
Consider horizontal motion during flight.

$$s = u.t + \frac{a.t^2}{2} \qquad \text{(Eq. 2.22),}$$

where

$s = s_r = s_0 - s_d = 19.85\,\text{m} - 0.25\,\text{m} = 19.60\,\text{m}$
u = horizontal component of release velocity
  $= v_h$
a = horizontal acceleration = 0
t = flight time = 1.92 s

By substitution and rearrangement,

$19.60\,\text{m} = v_h \times 1.92\,\text{s}$

i.e. $v_h = \dfrac{19.60\,\text{m}}{1.92\,\text{s}} = 10.21\,\text{m/s}$

2. Calculate the vertical component of velocity at release v_v
From Figure 2.93,

$$\frac{v_v}{v_h} = \tan \theta$$

where $v_h = 10.21\,\text{m/s}$ and $\theta = 39°$

i.e. $v_v = v_h.\tan \theta = 10.21\,\text{m/s} \times 0.8098$
  $= 8.27\,\text{m/s}$

3. Calculate release height s_l
Consider vertical motion during flight.

$$s = u.t + \frac{a.t^2}{2} \qquad \text{(Eq. 2.22),}$$

where

$s = s_l$
$u = v_v$ = vertical component of release velocity
  $= 8.27\,\text{m/s}$
a = vertical acceleration = $-9.81\,\text{m/s}^2$
t = flight time = 1.92 s

By substitution and rearrangement,

$$s_l = (8.26 \times 1.92) + \frac{(-9.81 \times 1.92^2)}{2}$$
$$= 15.87 - 18.08 = -2.21\,\text{m}$$

The negative result indicates, as expected, that the point where the shot landed was below the release point, i.e. a vertical displacement of 2.21 m below the release point.

4. Calculate flight height s_f

Consider vertical motion from release to maximum height.

$$v^2 - u^2 = 2a.s \qquad \text{(Eq. 2.23)},$$

where

$s = s_f$
$u = v_v$ = vertical component of release velocity
$\quad = 8.27\,\text{m/s}$
v = vertical velocity at maximum height $= 0$
a = vertical acceleration $= -9.81\,\text{m/s}^2$

By substitution and rearrangement,

$$0 - (8.27)^2 = -19.62.s_f$$

$$s_f = \frac{(8.27)^2}{19.62} = 3.48\,\text{m}$$

5. Calculate maximum height s_m

$$s_m = s_1 + s_f = 2.21\,\text{m} + 3.48\,\text{m} = 5.69\,\text{m}$$

v_v, v_h and flight time were used to calculate the horizontal and vertical displacement of the shot at 0.2 s intervals (Table 2.15). These data were used to plot the trajectory of the shot shown in Figure 2.93.

For a projectile launched from ground level and landing at ground level, the optimum release angle (to maximize range) is 45° (Fig. 2.91b). However, a shot is released from above ground level such that the optimal release angle is less than 45° (Lichtenberg & Wills 1978). Application of the equations of uniformly accelerated motion indicate that, for a fixed release speed and fixed release height, the optimal release angle is approximately 42°. For example, Figure 2.94 shows the relationship between release angle, flight time and range for a release velocity of 13.14 m/s and release height of 2.21 m (as in the put by Astrid Kumbernuss in Figure 2.93). The data corresponding to Figure 2.94 are shown in Table 2.16. Figure 2.94 indicates that maximum range (19.68 m) would be achieved with a release angle of 42°. However, the predicted relationships in Figure 2.94 are based on the assumption that release speed, release height and release angle are independent of each other, i.e. that changing one variable will not change the others. However, analysis of actual puts by elite athletes has shown that the three variables are not independent (Matheras 1998, Linthorne 2001). As the release angle and/or release height are increased above the optimum (to maximize

Table 2.15 Horizontal velocity, horizontal displacement, vertical velocity and vertical displacement of a shot during flight at 0.2 s intervals, Release velocity = 13.14 m/s; release angle = 39°; flight time = 1.92 s

Time (s)	Horizontal velocity (m/s)	Horizontal displacement (m)	Vertical velocity (m/s)	Vertical displacement (m)
0	10.21	0.25	8.27	2.20
0.2	10.21	2.92	6.31	3.66
0.4	10.21	4.33	4.35	4.72
0.6	10.21	6.38	2.38	5.40
0.8	10.21	8.42	0.42	5.68
1.0	10.21	10.46	−1.54	5.56
1.2	10.21	12.50	−3.50	5.06
1.4	10.21	14.54	−5.46	4.16
1.6	10.21	16.59	−7.43	2.87
1.8	10.21	18.63	−9.39	1.19
1.92	10.21	19.85	−10.56	0

Flight time, calculated from Equation 2.22 by consideration of vertical motion; horizontal velocity, constant; horizontal displacement, calculated from Equation 2.22 by consideration of horizontal motion; vertical velocity, calculated from Equation 2.20 by consideration of vertical motion; vertical displacement, calculated from Equation 2.22 by consideration of vertical motion.

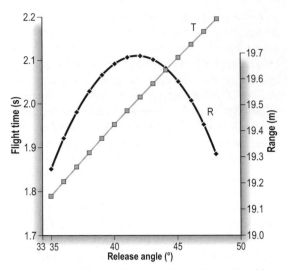

Fig. 2.94 Effect of release angle on flight time (T) and range (R) in the absence of air resistance for a shot with release velocity of 13.14 m/s and release height of 2.21 m. The data used to plot the graphs are shown in Table 2.16

Table 2.16 Effect of release angle on flight time and range for a shot with a release velocity of 13.14 m/s and release height of 2.21 m in the absence of air resistance

Angle (°)	Flight time (s)	Range (m)
35	1.79	19.25
36	1.82	19.37
37	1.85	19.46
38	1.89	19.55
39	1.92	19.61
40	1.95	19.65
41	1.98	19.68
42	2.02	19.68
43	2.05	19.67
44	2.08	19.64
45	2.11	19.58
46	2.14	19.51
47	2.17	19.42
48	2.19	19.30

range) for an athlete, the release speed that the athlete can produce decreases, which results in reduced range.

The range of release angles exhibited by elite shot putters is 26–45° with an average of 37°

(Susanka & Stepanek 1988, Tsirakos et al 1995). Release speed is the most important determinant of range. It is reasonable to assume that, through extensive training and practice, elite shot putters optimize their anthropometric (including height and arm length) and musculoskeletal (including strength and power) attributes in order to maximize the impulse of the propulsive thrust exerted on the shot and therefore maximize the release velocity of the shot. For most athletes this appears to be associated with a release angle in the region of 37°.

Effect of air resistance on the range of a shot put

In the above example of the shot put by Astrid Kumbernuss, the horizontal component of velocity at release was estimated to be 10.21 m/s. Consequently, using Equation 2.24 and the data in Table 2.11 for coefficient of drag (0.45), density of air (1.25 kg/m^3) and area (82.51 cm^2), the horizontal component of air resistance on the shot just after release is estimated to be 0.24 N, resulting in a horizontal deceleration of the shot of approximately 0.06 m/s^2. The vertical component of air resistance on the shot would retard the upward movement of the shot (from release to maximum height) and would also retard the downward movement of the shot (from maximum height to landing) such that the effect on flight time can be regarded as negligible. Consequently, the effect of the horizontal component of air resistance on the range of the shot can be estimated as follows.

1. Calculate the horizontal velocity of the shot on landing v_l

$$v = u + a.t \qquad \text{(Eq. 2.20),}$$

where

$v = v_l$
u = horizontal velocity of the shot at release = 10.21 m/s
a = −0.06 m/s^2
t = flight time = 1.92 s

By substitution,

$$v_1 = 10.21 - (0.06 \times 1.92) = 10.094\,\text{m/s}$$

2. Calculate range

$$s = \frac{(u + v)}{2}.t \qquad \text{(Eq. 2.21)},$$

where

s = range
u = horizontal velocity of the shot at release = 10.21 m/s
$v = v_l$ = horizontal velocity of the shot on landing = 10.094 m/s
t = flight time = 1.92 s

By substitution,

$$s = \frac{(10.21 + 10.094)}{2} \times 1.92 = 19.49\,\text{m}$$

Consequently air resistance is estimated to reduce the range of the shot by about 0.11 m (4¼ in) from 19.60 m (64 ft 3½ in) to 19.49 m (63 ft 11¼ in). This estimation is in agreement with Lichtenberg & Wills 1978, who estimated that air resistance reduces a 73 ft (22.25 m) shot put by a male athlete by about 6 in (0.15 m) in still air.

Variation in wind speed and direction will affect relative velocity and, therefore, the amount of air resistance acting on a shot during flight (Eq. 2.24). Whereas the effect of such wind variation on the trajectory of a shot is likely to be very small, the result of a competition, which might be decided by a few centimetres, could theoretically be affected by marked differences in wind speed or direction between throws.

Trajectory of a long jumper

As in shot put, the effect of air resistance on the trajectory of the centre of gravity of a long jumper is likely to be very small, largely because the duration of flight is so short, i.e. less than 1 s (Ward-Smith 1985). A long jump is measured as the perpendicular distance from the front edge of the take-off board to the nearest mark in the sand made by the jumper on landing. The surface of the sand in the landing area should be level with the top of the take-off board. The centre of gravity of the jumper is usually in front of the front edge of the board at take-off, referred to as the take-off distance s_d, and behind the feet on landing, referred to as the landing distance s_l. Consequently, the measured distance s_0 is the sum of s_d, s_l and the flight distance s_r (horizontal distance travelled during flight), i.e. $s_0 = s_d + s_r + s_l$ (Fig. 2.95). The maximum height of the centre of gravity during flight s_m is the sum of the take-off height s_t (height of the centre of gravity at take-off) and the flight height s_f (vertical displacement of the centre of gravity between take-off and maximum height), i.e. $s_m = s_t + s_f$. On landing, the centre of gravity is above as well as behind the heels. The height of the centre of gravity on landing is referred to as the landing height s_n. The relative height of the centre of gravity $s_v = s_t - s_n$, i.e. the vertical distance between the positions of the centre of gravity at take-off and landing.

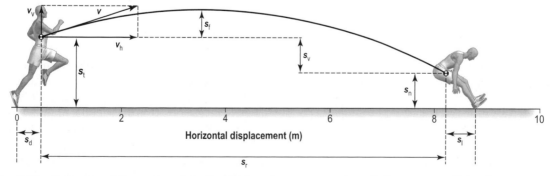

Fig. 2.95 Trajectory of the centre of gravity of a long jumper. s_d = take-off distance; s_r = flight distance; s_l = landing distance; s_t = take-off height; s_f = flight height; s_n = landing height; s_v = relative height; v = take-off velocity; v_h = horizontal component of take-off velocity; v_v = vertical component of take-off velocity. The data used to plot the trajectory are shown in Table 2.17

The men's long jump at the 1983 USA Track and Field Championships was won by Carl Lewis with a jump of 8.79 m (Hay et al 1986). The jump was made up of take-off, flight and landing distances of 0.46 m, 7.77 m and 0.56 m respectively and the vertical v_v and horizontal v_h components of velocity at take-off were 3.2 m/s and 9.5 m/s respectively. The height of the centre of gravity at take-off s_t was 1.33 m. Using this information, the complete trajectory of the jump can be described, as shown in Figure 2.95.

1. Calculate flight time t_f
Consider horizontal motion during flight.

$$s = u.t + \frac{a.t^2}{2} \qquad \text{(Eq. 2.22)},$$

where

$s = s_r = 7.77$ m
$u = v_h = 9.5$ m/s
$a = $ horizontal acceleration $= 0$
$t = t_f$

By substitution,

$7.77 = 9.5.t_f$

i.e. flight time $t_f = \dfrac{7.77}{9.5} = 0.818$ s

2. Calculate the landing height s_n
Consider vertical motion during flight.

$$s = u.t + \frac{a.t^2}{2} \qquad \text{(Eq. 2.22)},$$

where

$s = s_v$
$u = v_v = 3.2$ m/s
$a = -9.81$ m/s^2
$t = t_f = 0.818$ s

By substitution,

$$s_v = (3.2 \times 0.818) + \frac{(-9.81 \times 0.818^2)}{2}$$

$s_v = 2.62 - 3.28 = -0.66$ m

The negative result indicates, as expected, that the position of the centre of gravity on landing was below its position at take-off, i.e. a vertical displacement of 0.66 m below its position at the take-off point. As $s_v = s_t - s_n$, then,

$s_n = s_t - s_v = 1.33$ m $- 0.66$ m $= 0.67$ m

i.e. the landing height $s_n = 0.67$ m

3. Calculate flight height s_f
Consider vertical motion from take-off to maximum height.

$$v^2 - u^2 = 2a.s \qquad \text{(Eq. 2.23)},$$

where

$s = s_f$
$u = v_v = 3.2$ m/s
$v = $ vertical velocity at maximum height $= 0$
$a = -9.81$ m/s^2

By substitution and rearrangement,

$0 - 3.2^2 = -19.62.s_f$

$$s_f = \frac{3.2^2}{19.62} = 0.52 \text{ m}$$

i.e. flight heights $s_f = 0.52$ m

4. Calculate maximum height s_m

$s_m = s_t + s_f = 1.33$ m $+ 0.52$ m $= 1.85$ m

v_v, v_h and flight time were used to calculate the horizontal and vertical displacement of the centre of gravity at 0.1s intervals (Table 2.17). These data were used to plot the trajectory of the centre of gravity shown in Figure 2.95.

The height of the centre of gravity of a long jumper at take-off is higher than on landing. Consequently, the optimal release angle for maximum range is less than 45° (Linthorne et al 2005). Application of the equations of uniformly accelerated motion indicate that for a fixed take-off speed of 10.02 m/s and fixed relative height of −0.66 m, as in the jump by Carl Lewis in Figure 2.95, the optimal take-off angle is approximately 43°. However, the actual take-off angle by Carl Lewis was 18.6°. This is much lower than the predicted optimum angle, but consistent with the 15–27° range of take-off angles exhibited by elite long jumpers (Hay et al 1986, Lees et al 1993, 1994). There are two

Table 2.17 Horizontal velocity, horizontal displacement, vertical velocity and vertical displacement of the centre of gravity of a long jumper during flight at 0.1 s intervals: Take-off velocity = 10.02 m/s; release angle = 18.6°; flight time = 0.818 s

Time (s)	Horizontal velocity (m/s)	Horizontal displacement (m)	Vertical velocity (m/s)	Vertical displacement (m)
0	9.5	0.46	3.20	1.33
0.1	9.5	1.41	2.21	1.60
0.2	9.5	2.36	1.22	1.77
0.3	9.5	3.31	0.23	1.85
0.4	9.5	4.26	−0.76	1.82
0.5	9.5	5.21	−1.75	1.70
0.6	9.5	6.16	−2.75	1.48
0.7	9.5	7.11	−3.74	1.17
0.8	9.5	8.06	−4.73	0.75
0.818	9.5	8.23	−4.91	0.67

Flight time, calculated from range and horizontal velocity at take-off; horizontal velocity, constant; horizontal displacement, calculated from Equation 2.22 by consideration of horizontal motion; vertical velocity, calculated from Equation 2.20 by consideration of vertical motion; vertical displacement, calculated from Equation 2.22 by consideration of vertical motion.

main reasons why actual take-off angles are much smaller than predicted optimum angles.

1. Release velocity is the most important determinant of flight distance in shot put and long jump (and most other projectiles). Consequently, any variation in technique that reduces take-off velocity will almost certainly reduce flight distance. In order for the take-off angle to be 45°, the vertical component of velocity at take-off would have to be the same as the horizontal component. Even a 43° take-off angle would require the vertical component to be 90% of the horizontal component. However, the maximum vertical velocity that elite long jumpers can achieve at take-off is approximately 3.6 m/s (Hay et al 1986, Lees et al 1993). Even elite male high jumpers cannot generate more than about 4.3 m/s at take-off. A take-off angle of 43° with a vertical component of velocity v_v of 3.6 m/s would require a horizontal component v_h of 3.83 m/s and resultant take-off velocity of 5.28 m/s. This combination of take-off velocity and take-off angle would result in a flight time of 0.88 s and a flight distance of 3.43 m, which is less than half that normally achieved by elite male jumpers.

The difference, of course, is due to the much greater horizontal component of velocity generated by elite jumpers. Whereas the range of vertical velocity at take-off in elite long jumpers is approximately 2.4 m/s to 3.6 m/s in females and 3.0 m/s to 3.6 m/s in males, the range of horizontal velocity at take-off is approximately 7.2 m/s to 8.6 m/s in females and 8.5 m/s to 9.5 m/s in males (Hay et al 1986, Lees et al 1993). Since the horizontal component is usually more than double the vertical component, the take-off angle is usually in the range 15–27°. The small take-off angle is more than compensated by the large horizontal component of velocity.

2. At take-off, a long jumper would ideally like to maximize vertical velocity in order to maximize flight time and, simultaneously, maximize horizontal velocity in order to maximize flight distance. However, as in shot put, take-off velocity, take-off angle and take-off height in long jump are not independent of each other (Linthorne et al 2005). As the take-off angle and/or take-off height are increased above the optimum (for maximum range) for a jumper, the release speed that the jumper can produce decreases,

which results in reduced range. It is reasonable to assume that, through extensive training and practice, elite long jumpers optimize their anthropometric (including height and leg length) and musculoskeletal (including strength and power) attributes in order to achieve the optimal combination of take-off velocity and take-off height that, when properly executed, results in maximum flight distance. For most long jumpers this appears to be associated with a take-off angle in the range 15–27°.

Effect of air resistance on flight distance in the long jump

In the above example of the long jump by Carl Lewis, the horizontal component of velocity at take-off was 9.5 m/s. Consequently, using Equation 2.24 and the data in Table 2.11 for coefficient of drag (0.60), density of air (1.25 kg/m^3), area (4500 cm^2) and mass (85 kg), the horizontal component of air resistance on the jumper during flight is estimated to be 15.23 N, resulting in a horizontal deceleration of 0.18 m/s^2. The vertical component of air resistance on the jumper would retard upward movement (from take-off to maximum height) and would also retard downward movement (from maximum height to landing) such that the effect on flight time can be regarded as negligible. Consequently, the effect of the horizontal component of air resistance on the flight distance of the jumper can be estimated as follows.

1. Calculate the horizontal velocity of the jumper on landing v$_l$

$$v = u + a.t \qquad \text{(Eq. 2.20)},$$

where

$v = v_l$
u = horizontal velocity of the jumper at take-off = 9.5 m/s
$a = -0.18 \, \text{m/s}^2$
t = flight time = 0.818 s

By substitution,

$$v_1 = 9.5 - (0.18 \times 0.818) = 9.35 \, \text{m/s}$$

2. Calculate range s$_r$

$$s = \frac{(u + v)}{2}.t \qquad \text{(Eq. 2.21)},$$

where

$s = s_r$ = range
u = horizontal velocity of the jumper at take-off = 9.5 m/s
$v = v_l$ = horizontal velocity of the jumper on landing = 9.35 m/s
t = flight time = 0.818 s

By substitution,

$$s_r = \frac{(9.5 + 9.35)}{2} \times 0.818 = 7.71 \, \text{m}$$

Consequently air resistance is estimated to reduce flight distance by about 0.06 m (2½ in) from 7.77 m (25 ft 6 in) to 7.71 m (25 ft 3½ in). Variation in wind speed and direction will affect relative velocity and therefore the amount of air resistance acting on a jumper during flight (Eq. 2.24). Whereas the effect of such wind variation on the trajectory of a long jumper is likely to be very small, the result of a competition, which might be decided by a few centimetres could theoretically be affected by marked differences in wind speed or direction between jumps.

REVIEW QUESTIONS

Linear kinematics

1. Define/describe the following terms: force, mechanics, biomechanics, forms of motion, linear motion, rectilinear translation, curvilinear translation, distance, speed, linear displacement, linear velocity, linear acceleration, kinematics, kinetics.

2. With regard to human movement, give an example of rectilinear translation and an example of curvilinear translation.

3. A runner completes the first and second laps of an 800 m race (on a 400 m track) in 56 s and 52 s respectively. Calculate the average speed of the runner in each lap and over the whole race. Record the time, distance and average speed data in Table 2Q.1.

4. Middle-distance runners often train on a treadmill by running at different speeds.

Table 2Q.2 shows the leg length and time for 10 strides of an athlete running on a treadmill at speeds of 3.5 m/s and 5.5 m/s. Calculate the stride rate, stride length and relative stride length (RSL; with respect to leg length) of the athlete at the two speeds. Record the results in Table 2Q.2.

5. London Marathon: 18 April 1999
   Women's race: winner's time = 2 h 23 min 21 s
   Men's race: winner's time = 2 h 7 min 56 s
   Distance = 26 miles 385 yards
   1 mile = 1760 yd
   1 yd = 0.9144 m
   1 m = 1.0936 yd
   1 mile = 1609.34 m

   5.1 Use the data provided to complete Tables 2Q.3 and 2Q.4 for distance, time and average speed in the units indicated. (The letter m is the symbol for miles in the British imperial system and for metres in the SI system.)

Table 2Q.1: Average speed in laps 1 and 2 and in the whole race

Lap	Time (s)	Distance (m)	Average speed (m/s)
1			
2			
Total time			

Table 2Q.2: Leg length and stride parameters at 3.5 m/s and 5.5 m/s

Leg length (m)	Speed (m/s)	Time for 10 strides (s)	Stride rate (strides/s)	Stride length (m/stride)	RSL
0.9	3.5	6.94			
0.9	5.5	5.80			

Table 2Q.3: Distance, time and average speed for the winner of the women's race in different units (winner's time = 2 h 23 min 21 s)

Distance		Time		Average speed	
Miles (m)		Hours (h)		mph	
Kilometres (km)		Hours (h)		km/h	
Metres (m)		Seconds (s)		m/s	

Table 2Q.4: Distance, time and average speed for the winner of the men's race in different units (winner's time = 2h 7min 56s)

Distance		Time		Average speed	
Miles (m)		Hours (h)		mph	
Kilometres (km)		Hours (h)		km/h	
Metres (m)		Seconds (s)		m/s	

5.2 Calculate the average speed of the winner of the women's race as a percentage of the average speed of the winner of the men's race.

5.3 Calculate the average time in minutes to complete one mile and one kilometre by the winner of each race. Record the distance, time and average time data in Table 2Q.5.

Table 2Q.5: Average time per mile and average time per kilometre for the winner of the women's race and the men's race

	Distance (miles)	Distance (km)	Winner's time (min)	Per mile (min)	Per km (min)
Women's race					
Men's race					

Linear impulse and linear momentum

6. List the metric units and their abbreviations for the following variables

Variable	Units	Unit abbreviation
Force		
Time		
Impulse		
Mass		
Velocity		
Linear momentum		

7. If a soccer ball of mass 0.35 kg is at rest and then kicked such that its velocity when it separates from the kicker's foot is 42 m/s (94 mph), calculate the average force exerted on the ball during the kick if the contact time between boot and ball is 0.05 s. Give the force in N, kgf and lbf (1 kgf = 2.2046 lbf).

8. If a golf ball of mass 0.06 kg is at rest on a tee and is then driven such that its velocity when it separates from the club-head is 72 m/s (161 mph), calculate the average force exerted on the ball if the contact time between club-head and ball is 0.0005 s. Give the force in N, kgf, lbf and tons (1 ton = 2240 lbf).

9. In a shot put, if the impulse of the force exerted on the shot (mass = 7.26 kg) in the direction of release velocity is 159.72 N.s, calculate the release velocity of the shot. Assume that the shot was initially at rest.

10. If a gymnast of mass 55 kg lands on the mat following a vault with a downward velocity of 6.2 m/s and comes to rest in 0.2 s, calculate the average magnitude of the vertical component

of the ground reaction force exerted on the gymnast during the landing. Give the force in N, kgf, lbf and body weight (BW).

Vectors

11. Differentiate between vector and scalar quantities.

12. Define the terms sine, cosine and tangent with respect to a right-angled triangle.

13. If the angle θ in Figure 2Q.1 = 40° and the length of side c = 20 cm, calculate the lengths of sides a and b given that cos 40° = sin 50° = 0.766 and sin 40° = cos 50° = 0.643.

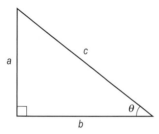

Fig. 2Q.1   A right angled triangle

14. In Figure 2Q.2, if the angle between the component force A and the resultant force F is 40° and the angle between the component force B and the resultant force F is 50°, calculate A and B given that F = 200 N, cos 40° = 0.766 and cos 50° = 0.643.

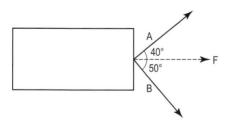

Fig. 2Q.2   Resultant of two forces pulling on a box

15. In Figure 2Q.3, if the force B exerted by the biceps brachii (assuming that this is the only active elbow flexor) = 100 N, calculate the

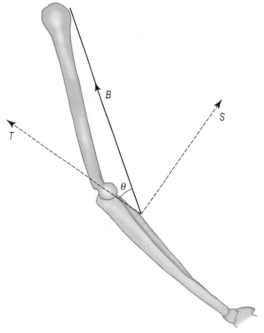

Fig. 2Q.3   Swing S and stabilization T components of the biceps brachii muscle force B

magnitude of the swing S and stabilization T components, given that sin 60° = 0.866 and cos 60° = sin 30° = 0.5. The swing and stabilization components are at right angles to each other.

16. Figure 2Q.4 shows the ground reaction force F exerted on a runner at an instant during the propulsion phase together with the x, y and z components of F (F_x, F_y, F_z). If body weight W = 70 kgf, F_x = 0.8 BW, F_y = 2.5 BW and F_z = 0.4 BW, determine the magnitude and direction (with respect to the horizontal) of:
i. F_{xy} (F in the sagittal plane)
ii. F_{yz} (F in the coronal plane)
iii. F_{xz} (F in the transverse plane)
iv. F (with respect to F_{xz}).

17. Figure 2Q.5 shows the anteroposterior F_x and vertical F_y components of the ground reaction force F exerted on an athlete running at 5 m/s.
i.   Use the force–time curves to determine (approximately) the magnitude of F_x and F_y in frames 2 and 4 of the stick-figure

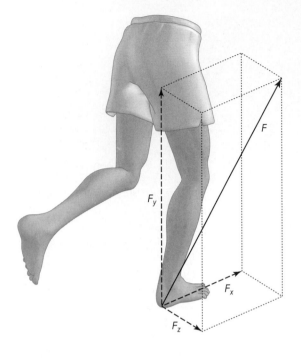

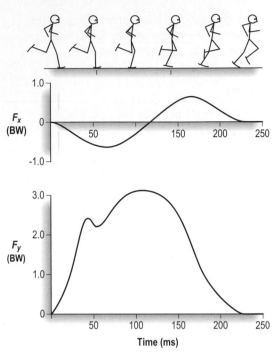

Fig. 2Q.5   Force–time graphs of the F_x (anteroposterior) and F_y (vertical) ground reaction force components

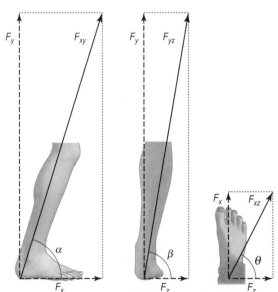

Fig. 2Q.4   Ground reaction force components

Table 2Q.6: Magnitude and direction of F_x, F_y and F_{xy}

	Frame 2	Frame 4
F_x (BW)		
F_y (BW)		
F_{xy} (BW)		
F_{xy} (°)		

sequence and record these values in Table 2Q.6. The point of application of the ground reaction force is indicated by the short vertical line underneath each frame.

ii.   Calculate the magnitude and direction (with respect to the horizontal) of the resultant force F_{xy} (resultant of F_x and F_y) in frames 2 and 4. Record the results in Table 2Q.6.

iii. Using a scale of 2 cm = 1 BW (body weight), draw the resultant force F_{xy} in frames 2 and 4 of the stick-figure sequence.

18.   Figure 2Q.6a shows the anterior aspect of the right knee complex, in particular, the quadriceps muscle group. Figure 2Q.6b shows the force vectors for vastus lateralis (L), combined rectus femoris and vastus

intermedius (F), and vastus medialis (M). Determine the resultant quadriceps force (magnitude and direction) by (i) vector chain method and (ii) calculation.

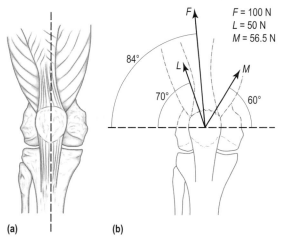

(a)   **(b)**

Fig. 2Q.6 Force components of the quadriceps muscle group

Ground reaction force

19. Define/describe the following terms: muscle latency, passive load, active load, passive phase, active phase, absorption phase, propulsion phase, stiffness, rate of loading.

20. Figure 2Q.7 shows the anteroposterior F_x and vertical F_y force–time components of the ground reaction force acting on the right foot of a rearfoot striker (mass = 70 kg) during ground contact while running in running shoes at approximately 3.5 m/s.

    i. Record the mass and weight of the subject in Table 2Q.7.
    ii. Use the graphs to determine the forces (N) and times (s) corresponding to the variables listed 1–5 in Table 2Q.7. Record the forces and times in the table.
    iii. Calculate the forces in units of body weight (BW) and record the forces in the table.

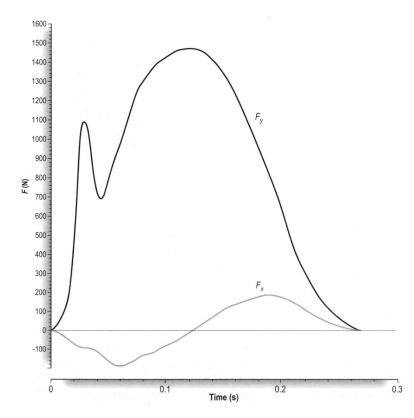

Fig. 2Q.7 Anteroposterior F_x and vertical F_y force–time components of the ground reaction force acting on the right foot of a rearfoot striker (mass = 70 kg) during ground contact while running in running shoes at approximately 3.5 m/s

Table 2Q.7: Analysis of the vertical component (F_y–time) of the ground reaction force acting on the right foot of a subject during contact time in running

Name of subject:		Mass (kg)		Weight (N)	
Mass of subject					
Key points on F_y–time graph		Time (s)	Force (N)	Force (BW)	
1. Heel contact (t_1, F_{y1})					
2. Impact force peak IFP (t_2, F_{y2})					
3. End of the passive phase (minimum force following IFP) (t_3, F_{y3})					
4. End of absorption phase (t_4, F_{y4}) (when $F_x = 0$)					
5. Toe-off (t_5, F_{y5})					
		Time (s)		Proportion of contact time (%)	
6. Contact time ($t_5 - t_1$)					
7. Time to IFP ($t_2 - t_1$)					
8. Duration of passive phase ($t_3 - t_1$)					
9. Duration of absorption phase ($t_4 - t_1$)					
10. Duration of propulsion phase ($t_5 - t_4$)					
		L_R (N/s)		L_R (BW/s)	
Rate of loading (L_R) during impact ($F_{y2}/(t_2 - t_1)$)					

iv. Using the time data in Table 2Q.7 for points 1–5, calculate and record the time variables 6–10 in the table.

v. Calculate and record in Table 2Q.7 the rate of loading (L_R) during impact in N/s and BW/s.

Uniformly accelerated motion

In all the questions in this section, assume that the effect of air resistance is negligible.

21. A high jumper takes off with an upward vertical velocity of 4.2 m/s. Calculate (i) how high his centre of gravity rises from take-off to maximum height, (ii) the length of time from take-off to the maximum height.

22. During the upward propulsion phase of take-off (upward velocity at the start of the propulsion phase = 0), the net upward impulse on a high jumper of mass 60 kg is 246 N.s. Calculate how high the jumper's centre of gravity rises from take-off to maximum height.

23. A stone is dropped from a height of 150 m. Calculate the time it takes for the stone to hit the ground and the velocity of the stone as it hits the ground.

24. A ball is thrown upward with a release velocity of 10 m/s from a release height of 2 m. Use the convention that upward is positive and downward is negative to (i) complete Table 2Q.8 to show the velocity and displacement of the ball at 0.2 s intervals and on landing and (ii) plot the displacement–time and velocity–time graphs of the motion of the ball. Suggestion: use a spreadsheet such as Microsoft Excel to calculate and plot the data.

25. A shot putter releases the shot from a height of 2.1 m with a velocity of 12.5 m/s at an angle of 38° with respect to the horizontal. Calculate the range of the put, the maximum height of the shot during its trajectory and the impulse responsible for the release velocity.

Table 2Q.8:
Displacement and velocity of a ball thrown upward with a release velocity of 10 m/s from a release height of 2 m

Time into flight (s)	Velocity (m/s)	Displacement (m)
0	10.0	2.0
0.2		
0.4		
0.6		
0.8		
1.0		
1.2		
1.4		
1.6		
1.8		
2.0		
2.2		
2.222		

References

Alexander R McN 1992 The human machine. Natural History Museum Publications, London.

Asken M J, Schwartz R C 1998 Heading the ball in soccer. Physician and Sportsmedicine 26(11): 37–42, 44.

Baumann W 1976 Kinematic and dynamic characteristics of the sprint start. In: Komi P V (ed) Biomechanics VB. University Park Press, Baltimore, p 194–199.

Castle F 1969 Five-figure logarithmic and other tables. Macmillan, London.

Cavanagh P R, Lafortune M A 1980 Ground reaction forces in distance running. Journal of Biomechanics 13: 397–406.

Cavanagh P R, Williams K W 1982 The effect of stride length variation on oxygen uptake in distance running. Medicine and Science in Sports and Exercise 14: 30–35.

Cavanagh P R, Pollock M L, Landa J 1977 A biomechanical comparison of elite and good distance runners. Annals of New York Academy of Sciences 301: 328–345.

Cavanagh P R, Valiant G A, Misevich K W 1984 Biological aspects of modelling shoe/foot interaction during running. In Frederick E C (ed) Sport shoes and playing surfaces. Human Kinetics, Champaign, IL, p 24–46.

Cutnell J D, Johnson K W 1995 Physics. 3rd Edn, Wiley, New York, p 315.

Czerniecki, J. M. 1988. Foot and ankle biomechanics in walking and running: a review. American Journal of Physical Medicine and Rehabilitation 67(6): 246–252.

Dagg A I 1977 Running, walking and jumping: the science of locomotion. Wykeham Publications, London.

Daish C B 1972 The physics of ball games. English University Press, London.

Davies C T M 1980 Effects of wind assistance and resistance on the forward motion of a runner. Journal of Applied Physiology 48: 702–709.

Elert G (ed) The physics factbook. Available on line at: http://hypertextbook.com/facts/2000/KatherineMalfucci.shtml.

Elliot B C, Blanksby B A 1979 Optimal stride length considerations for male and female recreational runners. British Journal of Sports Medicine 13: 15–18.

Filippone A 2005 Aerodynamic database: drag coefficients. Available on line at: http://aerodyn.org/Drag/tables.html.

Hay J G 2002 Cycle rate, length and speed of progression in human locomotion. Journal of Applied Biomechanics 18: 257–270.

Hay J G, Miller J A, Canterna R W 1986 The techniques of elite male long jumpers. Journal of Biomechanics 19: 855–866.

Heinert L D, Serfass R C, Stull G A 1988 Effect of stride length variation on oxygen uptake during level and positive grade treadmill running. Research Quarterly for Exercise and Sport 59: 127–130.

Hennig E M, Staats A, Rosenbaum D 1994 Plantar pressure distribution patterns of young children in comparison to adults. Foot and Ankle 15(10): 35–40.

International Amateur Athletic Federation 1984 Track and field athletics: a basic coaching manual. IAAF, London.

Jones A M, Whipp, B J 2002 Bioenergetic constraints on tactical decision making in middle distance running. British Journal of Sports Medicine 36: 102–104.

Kerr B A, Beauchamp L, Fisher B 1983 Foot-strike patterns in distance running. In Nigg B M, Kerr B A (eds) Biomechanical aspects of sports shoes and playing surfaces. University Printing, Calgary, p 34–45.

Kubaha K, Fiala D, Lomas K J 2003 Predicting human geometry-related factors for detailed radiation analysis in indoor spaces. VIIIth International IBPSA Conference, Eindhoven, Netherlands, p 681–688.

Kyrolainen H, Belli A, Komi P V 2001 Biomechanical factors affecting running economy. Medicine and Science in Sports and Exercise 33: 1330–1337.

Lees A, Fowler N, Derby, D 1993 A biomechanical analysis of the last stride, touch-down and take-off characteristics of the women's long jump. Journal of Sports Sciences 11: 303–314.

Lees A, Graham-Smith P, Fowler, N 1994 A biomechanical analysis of the last stride, touch-down and take-off characteristics of the men's long jump. Journal of Applied Biomechanics 10: 61–78.

Lichtenberg D B, Wills J G 1978 Maximising the range of the shot put. American Journal of Physics 46: 546–549.

Linthorne N P 1994 The effect of wind on 100 m sprint times. Journal of Applied Biomechanics 10: 110–131.

Linthorne N P 2001 Optimum release angle in the shot put. Journal of Sports Sciences 19: 359–372.

Linthorne N P, Guzman M S, Bridgett L A 2005 Optimal take-off angle in the long jump. Journal of Sports Sciences 23: 703–712.

Matheras A V 1998 Shot-put: optimum angles of release. Track & Field Coaches Review 72(2): 24–26.

Mero A, Komi P V 1986 Force-, EMG- and elasticity-velocity relationship at submaximal, maximal and supramaximal running speeds in sprinters. European Journal of Applied Physiology 55: 553–561.

Moravec P J, Ruzicka P, Susanka P et al 1988 The 1987 International Athletic Foundation/IAAF Scientific Project Report: time analysis of the 100 metres events at the II World Championships in Athletics. New Studies in Athletics 3: 61–96.

Murase Y, Hoshikawa T, Yasuda N et al 1976 Analysis of changes in progressive speed during 100-meter dash. In: Komi P V (ed.) Biomechanics VB. University Park Press, Baltimore, MD, p 200–207.

Mureika J R 2001 A realistic quasi-physical model of the 100 m dash. Canadian Journal of Physics 79: 697–713.

Nigg B M, Denoth B, Kerr, S et al 1984 Load, sports shoes and playing surfaces. In Frederick E C (ed.) Sport shoes and playing surfaces. Human Kinetics, Champaign, IL, p 1–23.

Roberts T D M 1995 Understanding balance: the mechanics of posture and locomotion. Chapman & Hall, London.

Serway R A, Jewett J W 2004 Physics for scientists and engineers. Harcourt College Publishers, Fort Worth, TX.

Susanka P, Stepanek J 1988 Biomechanical analysis of the shot put. In Scientific Report on the Second IAAF World Championships in Athletics. IAAF, Monaco, p 1–77.

Tsirakos D K, Bartlett R M, Kollias I A 1995 A comparative study of the release and temporal characteristics of shot put. Journal of Human Movement Studies 28: 227–242.

Wagner G 1998 The 100-meter dash: theory and experiment. Physics Teacher 36: 144–146.

Ward-Smith A J 1985 The influence on long jump performance of the aerodynamic drag experienced during the approach and aerial phases. Journal of Biomechanical Engineering 107: 336–340.

Watkins J 1999 Structure and function of the musculoskeletal system. Human Kinetics, Champaign, IL.

Watkins J 2000 The effect of body configuration on the locus of the whole-body centre of gravity. Journal of Sports Sciences 18: 10.

Watkins J 2001 Structure and function of the foot. In Lorimer D L, French G, O'Donnell et al (eds) Neale's disorders of the foot. Churchill Livingstone, Edinburgh, p 1–22.

Watt D G D, Jones G M 1971 Muscular control of loading from unexpected falls in man. Journal of Physiology 219: 729–737.

Weyland P G, Strenlight D B, Bellizza M J et al 2000 Faster top running speeds are achieved with greater ground reaction forces not more rapid leg movements. Journal of Applied Physiology 89: 1991–1999.

Williams K R, Cavanagh P R 1987 Relationship between distance running mechanics, running economy and performance. Journal of Applied Physiology 63: 1236–1245.

Winter D A 1990 Biomechanics and motor control of human movement, 2nd edn. John Wiley, New York.

Chapter 3

Angular motion

CHAPTER CONTENTS

Newton's laws of motion apply to angular motion as well as linear motion. The purpose of this chapter is to describe the fundamental mechanical concepts underlying the study of angular motion, in particular, the turning effect of a force, angular impulse and angular momentum.

MOMENT OF A FORCE

Consider a rectangular block of wood resting on a table, as shown in Figure 3.1a. The centre of gravity of the block of wood is located at its geometric centre and the line of action of its weight intersects the base of support ABCD. If the block is tilted over on one of the edges of the base of support, such as the edge BC, as in Figure 3.1b, the weight of the block W will tend to rotate the block about the supporting edge back to its original resting position in Figure 3.1a. The tendency to restore the block to its original position is the result of the moment (or turning moment) of W about the axis of rotation BC. The magnitude of the moment of W about the axis BC is equal to the product of W and the perpendicular distance d between the axis BC and the line of action of W (Fig. 3.1b), i.e.

moment of W about axis BC = $W.d$
    (W multiplied by d)

If $W = 2\,\text{kgf}$ and $d = 0.1\,\text{m}$, then

moment of W about axis BC
    $= 2\,\text{kgf} \times 0.1\,\text{m} = 0.2\,\text{kgf.m}$

As $2\,\text{kgf} = 19.62\,\text{N}$, then

moment of W about axis BC
    $= 19.62\,\text{N} \times 0.1\,\text{m} = 1.962\,\text{N.m}$

The N.m (newton metre) is the unit of moment of force in the SI system (Table 1.1).

In general, when a force F acting on an object rotates or tends to rotate the object about some specified axis, the moment of F is defined as the product of F and the perpendicular distance d between the axis of rotation and the line of action of F, i.e. moment of $F = F.d$. The axis of rotation is often referred to as the fulcrum and the perpendicular distance between the line of action of the force and the axis of rotation is usually referred to as the moment arm of the force. The moment of a force is sometimes referred to as torque. For a given moment of force, the greater the force, the smaller the moment arm of the force and vice versa. For example, in trying to push open a heavy door, much less force will be required if the force is applied to the side of the door furthest away from the hinges, i.e. a large moment arm, than if the force is applied to the door close to the hinges, i.e. a small moment arm (Fig. 3.2).

> The moment of a force is the product of the magnitude of the force and the perpendicular distance between the line of action of the force and the axis of rotation.

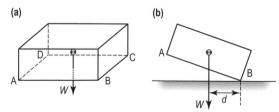

Fig. 3.1   The turning moment of a force. (a) Block of wood at rest on base of support ABCD. (b) Turning moment $W.d$ of the weight of the block W tending to restore to the block to its original resting position after being tilted over on edge BC; d = moment arm of W about edge BC

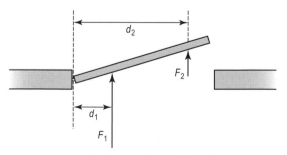

Fig. 3.2   Effect of length of moment arm on magnitude of force needed to produce a particular moment of force to open a door. $F_1.d_1 = F_2.d_2$. If $d_2 = 3d_1$, then $F_1 = 3F_2$

CLOCKWISE AND ANTICLOCKWISE MOMENTS

When an object is acted upon by two or more forces that tend to rotate the object, the actual amount and speed of rotation that occurs will depend upon the resultant moment acting on the object, i.e. the resultant of all the individual moments. For example, consider two boys A and B sitting on a seesaw S as shown in Figure 3.3. A seesaw is normally constructed so that its centre of gravity coincides with the fulcrum, i.e. in any position the line of action of its weight will pass through the fulcrum and the weight of the seesaw will therefore not exert a turning moment on the seesaw, since the moment arm of its weight about the fulcrum will be zero. Consequently, in Figure 3.3 the only moments tending to rotate the seesaw will be those exerted by the weights of the two boys. The weight of A will exert an anticlockwise moment $W_A \times d_A$ and the weight of B will exert a clockwise moment $W_B \times d_B$. When $W_A \times d_A$ is greater than $W_B \times d_B$, there will be a resultant anticlockwise moment acting on the seesaw such that B will be lifted as A descends. When $W_A \times d_A$ is equal to $W_B \times d_B$, i.e. when the clockwise moment is equal to the anticlockwise moment, the resultant moment acting on the seesaw will be zero and the seesaw will not rotate in either direction but will remain perfectly still in a balanced position. Consequently, if the weight of one of the boys was known, the weight of the other boy could be found by balancing the seesaw with one boy on each side of the fulcrum

with both boys off the floor and then equating the clockwise and anticlockwise moments. For example, if $W_A = 40\,\text{kgf}$ and in the balanced position $d_A = 1.5\,\text{m}$ and $d_B = 2.0\,\text{m}$, then by equating moments about the fulcrum,

anticlockwise moments (ACM)
  = clockwise moments (CM)

$$40\,\text{kgf} \times 1.5\,\text{m} = W_B \times 2.0\,\text{m}$$

$$W_B = \frac{40\,\text{kgf} \times 1.5\,\text{m}}{2.0\,\text{m}} = 30\,\text{kgf}$$

> When an object is acted upon by two or more forces that tend to rotate the object, the amount and speed of rotation that occurs will depend upon the resultant moment.

THE LOCATION OF THE JOINT CENTRE OF GRAVITY OF TWO MASSES

In order to balance an object on a knife-edge support, it is necessary to position the object so that its centre of gravity lies in the vertical plane through the knife-edge support. Therefore, in the above example of the seesaw, when the seesaw is in a balanced position with both boys off the floor the centre of gravity of the composite body consisting of the seesaw and the two boys must lie in the vertical plane through the fulcrum. However, since the centre of gravity of the seesaw coincides with the fulcrum in all positions of the seesaw, it follows that the joint centre of gravity of the two boys, i.e. the point at which the combined weight of the two boys can be considered to act, must also lie in the vertical plane through the fulcrum, otherwise the seesaw would rotate as a result of a non-zero resultant moment.

  If boy A sat further away from the fulcrum such that $d_A = 2.25\,\text{m}$ and boy B moved further away from the fulcrum in order to balance the seesaw, d_B could be found by equating the clockwise and anticlockwise moments as before, i.e.

$$W_A = 40\,\text{kgf}$$

$$W_B = 30\,\text{kgf}$$

$$d_A = 2.25\,\text{m}$$

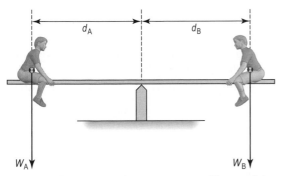

Fig. 3.3 Two boys sitting on a seesaw. W_A = weight of boy A; W_B = weight of boy B; d_A = moment arm of W_A; d_B = moment arm of W_B

ACM = CM

$40 \, \text{kgf} \times 2.25 \, \text{m} = 30 \, \text{kgf} \times d_B$

$$d_B = \frac{40 \, \text{kgf} \times 2.25 \, \text{m}}{30 \, \text{kgf}} = 3.0 \, \text{m}$$

In each of the above examples, the seesaw was in a balanced position, i.e. the joint centre of gravity of the two boys was directly above the fulcrum when

$$W_A \times d_A = W_B \times d_B$$

$$\frac{W_A}{W_B} = \frac{d_B}{d_A}$$

Therefore, whatever the distance between the centre of gravity of boy A and the centre of gravity of boy B, the ratio of the moment arms of the weights of the two boys about their joint centre of gravity will remain constant. In the first example,

$$\frac{d_B}{d_A} = \frac{2.0}{1.5} = 1.333$$

In the second example,

$$\frac{d_B}{d_A} = \frac{3.0}{2.25} = 1.333$$

For any two weights W_1 and W_2, the ratio of their moment arms d_1 and d_2 about their joint centre of gravity will be constant, i.e.

$$\frac{W_1}{W_2} = \frac{d_2}{d_1} = \text{a constant value} \qquad \text{Eq. 3.1}$$

In the above examples, it was not necessary to involve the weight of the seesaw in the calculations since it had no moment about the fulcrum. However, provided that both the weight of the seesaw and the position of its centre of gravity are known, the weight of boy B could be found by balancing the seesaw, with one boy each side of the fulcrum, about any point on its length and then equating the clockwise and anticlockwise moments as before. For example, Figure 3.4 shows the seesaw in a balanced position with the centre of gravity of the seesaw located a distance of 0.25 m to the right of the fulcrum. By

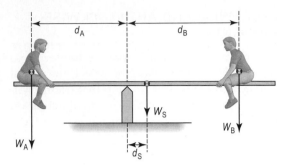

Fig. 3.4 Two boys sitting on a seesaw in a balanced position with the centre of gravity of the seesaw located a distance to the right of the fulcrum. W_A = weight of boy A = 40 kgf; d_A = moment arm of W_A = 1.25 m. W_S = weight of seesaw = 20 kgf; d_S = moment arm of W_S = 0.25 m. W_B = weight of boy B; d_B = moment arm of W_B = 1.5 m

equating the anticlockwise and clockwise moments,

$$W_A \times d_A = (W_S \times d_S) + (W_B \times d_B)$$

where W_S = weight of the seesaw = 20 kgf, and d_S = moment arm of W_S about the fulcrum = 0.25 m.

If W_A = 40 kgf, d_A = 1.25 m and d_B = 1.5 m, then

$$40 \, \text{kgf} \times 1.25 \, \text{m} = (20 \, \text{kgf} \times 0.25 \, \text{m}) + (W_B \times 1.5 \, \text{m})$$

$$50 \, \text{kgf.m} = 5 \, \text{kgf.m} + (1.5 \, \text{m} \times W_B)$$

$$W_B = \frac{45 \, \text{kgf.m}}{1.5 \, \text{m}} = 30 \, \text{kgf}$$

In the above example, the total clockwise moment was the sum of two component moments, i.e. the moment of W_S and the moment of W_B. The total clockwise moment could be exerted by a force equal to $W_S + W_B$ acting at the joint centre of gravity of W_S and W_B. For example, consider the plane containing the joint centre of gravity of W_S and W_B as shown in Figure 3.5. From Equation 3.1,

$$\frac{W_S}{W_B} = \frac{d_{BG}}{d_{SG}}$$

where

d_{BG} = moment arm of W_B about the joint centre of gravity of W_S and W_B

(a)

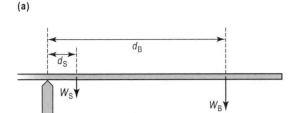

(b)

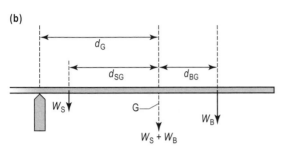

Fig. 3.5 The location of the joint centre of gravity of two masses. W_S = weight of seesaw; W_B = weight of boy B; G = vertical plane containing the joint centre of gravity of the seesaw and boy B; d_{SG} = moment arm of W_S about the joint centre of gravity of the seesaw and boy B; d_{BG} = moment arm of W_B about the joint centre of gravity of the seesaw and boy B; d_G = moment arm of the joint centre of gravity of the seesaw and boy B about the fulcrum

d_{SG} = moment arm of W_S about the joint centre of gravity of W_S and W_B.

As W_S = 20 kgf and W_B = 30 kgf, it follows that

$$\frac{d_{BG}}{d_{SG}} = \frac{2}{3}$$

i.e. $d_{BG} = \dfrac{2 \times d_{SG}}{3}$ Eq. 3.2

From Figure 3.5,

$$d_B = d_S + d_{SG} + d_{BG}$$

i.e. $d_{SG} + d_{BG} = d_B - d_S$
$$= 1.5\,m - 0.25\,m$$
$$= 1.25\,m \qquad \text{Eq. 3.3}$$

From Equations 3.2 and 3.3,

$$d_{SG} + \frac{2d_{SG}}{3} = 1.25\,m$$

i.e. $d_{SG} = 0.75\,m$

From Figure 3.5,

$$d_G = d_S + d_{SG} = 0.25\,m + 0.75\,m = 1.0\,m$$

Therefore the joint moment of $W_S + W_B$ is given by,

$$(W_S + W_B) \times d_G = 50\,kgf \times 1.0\,m = 50\,kgf.m$$

This is the same as the sum of the moments of W_S and W_B,

i.e. $(W_S \times d_S) + (W_B \times d_B) = (20\,kgf \times 0.25\,m)$
$$+ (30\,kgf \times 1.5\,m)$$
$$= 50\,kgf.m$$

Therefore, the sum of the moments of W_S and W_B is equivalent to the moment exerted by a single force of magnitude $W_S + W_B$ acting at the joint centre of gravity of W_S and W_B. This is an illustration of the principle of moments, i.e. the moment of the resultant of any number of forces about any axis is equal to the algebraic sum of the moments of the individual forces about the same axis. When all the forces are weights, such as the weights of the segments of the human body, the sum of the moments of the weights about any particular axis is equal to the moment of total body weight acting at the whole-body centre of gravity. As will be described shortly, this principle is used to determine the location of the whole-body centre of gravity in biomechanical analysis.

TWO CONDITIONS FOR A STATE OF EQUILIBRIUM

In the situations illustrated in Figures 3.3 and 3.4, the seesaw is in equilibrium, i.e. when in a balanced position the resultant force on the seesaw is zero. Consequently, the resultant downward force on the seesaw, i.e. the weights of the seesaw and the two boys, must be counteracted by one or more forces whose resultant is equal and opposite to the weights of the seesaw and the two boys. In the case of the seesaw, the counteracting force is a single force R exerted by the seesaw support through the fulcrum. Figure 3.6 shows the free body diagrams for the seesaw in the situations illustrated in Figure 3.3 and Figure 3.4 respectively. As

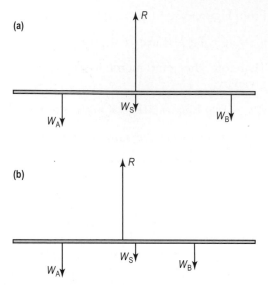

Fig. 3.6   Free body diagrams of the seesaw in the situations shown in Figures 3.3 and 3.4 respectively. W_A = weight of boy A; W_S = weight of seesaw; W_B = weight of boy B; R = force exerted by the seesaw support on the seesaw. In both cases, $R = W_A + W_S + W_B$

$W_A = 40\,\text{kgf}$, $W_B = 30\,\text{kgf}$ and $W_S = 20\,\text{kgf}$, then $R = W_A + W_B + W_S = 90\,\text{kgf}$.

With regard to linear motion, an object is in equilibrium when the resultant force acting on the object is zero. With regard to angular motion, an object is in equilibrium when the resultant moment acting on the object is zero. Both conditions, zero resultant force and zero resultant moment, are illustrated in the seesaw examples in Figures 3.3 and 3.4.

When the resultant moment of the forces acting on an object is zero, the sum of the clockwise and anticlockwise moments will be zero with respect to any reference axis of rotation. For example, consider the forces acting on the seesaw as shown in Figure 3.6b and re-drawn showing the distances between the individual forces in Figure 3.7. By taking moments about a horizontal axis (perpendicular to the plane of Figure 3.7) through the point of application of W_A,

CM = ACM

$(W_S \times 1.5\,\text{m}) + (W_B \times 2.75\,\text{m}) = R \times 1.25\,\text{m}$

As $W_S = 20\,\text{kgf}$ and $W_B = 30\,\text{kgf}$, then

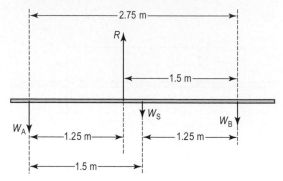

Fig. 3.7   Free body diagram of the seesaw in Figure 3.4 showing the distances between the forces

$$R = \frac{(20\,\text{kgf} \times 1.5\,\text{m}) + (30\,\text{kgf} \times 2.75\,\text{m})}{1.25\,\text{m}}$$

$$R = \frac{112.5\,\text{kgf.m}}{1.25\,\text{m}} = 90\,\text{kgf}$$

Alternatively, by taking moments about a horizontal axis (perpendicular to the plane of Fig. 3.7) through the point of application of W_B,

CM = ACM

$R \times 1.5\,\text{m} = (W_S \times 1.25\,\text{m}) + (W_A \times 2.75\,\text{m})$

$$R = \frac{(20\,\text{kgf} \times 1.25\,\text{m}) + (40\,\text{kgf} \times 2.75\,\text{m})}{1.5\,\text{m}}$$

$$R = \frac{135\,\text{kgf.m}}{1.5\,\text{m}} = 90\,\text{kgf}$$

> The moment of the resultant of any number of forces about any axis is equal to the algebraic sum of the moments of the individual forces about the same axis. This is referred to as the principle of moments.

LOCATION OF THE CENTRE OF GRAVITY OF THE HUMAN BODY

In all movements, the movement of the centre of gravity of the body and, therefore, the movement of the body as a whole, is determined by the impulse of the resultant force acting on the body during the movement. For example, in a long jump, take-off velocity is determined by the velocity of the centre of gravity generated

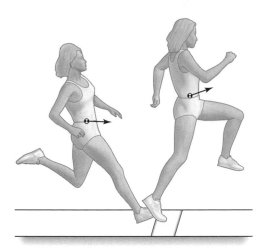

Fig. 3.8 Position and velocity of the whole body centre of gravity of a female long jumper at touchdown and take-off: velocity vectors based on mean data in Lees et al 1993

in the run-up and the impulse of the resultant force acting on the centre of gravity during the period from touchdown to take-off (Fig. 3.8). Provided that the velocity of the jumper at the instance of touchdown is known and the components of the ground reaction force have been recorded from touchdown to take-off, the take-off velocity of the jumper can be determined from the impulse of the resultant force acting on the jumper from touchdown to take-off. However, force platforms are not usually available. Furthermore, the position of the centre of gravity at take-off (take-off height and take-off distance in Fig. 2.95), as well as take-off velocity, would be needed in order to describe the trajectory of the centre of gravity during flight. In such situations, the position of the centre of gravity (take-off height and take-off distance) and velocity of the centre of gravity at take-off are determined from the distance–time graph of the movement of the centre of gravity (as described in the section on linear kinematics of a 100 m sprint in Ch. 2). In order to produce a distance–time graph of the movement of the centre of gravity, it is necessary to locate the position of the centre of gravity in each frame of video of the movement under consideration. There are two approaches to determining the position of the centre of gravity of the human body, the direct (whole-body) approach, in which the

body is considered as a whole, and the indirect (segmental) approach, in which the body is considered to consist of a number of segments (Hay 1973). In both approaches, the position of the centre of gravity is determined from the intersection of three non-parallel planes that contain the centre of gravity.

DIRECT APPROACH

There are, theoretically, three direct methods of determining the position of the centre of gravity of the human body: suspension, balancing, reaction board (equating the moment of the weight of the body about a horizontal support). The suspension method was described in Chapter 2 (Figs 2.18 & 2.19) and simply involves suspending the body from at least three points and noting the point of intersection of the lines of action of the weight of the body in the different positions. However, this method is impractical with regard to the human body since it would be difficult to suspend the body from three or more positions while the subject maintained the required body posture.

Balancing the body on a knife-edge support is a more practical method than suspension. The position of the centre of gravity may be estimated by balancing the body on a plane wooden board, as shown in Figure 3.9a. Initially, it would be necessary to balance the board so that its centre of gravity (as in a seesaw) was located in the vertical plane through the knife-edge support. The subject could then lie down on the board and move his/her body up and down the board until it balanced. The centre of gravity of the body must then lie in the vertical plane through the knife-edge support. By repeating the procedure with the body in two other orientations, as in Figure 3.9b and c, the position of the centre of gravity of the body could be estimated by finding the point of intersection of the three planes.

Whereas the balancing method involves locating the position in which the weight of the body has no moment about the single knife-edge support, the position of the centre of gravity can also be determined by equating the moment of body weight while resting on a plane wooden

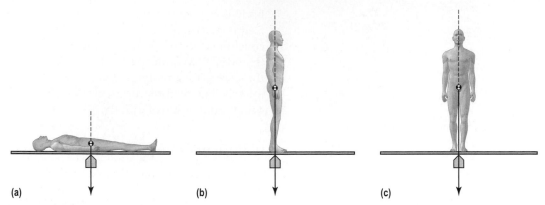

Fig. 3.9 Method of determining the position of the centre of gravity of the human body by balancing the body on a plane board

board supported by two parallel knife-edge supports. This method is referred to as the reaction board method. Figure 3.10a shows a plane wooden board (approximately $2.5\,\text{m} \times 0.5\,\text{m}$) supported in a horizontal position by two parallel knife-edge supports, one of which rests on a set of weighing scales. Figure 3.10b shows a free body diagram of the board. The weight of the board can be measured by simply weighing it. By taking moments about knife-edge support A,

$$CM = ACM$$

$$W_B \times d_1 = S_1 \times l \qquad \text{Eq. 3.4}$$

$$\text{i.e. } d_1 = \frac{S_1 \times l}{W_B}$$

where

W_B = weight of the board
l = distance between the knife-edge supports
S_1 = vertical force exerted by the scales on knife-edge support B
d_1 = horizontal distance between knife-edge support A and the vertical plane containing the centre of gravity of the board

Figure 3.10c shows a man lying on the board with the soles of his feet coincident with the vertical plane through knife-edge support A. Figure 3.10d shows a free body diagram of the board with the man lying on it. W_B, l and d_1 will be the same as before the man lay on the board but the vertical force exerted by the scales on the board will increase because of the weight of the man. By taking moments about knife-edge support A,

$$CM = ACM$$

$$(W_B \times d_1) + (W_S \times d_2) = S_2 \times l$$

where

W_S = weight of the man
S_2 = vertical force exerted by the scales on knife-edge support B
d_2 = horizontal distance between knife-edge support A and the vertical plane containing the centre of gravity of the man

i.e. $W_S \times d_2 = (S_2 \times l) - (W_B \times d_1)$

$\quad W_S \times d_2 = (S_2 \times l) - (S_1 \times l)$
$\qquad$ (by substitution of $W_B \times d_1$ from Eq. 3.4)

$$d_2 = \frac{l \times (S_2 - S_1)}{W_S} \qquad \text{Eq. 3.5}$$

For example, if

S_1 = 10 kgf
S_2 = 39.5 kgf
W_S = 72 kgf
l = 2.5 m

then $d_2 = \dfrac{2.5\,\text{m} \times (39.5\,\text{kgf} - 10\,\text{kgf})}{72\,\text{kgf}}$

$d_2 = 1.024\,\text{m}$

Therefore, the vertical plane containing the centre of gravity of the man would be at a distance of 1.024 m from knife-edge support A. If the height of the man was 1.83 m (6 ft) his centre of gravity would be located in the transverse plane at 55.9% of his stature (1.024 m/1.83 m × 100)

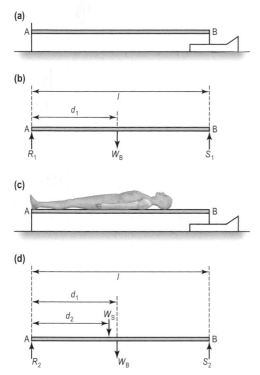

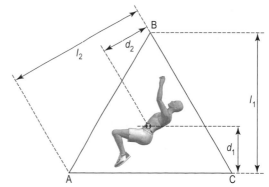

Fig. 3.11 Reaction board method of determining the position of the centre of gravity of the human body in two dimensions. W_S = weight of the subject lying on the board; A_1 = vertical force exerted on support A without the subject; A_2 = vertical force exerted on support A with the subject lying on the board; B_1 = vertical force exerted on support B without the subject; B_2 = vertical force exerted on support B with the subject lying on the board; l_1 = perpendicular distance between B and the line AC; l_2 = perpendicular distance between A and the line BC; d_1 = distance between the vertical plane through AC and the vertical plane containing the centre of gravity of the subject lying on the board in one of the positions recorded on a video of the subject performing a back somersault; $d_1 = (l_1 \times (B_2 - B_1))/W_S$; d_2 = distance between the vertical plane through BC and the vertical plane containing the centre of gravity of the subject; $d_2 = (l_2 \times (A_2 - A_1))/W_S$

Fig. 3.10 Reaction board method of determining the position of the centre of gravity of the human body. (a) A plane wooden board supported in a horizontal position by two parallel knife-edge supports A and B with edge B resting on a set of weighing scales. (b) A free body diagram of the board. (c) A man lying on the board with the soles of his feet coincident with the vertical plane through knife-edge support A. (d) A free body diagram of the board with the man lying on it. W_B = weight of the board; W_S = weight of the man; l = distance between the knife-edge supports; R_1 = vertical force exerted by edge A on the board without the man; R_2 = vertical force exerted by edge A on the board with the man lying on it; S_1 = vertical force exerted by the scales on the knife-edge support B without the man; S_2 = vertical force exerted by the scales on the knife-edge support B with the man lying on it; d_1 = horizontal distance between the knife-edge support A and the vertical plane containing the centre of gravity of the board; d_2 = horizontal distance between the knife-edge support A and the vertical plane containing the centre of gravity of the man

when standing upright. By repeating the procedure with the body in two other orientations, the position of the centre of gravity of the body could be estimated by finding the point of intersection of the three planes.

This method is referred to as the one-dimension reaction board method, since the orientation of the body has to be changed in order to locate each separate plane. By using a rectangular or triangular reaction board with three points of support and two sets of weighing scales, the location of the centre of gravity of the body in two planes can be determined in a single step. Figure 3.11 shows an overhead view of a triangular reaction board (length of each side is approximately 2.5 m) supported in a horizontal position by separate point supports (such as the rounded head of a metal bolt) at each of the three corners of the board. The supports can be underneath the board close to the corners rather than at the corners, but the vertical planes containing the two supports on two sides of board (AC and BC in Figure 3.11) must be marked on the upper surface of the board.

If corners A and B rest on separate sets of weighing scales, the vertical line (intersection of two vertical planes) containing the centre of gravity of the subject lying on the board can be determined by equating moments about AC and BC respectively, using Equation 3.5, as shown in Figure 3.11.

Whereas the balancing and reaction board methods are fairly accurate if carefully applied, they are of limited value for three main reasons:

- It is unlikely that the subject will be able to reproduce in a static position all the positions obtained during the movement under consideration and displayed in the separate frames of video of the movement

- Unless photographs of the subject are taken at each stage of the procedure, it is difficult to map the position of the centre of gravity on to the video image

- The methods are very time-consuming, especially when there are a lot of frames of video to be analysed.

Practical worksheet 4 involves the use of a one-dimension reaction board to examine the effect of changes in body position on the position of the whole-body centre of gravity.

INDIRECT APPROACH

In the indirect approach, the human body is considered to consist of a number of segments linked by joints. Each segment has its own weight and centre of gravity. Provided that the weight of each segment and the position of the centre of gravity of each segment can be determined, the position of the whole-body centre of gravity can be determined by application of the principle of moments, i.e. the sum of the moments of the weights of the segments about any particular axis is equal to the moment of the total weight. Figure 3.12 shows a female long jumper just before take-off, with the body divided into nine segments: combined trunk,

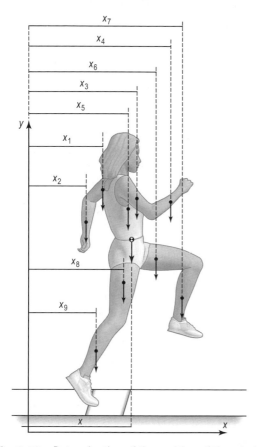

Fig. 3.12 Determination of the position of the whole body centre of gravity by application of the principle of moments. By taking moments about the Z axis in the X dimension,

$$W.x = W_1.x_1 + W_2.x_2 + W_3.x_3 + W_4.x_4 + W_5.x_5 + W_6.x_6 + W_7.x_7 + W_8.x_8 + W_9.x_9$$

where

W = total weight of the body; x = moment arm of W = X coordinate of the whole body centre of gravity; W_1 = weight of the left upper arm; x_1 = moment arm of W_1; W_2 = weight of combined left forearm and hand; x_2 = moment arm of W_2; W_3 = weight of the right upper arm; x_3 = moment arm of W_3; W_4 = weight of combined right forearm and hand; x_4 = moment arm of W_4; W_5 = combined weight of trunk, head and neck; x_5 = moment arm of W_5; W_6 = weight of the left thigh; x_6 = moment arm of W_6; W_7 = weight of combined left shank and foot; x_7 = moment arm of W_7; W_8 = weight of the right thigh; x_8 = moment arm of W_8; W_9 = weight of combined right shank and foot; x_9 = moment arm of W_9;

i.e. $x = \dfrac{W_1.x_1 + W_2.x_2 + W_3.x_3 + W_4.x_4 + W_5.x_5 + W_6.x_6 + W_7.x_7 + W_8.x_8 + W_9.x_9}{W}$

head and neck, left upper arm, combined left forearm and hand, right upper arm, combined right forearm and hand, left thigh, combined left shank (lower leg) and foot, right thigh, combined right shank and foot. The position of the centre of gravity of each segment is shown together with the position of the whole-body centre of gravity. The coordinate of the whole-body centre of gravity with respect to any axis of rotation and any dimension can be determined by applying the principle of moments, as shown in Figure 3.12.

The method is fairly straightforward and has been incorporated into a range of commercially available video motion analysis software. However, the accuracy of the method depends largely on the accuracy with which the weights of the segments and the positions of their centres of gravity can be determined. A number of studies have been undertaken to provide these data. The main studies may be classified as cadaver studies, immersion studies and anthropomorphic models (Hay 1973, Sprigings et al 1987).

Cadaver studies

The earliest reported cadaver study appears to be that of Harless (1860), who dissected two adult male cadavers. Braune & Fischer (1889) dissected four adult male cadavers. Each cadaver was frozen solid with the joints of the upper and lower limbs in mid-range position. The segments were then separated by sawing through each joint in a plane that bisected the angle between the segments. Each segment was then weighed and the position of its centre of gravity was determined by balancing and/or suspension. The most comprehensive and most frequently cited cadaver studies are those of Dempster (1955) and Clauser et al (1969), who used very similar methods to those of Braune & Fischer (1889). Dempster dissected eight white male cadavers (age range 52–83 years) and presented individual and average data on segmental weight (percentage of total weight), segmental centre of gravity position (as a proportion of the distance between defined segmental end points) and segment density. Loss of weight due to dismemberment, especially unknown quantities of body fluids, resulted in the sum of the average segment weights and,

therefore, the sum of the average segmental percentages (97.2%) being less than the corresponding whole-body data (which was measured prior to dissection). Dempster indicated that the weight loss was proportional to the weight of the segments. In the average segmental weight data presented in Table 3.1, the 2.8% weight discrepancy has been distributed in proportion to the segmental percentages so that the total percentage is 100% rather than 97.2%. For example, the percentage weight of each upper arm is given as 2.73%, which is equal to 2.65/97.2 × 100 where 2.65% is the average percentage weight of the upper arm reported by Dempster.

Clauser et al (1969) dissected 13 adult male cadavers (age range 28–74 years), selected to closely approximate a wide range of body types. Care was taken to minimize tissue loss during dismemberment. The average data for segmental weight and segmental centre of gravity locus from the Clauser et al study is shown in Table 3.1.

There do not appear to be any reported cadaver-based data on segment weights and segment centre of gravity loci in females.

Immersion studies

As mass is the product of volume and density, a number of studies have estimated segmental masses by measuring the volume of the segments by water displacement (carefully immersing each segment or segments in a tank of water and measuring the volume of water displaced) and multiplying the volume of the segment by the corresponding average segmental density reported by Dempster (1955). The most comprehensive immersion study carried out on living subjects would appear to be that of Plagenhoef et al (1983). Segmental volumes of 135 college-age athletes (100 women and 35 men) were measured. The corresponding average segmental weights are shown in Table 3.1 for men and Table 3.2 for women. Segmental centre of gravity loci were estimated using seven men and nine women (from the group of 135 subjects) using the immersion method described by Clauser et al (1969); this involves immersing the segment to a proportion of its volume (using average data presented by Clauser et al) that corresponds to the plane of the segmental

Table 3.1   Mean segment weights (% total weight) and centre of gravity locations (proportion of segment length in direction indicated) for adult males from Dempster 1955, Clauser et al 1969 and Plagenhoef et al 1983

Segment[§]	Dempster[*]		Clauser[†]		Plagenhoef[‡]	
	Weight	CG locus	Weight	CG locus	Weight	CG locus
Upper arm	2.73	0.436[a]	2.6	0.513[a]	3.25	0.436[a]
Forearm	1.59	0.430[b]	1.6	0.390[b]	1.87	0.430[b]
Hand	0.62	0.506[c]	0.7	0.480[c]	0.65	0.468[c]
Forearm and hand	2.21	0.677[d]	2.3	0.626[d]	2.52	0.671[d]
Whole upper limb	4.94	0.512[e]	4.9	0.413[e]	5.77	0.50[e]
Thigh	9.93	0.433[f]	10.3	0.372[f]	10.50	0.433[f]
Shank	4.63	0.433[g]	4.3	0.371[g]	4.75	0.434[g]
Foot	1.44	0.429[h]	1.5	0.449[h]	1.43	0.50[h]
Shank and foot	6.07	0.434[i]	5.8	0.475[i]	6.18	0.605[i]
Whole lower limb	16.00	0.434[j]	16.1	0.382[j]	16.68	0.436[j]
Trunk, head and neck	58.13	0.604[k]	58.0	0.604[m]	55.10	0.566[k]
Trunk, head and neck	58.13	0.346[n]	58.0	0.346[p]	55.10	0.370[n]
Head and neck	8.13	0.433[q]	7.3	0.433[r]	8.26	0.45[q]
Head	7.00[s]	0.545[t]	7.00[s]	0.545[t]	7.00[s]	0.545[t]
Trunk	50.00	0.620[v]	50.7	0.620[w]	46.48	0.630[v]

* Mean data from eight white male cadavers (age range 52–83 years). † Mean data from 13 white male cadavers (age range 28–74 years). ‡ Mean weight data from 35 living college-age men using water immersion method and density data from Dempster 1955 and mean CG locus data from seven living college-age men using water immersion method. § Segments in the anatomical position (Fig. 2.4).

[a] shoulder axis to elbow axis; [b] elbow axis to wrist axis. [c] wrist axis to first interphalangeal joint of the second finger; [d] elbow axis to styloid process of the ulna; [e] shoulder axis to styloid process of the ulna; [f] hip axis to knee axis; [g] knee axis to ankle axis; [h] intersection of the line joining the ankle axis and the ball of the foot and the vertical line perpendicular with the sole of the foot that divides the foot in the ratio 0.429 : 0.571 from heel to toe; [i] knee axis to medial malleolus; [j] hip axis to ankle axis; [k] Top of head to hip axis with head, neck and trunk in normal upright posture; [m] Top of head to hip axis with head, neck and trunk in normal upright posture (from Dempster 1955); [n] Shoulder axis to hip axis with trunk in normal upright posture; [p] Shoulder axis to hip axis with trunk in normal upright posture (from Dempster 1955); [q] Top of head to centre of body of 7th cervical vertebra; [r] Top of head to centre of body of 7th cervical vertebra (from Dempster 1955); [s] From Braune & Fischer 1889, reported by Hay 1973; [t] Top of head to occipital-atlas joint (from Braune & Fischer 1889; reported by Hay 1973); [v] shoulder axis to hip axis; [w] shoulder axis to hip axis (from Dempster 1955).

centre of gravity. The average segmental centre of gravity loci from the Plagenhoef et al study are shown in Table 3.1 for men and Table 3.2 for women. The studies referred to in Tables 3.1 and 3.2 did not all report data for the same segments. Consequently, to complete the data sets in Tables 3.1 and 3.2, data have been included from other studies as indicated.

Anthropomorphic models

In order to personalize the determination of segment weights and segment centre of gravity positions for a particular subject, a number of anthropomorphic models have been developed; these include Whitsett (1963), Hanavan (1964),

Hatze (1980) and Yeadon (1990). All the models are based on anthropometric measurements taken directly from the subject. The measurements are used to construct geometric representations of the body segments. The masses of segments are estimated from segment volume and average density and the positions of segmental centres of gravity are estimated by mathematical methods on the basis of the geometry of the segment shapes. The main disadvantages of anthropomorphic models are that anthropometric measurements have to be taken directly from the subject and the time required to take all the measurements may be considerable. For example, the time required to take the 242 measurements required for applying the Hatze (1980)

Table 3.2 Mean segment weights (% total weight) and centre of gravity locations (proportion of segment length in direction indicated) for adult females, from Plagenhoef et al 1983[†]

Segment[*]	Weight	CG locus
Upper arm	2.90	0.458[a]
Forearm	1.57	0.434[b]
Hand	0.50	0.468[c]
Forearm and hand	2.07	0.657[d]
Whole upper limb	4.97	0.486[e]
Thigh	11.75	0.428[f]
Shank	5.35	0.419[g]
Foot	1.33	0.50[h]
Shank and foot	6.68	0.568[i]
Whole lower limb	18.43	0.420[j]
Trunk, head and neck	53.20	0.603[k]
Trunk, head and neck	53.20	0.450[m]
Head and neck	8.20	0.45[n]
Head	7.00[p]	0.545[q]
Trunk	45.00	0.569[m]

[†] Mean weight data from 100 living college-age women using water immersion method and density data from Dempster (1955) and mean CG locus data from nine living college-age women using water immersion method

[*] Segments in the anatomical position (Fig. 2.4).

[a] shoulder axis to elbow axis; [b] elbow axis to wrist axis; [c]wrist axis to first interphalangeal joint of the second finger; [d] elbow axis to styloid process of the ulna; [e] shoulder axis to styloid process of the ulna; [f] hip axis to knee axis; [g] knee axis to ankle axis; [h] intersection of the line joining the ankle axis and the ball of the foot and the vertical line perpendicular with the sole of the foot that divides the foot in the ratio 0.429 : 0.571 from heel to toe; [i] knee axis to medial malleolus; [j] hip axis to ankle axis; [k] vertex (top of head) to hip axis with head, neck and trunk in normal upright posture; [m] shoulder axis to hip axis with trunk in normal upright posture; [n] vertex (top of head) to centre of body of 7th cervical vertebra; [p] from Braune & Fischer 1889, reported by Hay 1973; [q] top of head to occipital-atlas joint (from Braune & Fischer 1889, reported by Hay 1973).

model is about 80 min per subject (Sprigings et al 1987).

It is reasonable to expect that a personalized model would be more accurate than the application of average percent data from cadaver and immersion studies. However, the comparative data currently available are meagre (Sprigings et al 1987) and seem to indicate that the difference in the results of the different methods (in the estimated position of the whole-body centre of gravity) is unlikely to be significant in the analysis of whole-body movement.

The major advantage of using percentage data for segment weight and segment centre of gravity position is that the position of the whole-body centre of gravity of the subject can be determined from a video image without the need for any anthropometric information about the subject. Not surprisingly, the application of percent data for segment weight and segment centre of gravity position is the preferred method in most biomechanical analyses, especially those based on video analysis.

DETERMINATION OF THE WHOLE-BODY CENTRE OF GRAVITY BY THE APPLICATION OF THE PRINCIPLE OF MOMENTS

In undertaking segmental analysis, the analyst has to decide the number of segments that will comprise the segmental model. The more

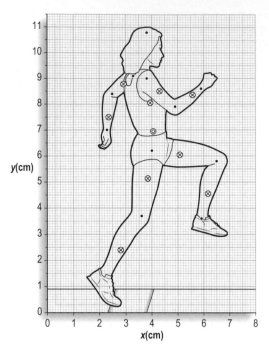

Fig. 3.13 Segment end points (●) defining a nine-segment model and the corresponding positions of the segment centres of gravity (⊗) and whole body centre of gravity (◎)

segments in the model, the greater the number of segmental end points and, therefore, the greater the time needed to digitize each frame of video. Digitization refers to the process of identifying and recording the coordinates of each point in the segmental model as well as reference points for the origin and axes of the reference axis system upon which the analysis will be based (Fig. 3.13). The number of segments in the model will largely depend on the purpose of the analysis. For example, if the description of ankle movement is an important objective, it will be necessary to have separate shank and foot segments for each leg. However, the weight of each foot is small relative to total body weight and the effect of movement of the foot relative to the shank on the position of the whole-body centre of gravity is likely to be insignificant. Consequently, if the main objective of the analysis is the movement of the whole-body centre of gravity, the analyst may decide to regard the shank and foot as a single segment. Similarly, the forearm and hand may be regarded as a single segment. In detailed biomechanical analyses

of elite long jumpers, researchers have used a number of segmental models ranging from an 11-segment model (Lees et al 1993) to a 16-segment model (Linthorne et al 2005).

Figure 3.13 shows the image of a female long jumper just before take-off taken from a frame of video and superimposed for the purpose of analysis onto a one centimetre grid. The segment end points defining a nine-segment model (defined in Figure 3.12) are shown. The first two columns of Table 3.3 show the x and y coordinates of the segment end points. Column 6 of Table 3.3 shows the corresponding x and y coordinates of the segment centres of gravity. These points are shown in Figure 3.13. Table 3.4 shows the coordinates of the segment centres of gravity and the coordinates of the whole-body centre of gravity determined by application of the principle of moments. In applying the principle of moments, it is not necessary to know the actual body weight of the subject. Use of the segment weight proportions rather than the segment weights in the calculation of segment and body weight moments will give the same result. However, since the proportion data have no unit (it is simply a number because it is the ratio of two weights) the units of the calculated moments will be cm rather than N.cm. This may be confusing to some students and so a nominal body weight of 63 kgf (618 N) has been used in the illustration in Table 3.4.

Practical worksheet 5 involves the use of a one-dimension reaction board to compare the direct and indirect methods of determining the position of the whole-body centre of gravity of the human body.

> There are two approaches to determining the position of the centre of gravity of the human body, the direct (whole-body) approach and the indirect (segmental) approach.

LEVERS

Whereas weight forces are always vertical, other external forces acting on a body are likely to be oblique. For example, consider using a claw hammer to pull out a nail from a piece of wood, as shown in Figure 3.14a. In this example, the

Table 3.3 Coordinates of the segment end points and segment centres of gravity of the female long jumper shown in Figure 3.13

Segment		Coordinates* (cm)		Length[†] (cm)	CG$_P$[‡]	CG$_S$[§] (cm)	CG$_O$[¶] (cm)
		a	b			c	
Right upper arm		Shoulder	Elbow				
	x	3.8	4.9	1.1	0.458	0.50	4.30
	y	9.0	7.9	−1.1	0.458	−0.50	8.50
Right forearm and hand		Elbow	Wrist				
	x	4.9	5.9	1.0	0.657	0.66	5.56
	y	7.9	8.6	0.7	0.657	0.46	8.36
Left upper arm		Shoulder	Elbow				
	x	3.3	2.5	−0.8	0.458	−0.37	2.93
	y	9.1	8.4	−0.7	0.458	−0.32	8.78
Left forearm and hand		Elbow	Wrist				
	x	2.5	2.3	−0.2	0.657	−0.13	2.37
	y	8.4	7.0	−1.4	0.657	−0.92	7.48
Trunk, head and neck		Vertex	Right hip[‖]				
	x	3.8	4.0	0.2	0.603	−0.12	3.92
	y	10.8	6.2	−4.6	0.603	−2.77	8.03
Right thigh		Hip	Knee				
	x	4.0	3.6	−0.4	0.428	−0.17	3.83
	y	6.2	3.7	−2.5	0.428	−1.07	5.13
Right shank and foot		Knee	Ankle				
	x	3.6	2.2	−1.4	0.568	−0.79	2.81
	y	3.7	1.4	−2.3	0.568	−1.31	2.39
Left thigh		Hip	Knee				
	x	4.0	6.5	2.5	0.428	1.07	5.07
	y	6.2	5.8	−0.4	0.428	−0.17	6.03
Left shank and foot		Knee	Ankle				
	x	6.5	5.9	−0.6	0.568	−0.34	6.16
	y	5.8	3.6	−2.2	0.568	−1.25	4.55

* x and y coordinates of segment end points a and b. † Length of segment in the dimension = b − a. ‡ Position of segmental centre of gravity as a proportion of segment length in direction a to b (from Table 3.2). § Position of segmental centre of gravity in the dimension in relation to a. ¶ Coordinate of the position of the centre of gravity of the segment = a + c. ‖ In this example, the coordinates of the left hip joint and right hip joint are the same. If the coordinates of the left hip and right hip had been different from each other, it would have been necessary to find the midpoint of the line linking the two joints as the hip reference point for determining the position of the centre of gravity of the trunk, head and neck segment.

line of contact between the claw of the hammer and the surface of the wood constitutes the fulcrum. E is the force exerted on the handle of the hammer and R is the resistance of the nail. Figure 3.14b shows a force–moment arm diagram, i.e. the forces E and R and their moment arms d_E and d_R are shown in relation to the fulcrum in order to more clearly illustrate the turning effects of the forces. The nail will be pulled out if the anticlockwise moment exerted by E is greater than the clockwise moment exerted by R, i.e. if $E.d_E > R.d_R$.

In this situation the hammer is being used as a lever, a rigid or quasi-rigid object that can be made to rotate about a fulcrum in order to exert a force on another object. As in the example of the hammer, a lever encounters a resistance force R in response to an effort force E. The simplest form of lever, which is actually the simplest form of machine, i.e. a powered mechanism designed to apply force (Dempster 1965), is exemplified by a crowbar as shown in Figure 3.15. In this case, the power is supplied by the person using the crowbar. The greater the moment arm of E

Table 3.4 Coordinates of the segment centres of gravity and whole-body centre of gravity (determined by the principle of moments) of the female long jumper shown in Figure 3.13

Segment	Coordinates* (cm)		Weight[†]	Weight[‡] (N)	Moment X[§] (N.cm)	Moment Y[¶] (N.cm)
	x	y				
Right upper arm	4.30	8.50	0.0290	17.92	77.06	152.32
Right forearm and hand	5.56	8.36	0.0207	12.79	71.13	106.92
Left upper arm	2.93	8.78	0.0290	17.92	37.47	157.34
Left forearm and hand	2.37	7.48	0.0207	12.79	30.31	95.67
Trunk, head and neck	3.92	8.03	0.5320	328.78	1288.80	2640.07
Right thigh	3.83	5.13	0.1175	72.61	278.11	372.51
Right shank and foot	2.81	2.39	0.0668	41.28	116.00	98.66
Left thigh	5.07	6.03	0.1175	72.61	368.13	437.84
Left shank and foot	6.16	4.55	0.0668	41.28	254.28	187.82
Totals				618.00	2521.29	4249.15
Coordinates of CG[‖]	4.08	6.87				

* x and y coordinates of the segmental centres of gravity from Table 3.3 (cm). [†] Weight of segments as a proportion of total body weight (from Table 3.2). [‡] Weight of segments in newtons (total body weight = 63 kgf = 618 N). [§] Moments of the segmental weights about z axis with respect to x dimension (N.cm). [¶] Moments of the segmental weights about z axis with respect to y dimension (N.cm). [‖] Moment of body weight = sum of moments of segments, i.e. $W.x_G$ = sum of Moment X, where W = body weight = 618 N and x_G = x coordinate of CG, i.e.

$$x_G = \frac{\text{sum of Moment X}}{W} = \frac{2521.29\,\text{N.cm}}{618\,\text{N}} = 4.08\,\text{cm.}$$

Similarly,

$$y_G = \frac{\text{sum of Moment Y}}{W} = \frac{4249.15\,\text{N.cm}}{618\,\text{N}} = 6.87\,\text{cm,}$$

where y_G = Y coordinate of CG.

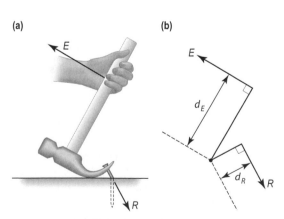

Fig. 3.14 (a) Pulling a nail out of a piece of wood using a claw hammer. (b) Corresponding force–moment arm diagram. E = force exerted on the handle of the hammer; d_E = moment arm of E; R = resistance force exerted by the nail; d_R = moment arm of R

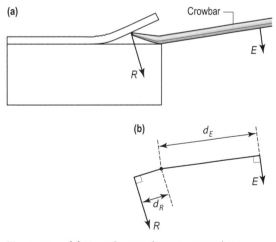

Fig. 3.15 (a) Use of a crowbar to open a box. (b) Corresponding force–moment arm diagram. E = force exerted on the crowbar by the person using it; d_E = moment arm of E; R = resistance force exerted on the crowbar by the lid of the box; d_R = moment arm of R

(d_E), i.e. the greater the leverage of the crowbar, the smaller will be the effort required to overcome the moment of the resistance force.

LEVER SYSTEMS

Levers are classified into three systems depending on the location of the points of application of the E and R forces in relation to the fulcrum. A lever can be any shape, as will be demonstrated in the section on lever systems in the human musculoskeletal system. However, in describing the different classes of levers it is usual to represent the lever as a straight line and the fulcrum as the vertex of a small triangle as shown in Figure 3.16a.

In a first-class lever system the fulcrum is between the E and R forces (Fig. 3.16a). The use of a crowbar is an example of a first-class lever system (Fig. 3.15), as is a seesaw (Fig. 3.3). Scissors are a pair of first-class levers that share the same fulcrum (Fig. 3.16b).

In a second-class lever system the R force is between the fulcrum and the E force as in, for example, a wheelbarrow (Fig. 3.17a and b). A crowbar may also take the form of a second-class lever (Fig. 3.17c). In a third-class lever system the E force is between the fulcrum and the R force as, for example, when holding a fishing rod (Fig. 3.18a and b). Tongs consist of a pair of third-class levers that share the same fulcrum (Fig. 3.18c).

> A lever is an object that can be made to rotate about a fulcrum in order to exert a force on another object.

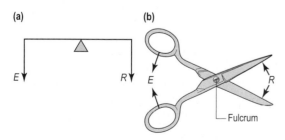

Fig. 3.16   (a) A first-class lever system. (b) Scissors are a pair of first-class levers that share the same fulcrum. E = effort force; R = resistance force

Mechanical advantage

The mechanical advantage (MA) of a lever system is a measure of its efficiency in terms of the amount of effort needed to overcome a particular resistance, i.e.

$$MA = \frac{\text{magnitude of resistance}}{\text{magnitude of effort}} = \frac{R}{E}$$
$$= \frac{\text{length of moment arm of } E}{\text{length of moment arm of } R} = \frac{d_E}{d_R}$$

Any machine with a mechanical advantage greater than 1.0 is regarded as very efficient.

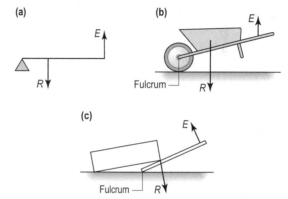

Fig. 3.17   (a) A second-class lever system. (b) A wheelbarrow is a second-class lever system. (c) A crowbar can take the form of a second-class lever system. E = effort force; R = resistance force

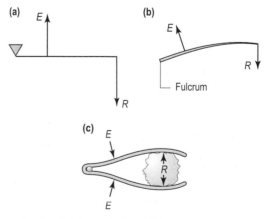

Fig. 3.18   (a) A third-class lever system. (b) A fishing rod is a third-class lever system. (c) Tongs consist of a pair of third-class levers that share the same fulcrum. E = effort force; R = resistance force

A first-class lever may have a mechanical advantage greater than 1.0 or less than 1.0. The first-class lever system in Figure 3.15 has a mechanical advantage much greater than 1.0 since d_E is much greater than d_R. All second-class lever systems have mechanical advantages greater than 1.0 since d_E is always larger than d_R. All third-class lever systems have mechanical advantages less than 1.0 since d_E is always smaller than d_R. In all three lever systems, the greater the length of d_E in relation to the length of d_R, the greater the leverage of the system.

LEVER SYSTEMS IN THE HUMAN MUSCULOSKELETAL SYSTEM

The bones of the skeleton are essentially levers and each joint constitutes a fulcrum. The muscles pull on the bones to control the movement of the joints. The resistance to movement exerted by a body segment is in the form of the segment's weight and any other external loads attached to the segment. Most, if not all, of the skeletal muscles of the body operate in first- or third-class lever systems. Like the third-class lever systems, most of the first-class lever systems have mechanical advantages less than 1.0 because the tendons of the muscles that operate within them tend to be inserted close to the joints they control and, as such, have shorter moment arms than the resistance forces they counteract.

External and internal forces

Figure 3.19a shows the position of the head in normal upright standing. In this position the line of action of the weight of the head passes in front of the vertebral column and, as such, exerts a clockwise moment that tends to rotate the head forward and downward about a mediolateral axis through the fulcrum, i.e. the joint between the occipital bone (at the base of the skull) and the atlas (the first cervical vertebra). The tendency of the weight of the head W to rotate the head forward and downward is counteracted by the neck extensor muscles.

Figure 3.19b shows a free body diagram of the head where F is the force exerted by the neck extensor muscles and J is the force exerted at the fulcrum, i.e. the joint reaction force exerted by the atlas on the occipital bone. Figure 3.19c

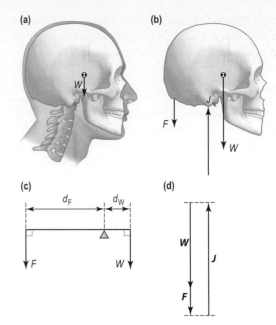

Fig. 3.19 Forces acting on the head when standing upright. (a) Location of the centre of gravity of the head. (b) Free body diagram of the head. (c) Force–moment arm diagram of the forces acting on the head. (d) Vector chain of the forces acting on the head. W = weight of the head; d_W = moment arm of W; F = force exerted by the neck extensor muscles; d_F = moment arm of F; J = joint reaction force exerted by the atlas on the occipital bone

shows the corresponding force–moment arm diagram. F and W constitute a first-class lever system. In this example, it is assumed that F acts vertically downward. The weight of the head of an adult is approximately 7.0% of total body weight (Table 3.1). Consequently, if total body weight is 70 kgf, the weight of the head will be approximately 4.9 kgf. The moment arms of W and F will be approximately 2 cm and 7 cm respectively. Since the head is in equilibrium, the resultant moment acting on the head will be zero and the resultant force acting on the head will be zero. Consequently, the forces F and J can be determined by equating moments and then equating forces as follows:

Equating moments:

$$W.d_W = F.d_F$$

where

$W = 4.9\,\text{kgf}$

d_W = moment arm of W = 2 cm

F = force exerted by the neck extensor muscles

d_F = moment arm of $F = 7\,\text{cm}$

$$F = \frac{W.d_W}{d_F} = \frac{4.9\,\text{kgf} \times 2\,\text{cm}}{7\,\text{cm}} = 1.4\,\text{kgf}$$

Equating forces:

Since F and W are vertical forces, J must also be vertical and the resultant force must be zero. Using the convention that upward is positive and downward is negative, then

$$\text{resultant force} = J - F - W = 0$$

$$J = F + W = 1.4\,\text{kgf} + 4.9\,\text{kgf}$$

$$J = 6.3\,\text{kgf}$$

Consequently, to counteract W, an external force, the musculoskeletal system has to exert two internal forces, F and J. Force F is an active force, a muscle force, and J is a passive force, a joint reaction force. This example illustrates the relationship between the internal and external forces that act on the body; the musculoskeletal system exerts internal forces to counteract the effects of gravity on body segments.

In the above example, all the forces acting on the head were vertical forces and, as such, the vector chain of the forces is a straight line (Fig. 3.19d). In most musculoskeletal lever systems, the internal and external forces are not usually parallel. For example, Figure 3.20a shows the head position of a person writing at a desk. In this situation the head and trunk are tilted forward such that d_W will be greater than when the head is in the upright position (about 4 cm rather than 2 cm). d_F will be approximately the same as when the head is in the upright position, i.e. about 7 cm, but the line of action of F will be at approximately 50° to the horizontal. Figure 3.20b shows a free body diagram of the head and Figure 3.20c shows the corresponding force–moment arm diagram. By taking moments about the fulcrum,

$$W.d_W = F.d_F$$

where

$W = 4.9\,\text{kgf}$, $d_W = 4\,\text{cm}$ and $d_F = 7\,\text{cm}$

$$\text{i.e } F = \frac{W.d_W}{d_F} = \frac{4.9\,\text{kgf} \times 4\,\text{cm}}{7\,\text{cm}} = 2.8\,\text{kgf}$$

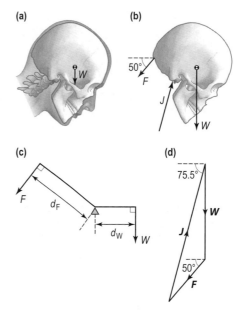

Fig. 3.20 Forces acting on the head while writing at a desk. (a) Location of the centre of gravity of the head. (b) Free body diagram of the head. (c) Force–moment arm diagram of the forces acting on the head. (d) Vector chain of the forces acting on the head. W = weight of the head; d_W = moment arm of W; F = force exerted by the neck extensor muscles; d_F = moment arm of F; J = joint reaction force exerted by the atlas on the occipital bone

The joint reaction force J can be found in two ways: constructing the vector chain and calculation by trigonometry. Figure 3.20d shows the vector chain solution; J has a magnitude of approximately 7.25 kgf and acts at an angle of approximately 75.5° to the horizontal. Figure 3.21 shows the solution by trigonometry. Figure 3.21a shows a free body diagram of the head (same as Fig. 3.20b). Figure 3.21b shows the force F resolved into its horizontal and vertical components, and Figure 3.21c shows the force J resolved into its horizontal and vertical components. Figure 3.21d shows the forces acting on the head in terms of their horizontal and vertical components. Since the head is in equilibrium, the resultant force on the head will be zero. Consequently, the resultant of the horizontal forces will be zero and the resultant of the vertical forces will be zero. Using the convention that forces acting to the right or upward are positive and that forces acting to the left or downward (with respect to Fig. 3.21) are negative, it follows

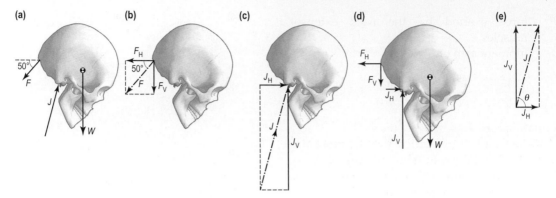

Fig. 3.21 Determination of the joint reaction force by trigonometry. (a) Free body diagram of the head. (b) Horizontal and vertical components of F. (c) Horizontal and vertical components of J. (d) Free body diagram of the head with forces resolved into their horizontal and vertical components. (e) Angle of J with respect to the horizontal (θ)

that, with regard to the horizontal forces,

$$J_H - F_H = 0$$

where J_H = horizontal component of J and F_H = horizontal component of F, i.e.

$$J_H = F_H$$

$$J_H = F.\cos 50° = 2.8\,\text{kgf} \times 0.6428$$

$$J_H = 1.8\,\text{kgf}$$

With regard to the vertical forces,

$$J_V - F_V - W = 0$$

where J_V = vertical component of J and F_V = vertical component of F, i.e.

$$J_V = F_V + W$$

$$J_V = F.\sin 50° + W$$

$$J_V = 2.8\,\text{kgf} \times 0.7664 + 4.9\,\text{kgf}$$

$$J_V = 2.15\,\text{kgf} + 4.9\,\text{kgf}$$

$$J_V = 7.05\,\text{kgf}$$

Since J_V and J_H are at right angles to each other, the magnitude of their resultant J can be found by applying Pythagoras' theorem, i.e.

$$J^2 = J_V^2 + J_H^2 = (7.05^2 + 1.8^2)\text{kgf}^2$$

$$J^2 = 52.94\,\text{kgf}^2$$

$$J = 7.27\,\text{kgf}$$

If J makes an angle of θ with respect to the horizontal (Fig. 3.21e), then

$$\tan \theta = J_V/J_H = 7.05/1.8 = 3.914$$

$$\theta = 75.7°$$

As expected, the vector chain method and calculation by trigonometry method produce almost exactly the same result for the magnitude and direction of J.

> Most of the skeletal muscles of the human body operate in first- or third-class lever systems with mechanical advantages of less than 1.

Effect of increasing the moment arm of external forces on the magnitude of internal forces

The examples of the forces acting on the head in the upright (Fig. 3.19) and writing positions (Fig. 3.20) show that an increase in the moment arm of an external force results in an increase in the magnitude of the counteracting muscle forces, which, in turn, results in an increase in the associated joint reaction forces. This is illustrated in Figure 3.22, which shows a 6 m long beam of wood of weight W balanced in three positions on a knife-edge support. In Figure 3.22a, the beam is balanced with the line of action of its weight passing through the knife-edge support, i.e. the moment of W about the fulcrum is zero. In this situation the reaction force R is sufficient to counteract W and maintain equilibrium; Figure 3.22b shows a free body diagram of the beam. In Figure 3.22c, the beam has been displaced 1 m to the right such that W

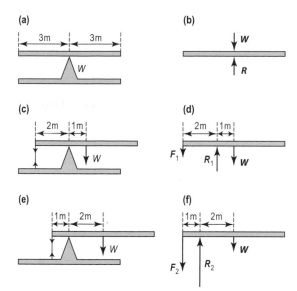

Fig. 3.22 Effect of increasing the moment arm of the weight W of a beam on the magnitude of the restraining forces needed to maintain equilibrium. (a) Beam balanced with the line of action of W acting through the fulcrum. (b) Free body diagram of the beam in (a). (c) Beam in equilibrium with line of action of W displaced 1 m to the right. (d) Free body diagram of the beam in (c). (e) Beam in equilibrium with line of action of W displaced 2 m to the right. (f) Free body diagram of the beam in (e)

exerts a clockwise turning moment on the beam of $W \times 1\,\mathrm{m}$. The beam is held in equilibrium by the reaction force R_1 and a force F_1 exerted by a tie that attaches the left end of the beam to the base of support. If it is assumed that F_1 acts vertically, R_1 will also act vertically. Figure 3.22d shows a free body diagram of the beam. By equating moments about the fulcrum,

$$W \times 1\,\mathrm{m} = F_1 \times 2\,\mathrm{m}$$

i.e. $F_1 = \dfrac{W \times 1\,\mathrm{m}}{2\,\mathrm{m}} = 0.5\,W$

By equating the forces,

$$R_1 = F_1 + W = 0.5W + W = 1.5W$$

In Figure 3.22e, the beam has been displaced 2 m to the right with respect to its original position such that W exerts a clockwise turning moment on the beam of $W \times 2\,\mathrm{m}$. The beam is held in equilibrium by the reaction force R_2 and a force

F_2 exerted by the tie. Assuming that F_2 and, consequently, R_2 act vertically, Figure 3.22f shows a free body diagram of the beam. By equating moments about the fulcrum,

$$W \times 2\,\mathrm{m} = F_2 \times 1\,\mathrm{m}$$

i.e. $F_2 = \dfrac{W \times 2\,\mathrm{m}}{1\,\mathrm{m}} = 2W$

By equating the forces,

$$R_2 = F_2 + W = 2W + W = 3W$$

Forces at the hip in single leg stance

The distribution of load on the beam in Figure 3.22e is similar to that on the pelvis during single-leg support during standing or walking (Fig. 3.23a–c). In this position the pelvis acts as a first-class lever and rotates about the hip joint under the action of the weight of the body and the force exerted by the hip abductor muscles. Figure 3.23c shows a free body diagram of the pelvis in this situation and Figure 3.23d shows the corresponding force–moment arm diagram. W is the weight of the body less the weight of the grounded leg. For a man of total body weight of 70 kgf, W is approximately 59 kgf (84% of total body weight; see Dempster data in Table 3.1). A is the force exerted by the hip abductor muscles. W will tend to rotate the pelvis clockwise about the hip joint and A will normally maintain the pelvis in a horizontal position by exerting an equal and opposite moment. Force J is the joint reaction force, i.e. the force exerted by the head of the femur on the pelvis via the acetabulum. When the pelvis is in equilibrium, the resultant of W, A and J will be zero. The line of action of A will be approximately 80° to the horizontal. The moment arms of A and W with respect to the hip joint axis of rotation will be approximately 6 cm and 11 cm respectively. By taking moments about the fulcrum (the point of application of J),

$$W.d_W - A.d_A = 0,$$

where $W = 59$ kgf, $d_W = 11$ cm and $d_A = 6$ cm, i.e.

$$A = \frac{W.d_W}{d_A} = \frac{(59\,\mathrm{kgf} \times 11\,\mathrm{cm})}{6\,\mathrm{cm}} = 108\,\mathrm{kgf}$$

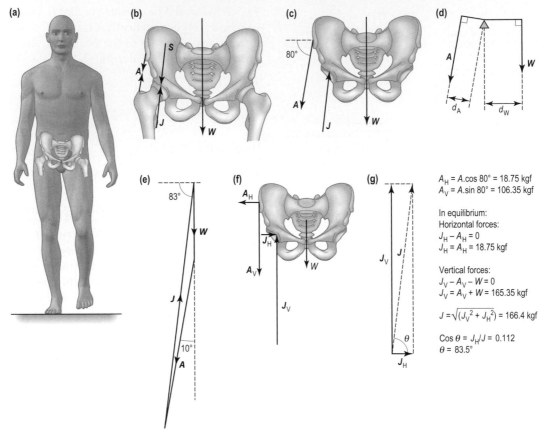

(a)

(b) S, A, J, W

(c) 80°, A, J, W

(d) A, W, d_A, d_W

(e) 83°, W, J, 10°, A

(f) A_H, J_H, A_V, W, J_V

(g) J_V, J, J_H, θ

$A_H = A.\cos 80° = 18.75$ kgf
$A_V = A.\sin 80° = 106.35$ kgf

In equilibrium:
Horizontal forces:
$J_H - A_H = 0$
$J_H = A_H = 18.75$ kgf

Vertical forces:
$J_V - A_V - W = 0$
$J_V = A_V + W = 165.35$ kgf

$J = \sqrt{(J_V^2 + J_H^2)} = 166.4$ kgf

$\cos \theta = J_H/J = 0.112$
$\theta = 83.5°$

Fig. 3.23   Forces at the hip in single leg stance. (a) Single-leg support on the right leg during the walking cycle. (b) Forces on the pelvis and hip joint. (c) Free body diagram of the pelvis. (d) Force–moment arm diagram. (e) Vector chain determination of hip joint reaction force. (f, g) Determination of the hip joint reaction force by trigonometry

The vector chain determination of J is shown in Figure 3.23e; $J = 166$ kgf at an angle of 83° to the horizontal. The determination of J by trigonometry is shown in Figure 3.23f and g; $J = 166.4$ kgf at an angle of 83.5° to the horizontal. The results show that the joint reaction force in one-legged stance is in the region of 2.4 times body weight.

The force S exerted by the pelvis on the head of the femur is equal and opposite to J (Fig. 3.23b). When someone is recovering from a serious leg injury such as a broken femur, it is necessary to reduce S during weight-bearing activities such as standing and walking by using crutches and walking sticks. Figure 3.24a shows a man walking with the aid of a stick in his left hand. During the right leg single-support

phase of the walking cycle the stick helps to support the weight of the body and, therefore, reduces the load on the right leg. In this situation, the stick is, in effect, an extension of the left arm, enabling the left arm to support the weight of the body by pushing against the floor. In this example the left arm can be considered to be a lateral extension of the pelvis, such that the free body diagram of the pelvis can be represented as in Figure 3.24b (Watkins 1999). The corresponding force–moment arm diagram is shown in Figure 3.24c.

When walking without a stick, as in Figure 3.23, the moment of W is counteracted by the moment of A on its own. When walking with a stick the moment of W is counteracted by the combined moment of A and the force B exerted

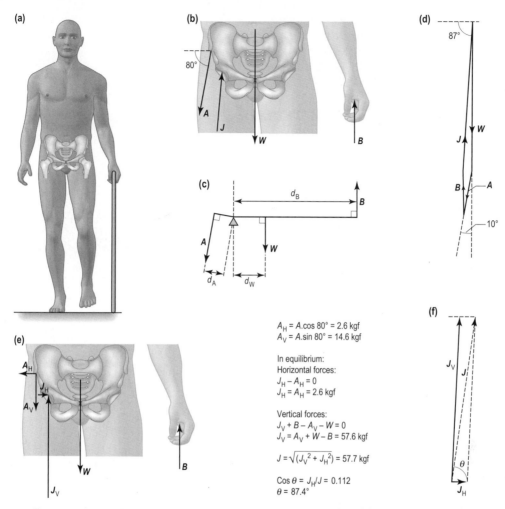

Fig. 3.24 Forces at the hip in single-leg stance while using a walking stick. (a) Single-leg support on the right leg during the walking cycle. (b) Free body diagram of the pelvis. (c) Force–moment arm diagram. (d) Vector chain determination of hip joint reaction force. (e, f) determination of the hip joint reaction force by trigonometry

by the stick on the man's left hand. When the pelvis is in equilibrium, the resultant of W, A, B and J will be zero. For a man of total body weight 70 kgf, B will be about 16 kgf with a moment arm of approximately 35 cm with respect to the hip joint axis of rotation; it is assumed that B acts vertically. By taking moments about the fulcrum,

$$W.d_W - A.d_A - B.d_B = 0$$

where $W = 59$ kgf, $d_W = 11$ cm, $B = 16$ kgf, $d_B = 35$ cm and $d_A = 6$ cm

i.e. $A = \dfrac{W.d_W - B.d_B}{d_A}$

$$A = \frac{(59 \text{ kgf} \times 11 \text{ cm}) - (16 \text{ kgf} \times 35 \text{ kgf})}{6 \text{ cm}}$$

$$= 14.8 \text{ kgf}$$

The vector chain determination of J is shown in Figure 3.24d; $J = 57.5$ kgf at an angle of 87° to the horizontal. The determination of J by trigonometry is shown in Figure 3.24e and f; $J = 57.7$ kgf at an angle of 87.4° to the horizontal.

The results indicate that using a walking stick considerably reduces the force exerted by the hip abductor muscles in single-leg stance (108 kgf to 14.8 kgf), which in turn considerably reduces the hip joint reaction force (166 kgf to 57.7 kgf).

Forces at the knee in knee extension from a sitting position

Many of the muscles of the body, especially those in the limbs, operate in third-class lever systems. A typical example of a third-class lever system in the leg is the action of the quadriceps in extending the knee. The distal ends of the quadriceps muscles all insert on to the quadriceps tendon. The quadriceps tendon encloses the anterior surface of the patella and is continuous with the patellar ligament, which inserts on to the tibial tuberosity. When the quadriceps muscles contract, the force is transmitted to the tibia, which tends to extend the knee. The patella increases the moment arm of the quadriceps tendon about the axis of knee flexion/extension and, as such, increases the moment of the quadriceps muscle force. During knee flexion/extension the posterior aspect of the patella slides on the patellar surface of the femur. The contact force between the patella and femur is referred to as the patellofemoral joint reaction force. The contact force between the tibia and femur is referred to as the tibiofemoral joint reaction force.

Figure 3.25a shows the foot, shank and distal end of the thigh while in a sitting position with the shank and foot held off the floor at an angle of 42° with respect to the horizontal and the foot at a right angle to the shank. In this position, the weight W of the shank and foot will exert an anticlockwise moment about the mediolateral axis through the knee that tends to flex the knee, but the shank and foot will be held in equilibrium by a clockwise moment exerted by the force L in the patellar ligament. The magnitude of the moment of L will depend upon the moment exerted by the hamstrings, which will tend to flex the knee. In this example, it will be assumed that the force in the hamstrings is zero and, therefore, the moment exerted by the hamstrings is zero. Consequently, the moment of L will be equal and opposite to that of W. Figure

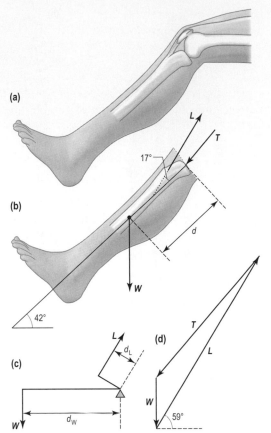

Fig. 3.25 Patellar ligament force and tibiofemoral joint reaction force while holding the shank and foot off the ground in a sitting position. (a) Sitting with shank and foot held at an angle of 42° to the horizontal. (b) Free body diagram of the shank and foot segment. (c) Force–moment arm diagram with respect to the mediolateral axis through the point of application of the tibiofemoral joint reaction force. (d) Vector chain determination of the tibiofemoral joint reaction force

3.25b shows the corresponding free body diagram of the combined shank and foot. Figure 3.25c shows the corresponding force–moment arm diagram. Force T is the tibiofemoral joint reaction force. When the shank and foot segment is in equilibrium, the resultant of W, L and T will be zero.

In women, the length of the shank (distance between the knee joint centre and the ankle joint centre) is approximately 25% of height (Plagenhoef et al 1983). Consequently, for a woman of height 170 cm, the length of the shank will be approximately 42.5 cm and the corresponding distance d between the point of application of T and the location of the centre of gravity of the combined shank and foot will be approximately 21 cm (assuming that the distance between the knee joint centre and the point of application of T is approximately 3 cm and that the knee joint centre, point of application of T and centre of gravity of the shank and foot all lie on the same line with respect to Figure 3.25b). Consequently, with the shank and foot held at an angle of 42°, the moment arm d_W of W about the mediolateral axis through the point of application of T will be approximately 15.6 cm. The line of action of L will be approximately 17° with respect to the line joining the point of application of T and the centre of gravity of the shank and foot, i.e. approximately 59° with respect to the horizontal and the length of the moment arm d_L of L will be approximately 4 cm through the 0–90° range of knee flexion (Chow 1999). For a woman of weight 62 kgf, W will be approximately 4.14 kgf (Table 3.2). By taking moments about the mediolateral axis through the point of application of T,

$$W.d_W - L.d_L = 0$$

where

$$W = 4.14 \text{ kgf}$$
$$d_W = d.\cos 42° = 15.6 \text{ cm}$$
$$d_L = 4 \text{ cm}$$

i.e. $L = \dfrac{W.d_W}{d_L} = \dfrac{(4.14 \text{ kgf} \times 15.6 \text{ cm})}{4 \text{ cm}}$

$$= 16.15 \text{ kgf}$$

The vector chain determination of T is shown in Figure 3.25d; $T = 12.8$ kgf at an angle of 49° to the horizontal. The determination of T by trigonometry is shown in Figure 3.26; $J = 12.78$ kgf at an angle of 49.4° to the horizontal.

Figure 3.27a shows a free body diagram of the patella corresponding to the position of the shank and foot in Figure 3.25a. In this position, the patella is held in equilibrium under the action of the force L in the patellar ligament (equal in magnitude but opposite in direction to L in Figure 3.25b), the force Q in the quadriceps tendon (which can be assumed to be equal

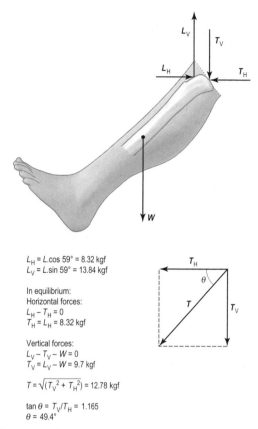

$L_H = L.\cos 59° = 8.32 \text{ kgf}$
$L_V = L.\sin 59° = 13.84 \text{ kgf}$

In equilibrium:
Horizontal forces:
$L_H - T_H = 0$
$T_H = L_H = 8.32 \text{ kgf}$

Vertical forces:
$L_V - T_V - W = 0$
$T_V = L_V - W = 9.7 \text{ kgf}$

$T = \sqrt{(T_V^2 + T_H^2)} = 12.78 \text{ kgf}$

$\tan \theta = T_V/T_H = 1.165$
$\theta = 49.4°$

Fig. 3.26 Determination of the tibiofemoral joint reaction force by trigonometry

in magnitude to L) acting at an angle of 8° to the horizontal and the patellofemoral joint reaction force P. The vector chain determination of P is shown in Figure 3.27b; $P = 13.9$ kgf at an angle of 56° to the horizontal. The determination of P by trigonometry is shown in Figure 3.27c and d; $P = 13.90$ kgf at an angle of 56.5° to the horizontal.

The results show that, to hold the shank and foot, weight approximately 4 kgf, at an angle of 42° to the horizontal requires a quadriceps muscle force of approximately 16 kgf, which, in turn, results in a patellar ligament force of approximately 16 kgf, a tibiofemoral joint reaction force of approximately 13 kgf and a patellofemoral joint reaction force of approximately 14 kgf. This illustrates the price that the body pays for the open-chain arrangement of the bones of the skeleton. The arms and legs form four peripheral chains, free at their extremities,

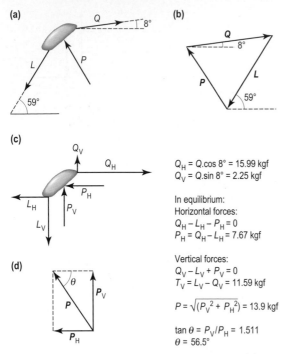

$Q_H = Q.\cos 8° = 15.99$ kgf
$Q_V = Q.\sin 8° = 2.25$ kgf

In equilibrium:
Horizontal forces:
$Q_H - L_H - P_H = 0$
$P_H = Q_H - L_H = 7.67$ kgf

Vertical forces:
$Q_V - L_V + P_V = 0$
$T_V = L_V - Q_V = 11.59$ kgf

$P = \sqrt{(P_V^2 + P_H^2)} = 13.9$ kgf

$\tan \theta = P_V/P_H = 1.511$
$\theta = 56.5°$

Fig. 3.27 Patellofemoral joint reaction force. (a) Free body diagram of the patella. (b) Vector chain determination of the patellofemoral joint reaction force. (c, d) Determination of the patellofemoral joint reaction force by trigonometry

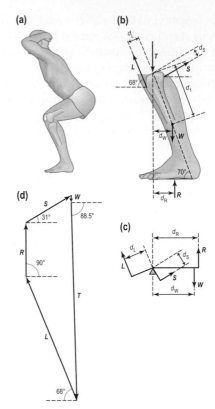

Fig. 3.28 Patellar ligament force and tibiofemoral joint reaction force in a half-squat standing position. (a) Half-squat standing position. (b) Free body diagram of the shank and foot segment of one leg. (c) Force–moment arm diagram with respect to the mediolateral axis through the point of application of the tibiofemoral joint reaction force. (d) Vector chain determination of the tibiofemoral joint reaction force

which attach on to a central chain (the vertebral column). This open chain arrangement allows any part of the body to move more or less independently of the rest and, as such, allows the body to adopt a very wide range of postures. However, this movement capability is only possible because the muscles are attached to the skeleton close to the joints that they control, i.e. the muscles have very low mechanical advantages and, as such, generally have to exert much larger forces than the weights of the body segments that they control. Furthermore, the larger the muscle forces, the larger the associated joint reaction forces (Watkins 1999).

Forces at the knee in knee extension from a standing position

Knee extension exercise from a sitting position, with and without additional load (such as resistance training equipment), is widely used in rehabilitation programmes following knee

injury. As illustrated in the previous section, the quadriceps muscle force and the tibiofemoral and patellofemoral forces are relatively small when there is no additional load (in the form of resistance training equipment) on the shank and foot segment. In a rehabilitation strength training programme, the load on the quadriceps muscles can be progressively increased by increasing the load on the shank and foot. Figure 3.28a shows a man performing a knee flexion/extension exercise from a standing position. In this situation, the load on each leg tending to flex the knee is half of body weight, i.e. if the exercise is performed slowly, avoiding high acceleration and deceleration at the start and end of each downward (knee flexion) and upward (knee extension) phase, the ground reaction force on each leg during the exercise will be approximately half of body weight. Figure 3.28b shows a free body diagram of one shank and foot corresponding to the position in Figure 3.28a.

In men, the length of the shank (distance between the knee joint centre and the ankle joint centre) is approximately 25% of height (Plagenhoef et al 1983). Consequently, for a man of height 180 cm, the length of the shank will be approximately 45 cm and the corresponding distance d_1 between the point of application of the tibiofemoral joint reaction force T and the location of the centre of gravity of the combined shank and foot will be about 24 cm (assuming that the distance between the knee joint centre and the point of application of T is about 3.2 cm and that the knee joint centre, point of application of T and centre of gravity of the shank and foot all lie on the same line with respect to Figure 3.28b). In the position shown in Figure 3.28a the long axis of the shank (line joining the point application of the T and the ankle joint centre) is approximately 70° to the horizontal and the line of action of the patellar ligament will be approximately 68° to the horizontal (based on Van Eijden et al 1985). The moment arm d_L of the patellar ligament force L about the mediolateral axis through the point of application of T will be approximately 4.5 cm (based on Chow 1999). The moment arm of the ground reaction force R will be approximately 9 cm (based on Wallace et al 2002). For a man of weight 80 kgf, the weight of the shank and foot W will be approximately 4.94 kgf (see Table 3.1, Plagenhoef data). In this example, it must be assumed that the hamstrings are active, since they normally work with the quadriceps to stabilize the knee joint. In the position shown in Figure 3.28a, the moment arm d_S of the force S exerted by hamstring muscles about the mediolateral axis through the point of application of T will be about 3 cm (based on Lieber 1992). It will be assumed that S is 40% of L (based on the ratio of the cross-sectional areas of the quadriceps and hamstring muscle groups; Lieber 1992). When the shank and foot segment is in equilibrium, the resultant of W, R, L, S and T will be zero. Figure 3.28c shows the corresponding

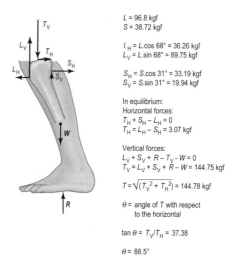

$L = 96.8$ kgf
$S = 38.72$ kgf

$L_H = L.\cos 68° = 36.26$ kgf
$L_V = L.\sin 68° = 89.75$ kgf

$S_H = S.\cos 31° = 33.19$ kgf
$S_V = S.\sin 31° = 19.94$ kgf

In equilibrium:
Horizontal forces:
$T_H + S_H - L_H = 0$
$T_H = L_H - S_H = 3.07$ kgf

Vertical forces:
$L_V + S_V + R - T_V - W = 0$
$T_V = L_V + S_V + R - W = 144.75$ kgf

$T = \sqrt{(T_V^2 + T_H^2)} = 144.78$ kgf

θ = angle of T with respect to the horizontal

$\tan \theta = T_V/T_H = 37.38$

$\theta = 88.5°$

Fig. 3.29   Determination of the tibiofemoral joint reaction force by trigonometry

force–moment arm diagram. By taking moments about the mediolateral axis through the point of application of T,

$$L.d_L + W.d_W - S.d_S - R.d_R = 0$$

where

$d_L = 4.5$ cm
$W = 4.94$ kgf
$d_W = d_1.\cos 70° = 8.21$ cm
$S = 0.4L$
$d_S = 3$ cm
$R = 40$ kgf
$d_R = 9.0$ cm

i.e. $L(d_L - 0.4d_S) = R.d_R - W.d_W$

$$
\begin{aligned}
L &= \frac{R.d_R - W.d_W}{d_L - 0.4d_S} \\
&= \frac{(40 \text{ kgf} \times 9 \text{ cm}) - (4.94 \text{ kgf} \times 8.21 \text{ cm})}{4.5 \text{ cm} - 1.2 \text{ cm}} \\
&= 96.8 \text{ kgf}
\end{aligned}
$$

As $L = 96.8$ kgf, $S = 38.72$ kgf

The vector chain determination of T is shown in Figure 3.28d; $T = 145$ kgf at an angle of 88.5° to the horizontal. The determination of T by trigonometry is shown in Figure 3.29; $T = 144.78$ kgf at an angle of 88.5° to the horizontal.

Figure 3.30a shows a free body diagram of the patella corresponding to the position of the shank and foot in Figure 3.28a. In this position,

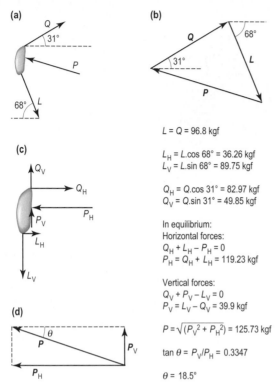

(a)

(b)

$L = Q = 96.8$ kgf

$L_H = L.\cos 68° = 36.26$ kgf
$L_V = L.\sin 68° = 89.75$ kgf

$Q_H = Q.\cos 31° = 82.97$ kgf
$Q_V = Q.\sin 31° = 49.85$ kgf

In equilibrium:
Horizontal forces:
$Q_H + L_H - P_H = 0$
$P_H = Q_H + L_H = 119.23$ kgf

(c)

Vertical forces:
$Q_V + P_V - L_V = 0$
$P_V = L_V - Q_V = 39.9$ kgf

$P = \sqrt{(P_V{}^2 + P_H{}^2)} = 125.73$ kgf

(d)

$\tan \theta = P_V/P_H = 0.3347$

$\theta = 18.5°$

Fig. 3.30 Patellofemoral joint reaction force.
(a) Free body diagram of the patella. (b) Vector chain
determination of the patellofemoral joint reaction
force. (c, d) Determination of the patellofemoral joint
reaction force by trigonometry

required at the knee: quadriceps muscle force
(approximately 1.2 BW), patellar ligament
force (approximately 1.2 BW), hamstrings muscle force (approximately 0.5 BW), tibiofemoral
joint reaction force (approximately 1.8 BW) and
patellofemoral joint reaction force (approximately 1.6 BW).

THE USE OF BODY SEGMENTS AS LEVERS IN STRENGTH AND ENDURANCE TRAINING

In any training exercise, such as a pull-up, sit-up
or press-up, the muscles involved are required
to overcome the moment of resistance exerted
by the resistance force. The moment of resistance
and, therefore, the load on the muscles can be
varied by changing the resistance force and/or
the moment arm of the resistance force. This is
the basis of progressive strength and local (muscular) endurance training. Whereas strength
training for sport is likely to involve the use of
resistance equipment to increase the load and,
therefore, the training effect on the muscles,
subtle changes in body posture can provide adequate resistance for the development of strength
and endurance that is consistent with good
health without the need for additional load.

Trunk curl and sit–up

Consider a man lying on his back with his arms
straight and hands, palms down, on the front
of his thighs (Fig. 3.31a). To sit up, the abdominal muscles and hip flexor muscles must overcome the moment of upper body weight about
the mediolateral axis a_H through the hip joints.
The first stage in the sit-up exercise usually
involves what is called a trunk curl, i.e. flexion
of the neck and thoracic region by the neck
and trunk flexor muscles. This movement
results in a decrease in the moment arm of upper
body weight about a_H (Fig. 3.31b). The sit-up is
completed by the action of the hip flexors, which
rotate the upper body about the hips. As the
upper body moves from the lying to the sit-up
position, the moment arm of upper body weight
about a_H gradually decreases (Fig. 3.31b, c).
Therefore, the moment of force required to raise

the patella is held in equilibrium by the action
of the force L in the patellar ligament (equal in
magnitude but opposite in direction to L in
Figure 3.28b), the force Q in the quadriceps tendon (which can be assumed to be equal in magnitude to L) acting at an angle of 31° to the
horizontal and the patellofemoral joint reaction
force P. The vector chain determination of P is
shown in Figure 3.30b; $P = 126$ kgf at an angle
of 18.5° to the horizontal. The determination of
P by trigonometry is shown in Figure 3.30c and
d; $P = 125.73$ kgf at an angle of 18.5° to the
horizontal.

In the half-squat position shown in Figure
3.28a, the external forces acting on the shank
and foot segment of each leg are the weight
of the shank and foot (approximately 0.062
body weight (BW)) and the ground reaction
force (approximately 0.5 BW). In order to
maintain equilibrium, five internal forces are

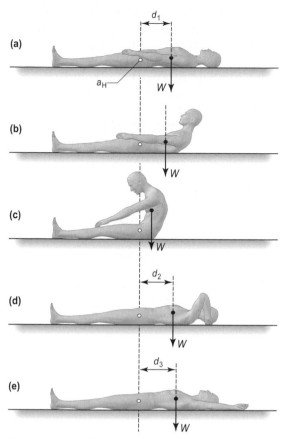

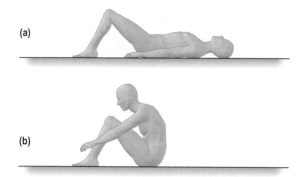

Fig. 3.32   Bent-leg sit-up

Fig. 3.31   (a–b) Trunk curl. (a–c) Sit-up. (d) Effect of putting the hands behind the head on the moment arm of upper body weight. (e) Effect of putting the arms by the side of the head on the moment arm of upper body weight. W = weight of trunk, head and neck

the upper body into the sitting position also gradually decreases. Since the moment arm of the hip flexor muscles gradually increases throughout the range of hip movement from lying to sitting up, the force exerted by the hip flexors gradually decreases as the upper body assumes the sit-up position. It follows that the most strenuous part of the whole sit-up movement occurs just after the start of hip flexion as the upper body is raised clear of the floor. The sit-up exercise can be made more strenuous by starting with the hands behind the head, as shown in Figure 3.31d. The movement of the arms redistributes upper body weight such that the moment arm of upper body weight

about a_H is increased (Fig. 3.31a, d; $d_2 > d_1$). Consequently, in raising the upper body into the sitting position, the hip flexors would need to exert a greater force than would be necessary from the starting position shown in Figure 3.31a. The exercise could be made even more strenuous by starting with the arms extended by the side of the head (Fig. 3.31d, e; $d_3 > d_2$).

Bent leg sit–up

If the abdominal and hip flexor muscles are not strong enough for the person to perform a sit-up from the straight leg starting position (Fig. 3.31a), it may be possible for the person to perform a bent leg sit-up (Fig. 3.32). With the hips flexed at 45° to the horizontal in the starting position (Fig. 3.32a), the moment arm of the hip flexors will be greater than in the straight leg starting position. Consequently, the hip flexors will be able to raise the upper body into the sitting position with less force than that required in the straight leg starting position. The moment arm of the abdominal muscles will be about the same in both starting positions.

Leg raise

When the hip flexor and abdominal muscles are very weak, such that the person cannot perform a bent leg sit-up, a suitable exercise to start training these muscles is alternate single leg raises (Fig. 3.33a, b). The moment arm of the weight of each leg about a_H is about the same as that of the upper body about a_H after the trunk curl stage of the sit-up (Figs 3.31b & 3.33a). However,

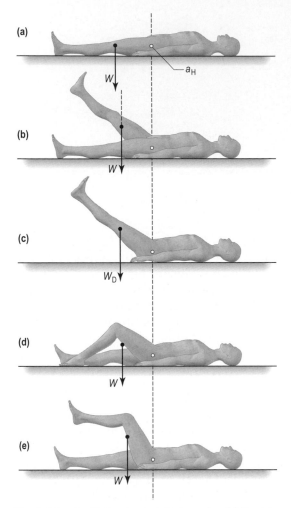

Fig. 3.33 (a–b) Single straight leg raise. (c) Double straight leg raise. (d, e) Single bent leg raise.
W = weight of one leg; W_D = weight of both legs

as the upper body (trunk, head, neck and arms) and each leg constitute about 68% and 16% respectively of total body weight (Table 3.1), the moment of resistance that the hip flexors of each leg are required to overcome when performing a single leg raise is much less than that required to perform a bent leg sit-up. Furthermore, the load on the abdominal muscles is much less in a single leg raise than in a bent leg sit-up. It might be assumed that a reasonable progression from alternate single leg raises is to raise both legs together (Fig. 3.33c). However, in order to perform this exercise correctly, i.e. without the risk of injury to the low back, the abdominal

muscles must exert considerable force in order to prevent the pelvis from rotating forward (anti-clockwise with respect to Figure 3.33c). The sacrum forms the lower end of the vertebral column and the rear part of the pelvis. Forward rotation of the pelvis increases the curvature of the lumbar region of the vertebral column (con-tinuous with the sacrum), which may result in low back pain due to strain of the lumbosacral plexuses, i.e. the peripheral nerves of the lumbar region (Watkins 1999).

The single leg raise can be made less strenu-ous by flexing the knee before raising the leg (Fig. 3.33d, e). Flexing the knee reduces the moment arm of the weight of the leg about a_H, thereby reducing the moment of resistance that the hip flexors need to overcome. A suitable progression of exercises for increasing the strength and endurance of the hip flexors and abdominal muscles would be:

1. Trunk curls
2. Alternate single bent leg raises
3. Double bent leg raises
4. Single straight leg raises
5. Bent leg sit-up
6. Straight leg sit-up.

Press–up

During a press-up from the floor, as shown in Figure 3.34a and b, the body segment consisting of head, neck, trunk and legs is held in line and rotated about the balls of the feet by the action of the arms. To complete a press-up, the elbow extensors and shoulder flexors must overcome the moment of body weight about the medio-lateral axis a_F through the points of contact between the feet and the floor. Provided that the head, neck, trunk and legs are held in line, the moment arm d_A of the force A exerted by the arms about a_F will be more or less the same irrespective of the inclination of the head, neck, trunk and legs (Fig. 3.34f). However, the greater the inclination of the head, neck, trunk and legs to the vertical, the greater the moment arm d_W of body weight W about a_F and, therefore, the greater the force A required to extend the arms. Therefore, in order to gradually increase the

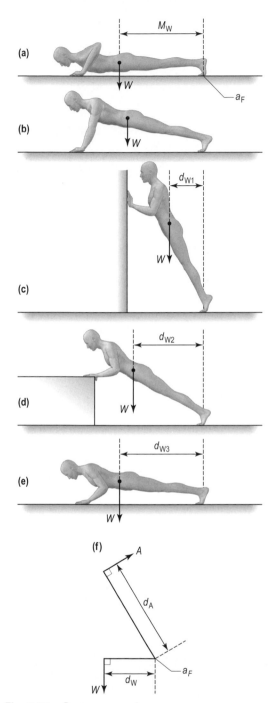

Fig. 3.34   Press-up exercise

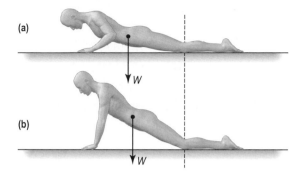

Fig. 3.35   Modified press-up using the knees rather than the feet as the fulcrum

reasonable progression would be to start with a press-up against a wall followed by the edge of a table, then a low box or bench and finally the floor (Fig. 3.34c–e; $d_{W1} < d_{W2} < d_{W3}$).

Press-ups against the floor can be made less strenuous by using the knees as fulcrum (with suitable cushioning) rather than the feet, as shown in Figure 3.35. In this form of press-up, the moment of resistance about the mediolateral axis through the knees–floor fulcrum is considerably less than the moment of resistance about the feet–floor fulcrum in Figure 3.34a.

Squat

The half squat with a barbell weight across the shoulders, as shown in Figure 3.36, is one of the most frequently used weight training exercises for increasing the strength of the leg extensor muscles, i.e. hip extensors, knee extensors and ankle plantar flexors. The effect that the exercise has on these three groups of muscles depends upon the moment of resistance about each corresponding joint. The resistance W is the combined weight of the body and the barbell. Since W is the same in positions 1 and 2, the effect on each muscle group depends upon the moment arm of W about each joint. In position 1, the trunk is inclined forward at about 45° to the horizontal such that the moment arm d_{K1} of W about the mediolateral axis a_K through the knee joint is less than the moment arm d_{H1} of W about the mediolateral axis a_H through the hip joint. In position 2, the trunk is more upright (inclination of about 63° to the horizontal) such that the moment arm d_{K2} of W about a_K is greater than

training effect of the exercise, it is necessary to gradually increase d_W. This can be achieved by gradually lowering the position of the hand support with respect to the feet. For example, a

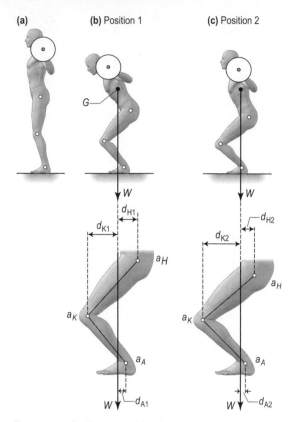

Fig. 3.36 Half squat with a barbell

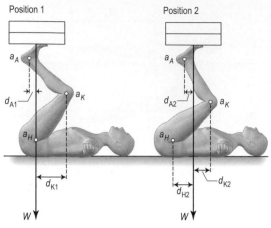

Fig. 3.37 Leg press

the moment arm d_{H2} of W about a_H. Consequently, the training effect on the hip extensors will be greater in position 1 than in position 2 and the training effect on the knee extensors will be greater in position 2 than in position 1. Similarly, as the moment arm of W about the mediolateral axis a_A through the ankle joint is greater in position 1 than in position 2, the training effect on the ankle plantar flexors will be greater in position 1 than in position 2.

Leg press

The leg press, like the half squat, is also a popular weight training exercise for strengthening the leg extensors. One form of leg press is shown in Figure 3.37. In this exercise the trainer lies on his/her back and lifts and lowers a weight vertically by extending and flexing the legs. In position 1, the line of action of the weight W passes through the mediolateral axis a_H through the hip joint. Consequently, the moment

of W about a_H is zero and there will be little training effect on the hip extensors. However, the moment arm of W about the mediolateral axis a_K through the knee joint and the mediolateral axis a_A through the ankle joint is relatively large such that the training effect on the knee extensors and ankle plantar flexors is likely to be significant. In position 2, W exerts a moment of resistance about all three joints, with the largest moment about the hip joint. The half squat and leg press show that slight changes in body posture can significantly alter the way in which the musculoskeletal system responds to a particular external load on the body.

> Appropriate changes in body posture in training exercises can provide adequate resistance for the development of strength and endurance consistent with good health without the need for resistance equipment.

ANGULAR DISPLACEMENT, ANGULAR VELOCITY AND ANGULAR ACCELERATION

Figure 3.38 shows a man performing a single leg raise from a lying position. In raising his left leg from position 1 to position 2, the centre of gravity of his leg moves a linear distance s, i.e. the arc of the circle of radius r about the

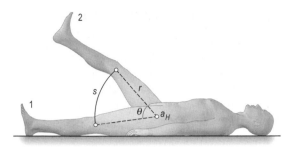

Fig. 3.38 Linear movement (s) of the centre of gravity of the leg and angular movement (θ) of the leg in a single leg raise. a_H = mediolateral axis through the hip joint; r = distance between a_H and the centre of gravity of the leg

mediolateral axis a_H through the left hip joint. Simultaneously, his leg rotates an angular distance θ (Greek letter theta) about a_H.

In trigonometry, angular distance is usually measured in degrees. There are 360° in one complete revolution. Figure 3.39a shows a gymnast performing a giant circle on the high bar. By rotating about the bar, i.e. the axis a_B, from position A to position D the gymnast will rotate an angular distance of 180° and an angular displacement (angular distance in a clockwise direction) of 180°. By rotating from position A back to position A the gymnast will have travelled an angular distance of 360°, i.e. one revolution. Angular displacement must reflect the number of revolutions between the initial and final positions of the object following a period of rotation.

In mechanics, angular distance is usually measured in radians (rad). One radian is the angle subtended at the centre of a circle by an arc of the circle that is the same length as the radius of the circle (Fig. 3.40). The circumference of a circle = $2\pi r$ where r is the radius of the circle, i.e.

$360° = 2\pi r/r$ rad = 2π rad = 6.2832 rad
(as π = 3.1416)

Therefore,

$1° = 0.017\,45$ rad (6.2832/360)
1 rad = 57.3° (360/6.2832)

Angular speed is the rate of change of angular distance. In mechanics, angular speed is usually

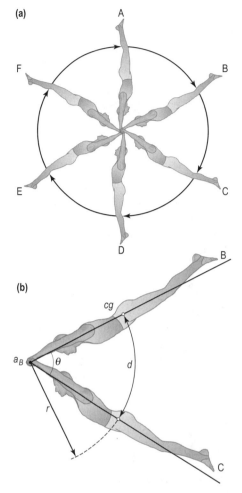

Fig. 3.39 A gymnast performing a giant circle on the high bar. cg = centre of gravity; a_B = horizontal axis along the centre of the bar; r = distance between a_B and cg = radius of the circle followed by the cg; d = linear distance travelled by the cg; θ = angular distance travelled by the body

measured in rad/s (radians per second). When the direction of rotation is specified, the term angular velocity is used rather than angular speed. The symbol for angular velocity is ω (Greek letter omega). Figure 3.39b shows the movement of the gymnast between positions B and C. The average angular velocity of the gymnast between positions B and C is given by

$$\omega = \frac{\theta_c - \theta_B}{t_C - t_B}$$ Eq. 3.6

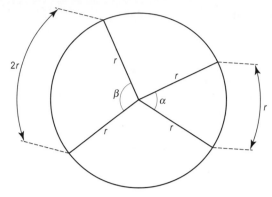

Fig. 3.40 A radian is the angle subtended at the centre of a circle by an arc on the circumference of the circle that is the same length as the radius of the circle. r = radius of the circle; α = 1 radian; β = 2 radians

where

θ_B = angular displacement of position B relative to position A

θ_C = angular displacement of position C relative to position A

t_B = time at position B with respect to position A

t_C = time at position C with respect to position A

If $\theta_B = 60°$, $\theta_C = 125°$, $t_B = 1.43\,s$, $t_C = 1.69\,s$, then

$$\omega = \frac{125° - 60°}{1.69\,s - 1.43\,s}$$

$$= 250°/s \text{ (degrees per second)} = 4.36\,rad/s$$

Angular acceleration is the rate of change of angular velocity. In mechanics, angular acceleration is usually measured in rad/s^2 (radians per second per second). The symbol for angular acceleration is α (Greek letter alpha). The average angular acceleration of the gymnast between positions B and C is given by

$$\alpha = \frac{\omega_C - \omega_B}{t_C - t_B} \qquad \text{Eq. 3.7}$$

where

ω_B = angular velocity at position B

ω_C = angular velocity at position C

t_B = time at position B with respect to position A

t_C = time at position C with respect to position A

If $\omega_B = 3.13\,rad/s$, $\omega_C = 5.55\,rad/s$, $t_B = 1.43\,s$, $t_C = 1.69\,s$, then

$$\alpha = \frac{5.55\,rad/s - 3.13\,rad/s}{1.69\,s - 1.43\,s} = 9.31\,rad/s^2$$

RELATIONSHIP BETWEEN LINEAR VELOCITY AND ANGULAR VELOCITY

In Figure 3.39b, if the orientation of the gymnast's body segments to each other remains the same between positions B and C, i.e. if the centre of gravity moves along the arc d of a circle of radius r in a time t, then the average linear velocity v of the centre of gravity during this period is given by

$$v = \frac{d}{t} \qquad \text{Eq. 3.8}$$

If the body rotates through an angle θ during the same period, then the average angular velocity of the body is given by

$$\omega = \frac{\theta}{t} \qquad \text{Eq. 3.9}$$

Since θ degrees = d/r radians, then

$$d = r.\theta \qquad \text{Eq. 3.10}$$

By substitution of d from Equation 3.10 into Equation 3.8,

$$v = \frac{r.\theta}{t} \qquad \text{Eq. 3.11}$$

By substitution of θ/t from Equation 3.9 into Equation 3.11,

$$v = r.\omega \qquad \text{Eq. 3.12}$$

i.e. the linear velocity of the centre of gravity is equal to the product of the radius of the circle (distance from the axis of rotation to the centre of gravity) and the angular velocity of the body. The radian is a dimensionless variable, i.e. it has no unit because it is the ratio of two distances (the arc of the circle and the radius of the circle). Consequently, the product $r.\omega$ is in m/s (where r is in metres and ω is in rad/s). For example, in Figure 3.39b, if $r = 1\,m$ and $\omega = 3.13\,rad/s$ at position B, then v at B = 3.13 m/s.

RELATIONSHIP BETWEEN LINEAR ACCELERATION AND ANGULAR ACCELERATION

From Equation 3.12, it follows that $v_B = r.\omega_B$ and $v_C = r.\omega_C$ where v_B, v_C and ω_B, ω_C are the linear and angular velocities of the centre of gravity of the gymnast at positions B and C in

Figure 3.39b. Consequently, the average linear acceleration a of the centre of gravity between positions B and C is given by

$$a = \frac{v_C - v_B}{t} = \frac{r(\omega_C - \omega_B)}{t}$$

As $(\omega_C - \omega_B)/t = \alpha$ = angular acceleration (Eq. 3.7), it follows that

$$a = r.\alpha \qquad\qquad \text{Eq. 3.13}$$

i.e. the linear acceleration of the centre of gravity in the direction of v is equal to the product of the radius of the circle (distance from the axis of rotation to the centre of gravity) and the angular acceleration of the body. As the direction of a is perpendicular to r, i.e. tangent to the circle, a is referred to as tangential acceleration and sometimes denoted a_T. In Figure 3.39b, if $r = 1$ m and $\alpha = 9.31$ rad/s^2 at position C, then $a_T = 9.31$ m/s^2.

CENTRIPETAL AND CENTRIFUGAL FORCE

It is clear from Figure 3.39b that the direction of the centre of gravity is continuously changing in order to maintain its circular path. In accordance with Newton's first law of motion, there must be a force acting on the centre of gravity that is responsible for its continuous change of direction. This force cannot be the weight of the body because weight acts vertically downward. Consequently, there must be another force acting on the centre of gravity. Intuitively, this force is the force exerted by the bar on the body, i.e. the equal and opposite reaction to the force exerted by the gymnast on the bar. To derive the magnitude and direction of this force, it is better to use an example, unlike a giant circle, where the force is not influenced by the weight of the moving body. Consider, for example, the movement of a small weight such as a plumb-bob attached to a piece of string which is being swung around with constant linear velocity v in a horizontal plane (Fig. 3.41a; Ninio 1993). If the object is rotating anticlockwise with respect to Figure 3.41a, the components of velocity v_X and v_Y at the point A

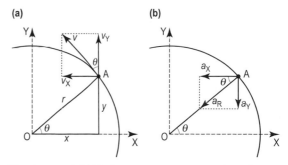

Fig. 3.41   (a) Velocity components v_X and v_Y of an object moving in a circle with constant velocity v. (b) Components a_X and a_Y of centripetal acceleration a_R. O = centre of the circle

in the directions of X (positive to the right) and Y (positive upward) respectively are given by

$$v_X = -v.\sin\theta = -\frac{v.y}{r} \quad (\sin\theta = y/r) \quad \text{Eq. 3.14}$$

$$v_Y = v.\cos\theta = \frac{v.x}{r} \quad (\cos\theta = x/r) \qquad \text{Eq. 3.15}$$

As v/r is constant, it follows from Equation 3.14 that the rate of change of v_X is the product of v/r and the rate of change of y. Since the rate of change of v_X is a_X = linear acceleration of the object in the X direction and the rate of change of y is v_Y = linear velocity of the object in the Y direction, then

$$\alpha_X = (-v/r).v_Y = (-v/r).(v.x/r)$$
$$= -(v^2/r).\cos\theta$$

Similarly, it follows from Equation 3.15 that the rate of change of v_Y is the product of v/r and the rate of change of x. Since the rate of change of v_Y is a_Y = linear acceleration of the object in the Y direction and the rate of change of x is v_X = linear velocity of the object in the X direction, then

$$\alpha_Y = (v/r).v_X = (v/r).(-v.y/r)$$
$$= -(v^2/r).\sin\theta$$

The resultant linear acceleration a of the object is given by Pythagoras' theorem,

$$a^2 = a_X^2 + a_Y^2 = (v^4/r^2.\cos^2\theta) + (v^4/r^2.\sin^2\theta)$$
$$a^2 = (v^4/r^2).(\cos^2\theta + \sin^2\theta)$$
$$a^2 = v^4/r^2.(\cos^2\theta + \sin^2\theta = 1)$$
$$a = v^2/r$$

The direction of a with respect to the horizontal is given by the angle β, where

$$\tan \beta = \frac{a_Y}{a_X} = \frac{-(v^2/r).\sin \theta}{-(v^2/r).\cos \theta}$$
$$= \tan \theta \; (\sin \theta / \cos \theta = \tan \theta)$$

i.e. $\beta = \theta$

Therefore, the magnitude of a is v^2/r and its direction is toward the centre of the circle. As a is directed along the radius of the circle, it is referred to as radial acceleration and sometimes denoted a_R to distinguish it from the tangential acceleration a_T. Figure 3.41b shows a_R, a_X and a_Y. From Newton's second law of motion, a_R is due to a force of magnitude $m.v^2/r$ where m is the mass of the object. This force is called the centripetal (centre-seeking) force, since it is directed toward the centre of the circle. Any object that moves on a curve (a circle is a regular curve) will do so as a result of the centripetal force F_C acting on it. As $F_C = m.v^2/r$ and $v = r.\omega$ (Eq. 3.12), it follows that

$$F_C = m.v^2/r = m.r.\omega^2 \qquad \text{Eq. 3.16}$$

In the above example, the centripetal force is applied to the plumb-bob by the string. In accordance with Newton's third law of motion, the plumb-bob will exert an equal and opposite force on the string. This force is called the centrifugal (centre-fleeing) force.

The centrifugal force is due to the inertia of the plumb-bob resisting the change in its direction of motion by the centripetal force. As soon as the centripetal force disappears, so does the centrifugal force. Consequently, if the string attached to the plumb-bob breaks, the plumb-bob will continue to move (with respect to the plane of rotation) in the direction it had at the instant that the string broke, i.e. in a straight line, tangent to the circle (Fig. 3.41a).

CENTRIPETAL FORCE IN THROWING THE HAMMER

In the hammer event in track and field athletics, the hammer consists of a metal ball (mass = 4 kg and diameter = 10 cm for women; mass = 7.26 kg and diameter = 12 cm for men) attached to a handle by a flexible wire (total length of handle and wire approximately 1.13 m for women and men). The aim of the athlete is to maximize the range of the hammer, i.e. the horizontal distance travelled by the hammer following release.

As in shot put, the main influences on the range of the hammer are release speed, release angle, release height and air resistance. Air resistance will have a greater effect on the range of a hammer throw (about 1.5% reduction in range) than on the range of a shot put (about 0.5% reduction in range) largely because of the greater release velocity of the hammer. Most elite male athletes release the hammer at about shoulder height with a release angle of about 45° to the horizontal (Dapena 1984). Consequently, the main determinant of range is release speed. The angular and linear velocity of the hammer is built up over a period of about 4 seconds by a swinging–turning action performed within a circle 2.135 m (7 ft) in diameter. With the thrower standing in the back of the circle, facing in the opposite direction to that of the throw, the action is usually initiated by two or three swings (lasting about 2.5 s) in which the hammer is swung overhead around the body. This is followed by three or four increasingly rapid whole-body turns (each turn lasting about 0.5 s) in which the hammer is swung around the body as the body rotates about a vertical axis and simultaneously moves to the front of the circle. During the turns, the plane of motion of the hammer progressively increases so that the release angle is about 45°. The hammer is launched, ideally with maximum linear velocity, at the end of the final turn.

The current men's world record is 86.74 m (Yuriy Sedykh, Russia, mass = 110 kg, height = 1.85 m). Assuming a release height of 1.65 m and release angle of 45°, a release speed of approximately 29 m/s would be required for a throw of 86.74 m. The radius of curvature of the hammer (the distance from the instantaneous axis of rotation to the centre of gravity of the metal ball) at release for a male athlete of mass 110 kg and height 1.85 m will be approximately 1.80 m (Dyson 1977; Fig. 3.42). Consequently, from Equation 3.16, the centripetal force F_C acting on the hammer immediately before release will be

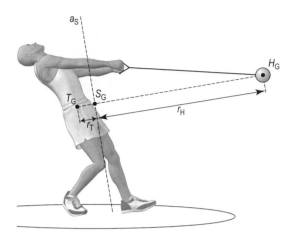

Fig. 3.42 Position of thrower and hammer just before release. T_G = centre of gravity of the thrower; H_G = centre of gravity of the hammer; S_G = centre of gravity of the combined thrower and hammer; a_S = axis that passes through the centre of gravity of the combined thrower and hammer and is perpendicular to the plane of rotation; r_H = radius of curvature of the hammer; r_T = radius of curvature of the thrower

approximately 3392 N, which is equivalent to 3.14 times the body weight (BW) of the athlete:

$$F_C = \frac{m.v^2}{r} = \frac{7.26 \text{ kg} \times (29 \text{ m/s})^2}{1.80 \text{ m}}$$
$$= 3392 \text{ N} = 345.8 \text{ kgf} = 3.14 \text{ BW}$$

Since the thrower pulls on the hammer with a force of 3.14 BW, the hammer will exert an equal and opposite force on the thrower, tending to pull him off balance. In order to maintain the centripetal force on the hammer and, therefore, the linear velocity (magnitude and direction) of the hammer, the thrower must counteract this force. The only way that this can be achieved is for the thrower to rotate his body in the same direction as the hammer about the same axis of rotation and thereby create a centripetal force on his centre of gravity that is equal and opposite to the centripetal force on the hammer, i.e. the thrower and hammer rotate at the same angular velocity on opposite sides of the axis that passes through the centre of gravity of the combined thrower and hammer and is perpendicular to the plane of rotation (Fig. 3.42). In this situation, the centrifugal force on the thrower will be equal and opposite to the centrifugal force on the

hammer so that the thrower can maintain his balance. It should be clear that the technique of throwing the hammer (usually referred to as throwing, but it is really a slinging action) requires not only great strength to produce and maintain such a large centripetal force on the hammer, especially in the final turn, when the linear velocity of the hammer rapidly increases, but also a very high level of coordination and timing.

Since the mass of the thrower is much greater than the mass of the hammer, the radius of curvature of the centre of mass of the thrower will be much smaller than the radius of curvature of the centre of mass of the hammer. A reasonable estimate of the radius of curvature of the centre of mass of the thrower can be made by considering the components of the centripetal forces on the hammer and thrower. Immediately prior to release, the centripetal force on the hammer will be more or less equal and opposite to the centripetal force on thrower. Consequently, from Equation 3.16,

$$m_H.r_H.\omega^2 = m_T.r_T.\omega^2 \qquad \text{Eq. 3.17}$$

where

m_H = mass of the hammer
r_H = radius of curvature of the hammer
m_T = mass of the thrower
r_T = radius of curvature of the thrower
ω = angular velocity of the hammer and the thrower

It follows from Equation 3.17 that

$$m_H.r_H = m_T.r_T \qquad \text{Eq. 3.18}$$

If m_H = 7.26 kg, r_H = 1.8 m and m_T = 110 kg, then it follows from Equation 3.18 that

$$r_T = \frac{m_H.r_H}{m_T} = \frac{7.26 \text{ kg} \times 1.8 \text{ m}}{110 \text{ kg}} = 0.119 \text{ m}$$

i.e. the radius of curvature of the centre of mass of the thrower is approximately 12 cm (Fig. 3.42).

CENTRIPETAL FORCE IN CYCLING AROUND A CURVED TRACK

In order to cycle around a curve, the cyclist must create centripetal force between the wheels of the bike and the road. This is achieved by leaning toward the centre of curvature so that the

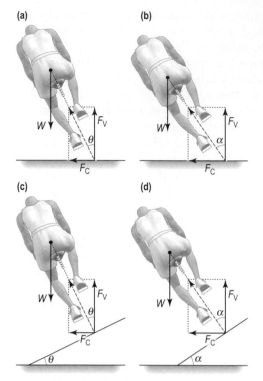

Fig. 3.43   Rear view free body diagram of a cyclist riding around a left hand bend with linear velocity 13.41 m/s (30 mph). (a) Horizontal surface, radius of curvature = 37 m. (b) Horizontal surface, radius of curvature = 27 m. (c) Banked curve of slope θ, radius of curvature = 37 m. (d) Banked curve of slope α, radius of curvature = 27 m. θ = 26.3°; α = 34.2°; W = weight of rider and bike; F_C = horizontal component of the ground reaction force = centripetal force; F_V = vertical component of the ground reaction force = W

horizontal component of the ground reaction force (in the plane of the radius of curvature) creates the required centripetal force. Figure 3.43a shows a rear view free body diagram of a cyclist moving around a left-hand bend. As the cyclist and bike will be in rotational equilibrium with respect to the plane of the radius of curvature (as in Figure 3.43a), the ground reaction force F (resultant of F_V and F_C) will act through the combined centre of gravity of the cyclist and bike. In order to maintain this situation, the cyclist and bike must lean at an angle θ, which is given by

$$\tan \theta = \frac{F_C}{F_V} \qquad \qquad \text{Eq. 3.19}$$

If the combined mass of the cyclist and bike is 72 kg, moving with linear velocity of 13.41 m/s (30 mph) around a curve with radius of curvature of 37 m (similar to a bend on a standard 400 m running track) the centripetal force F_C on the cyclist and bike will be

$$F_C = \frac{m.v^2}{r} = \frac{72 \text{ kg} \times (13.41 \text{ m/s})^2}{37 \text{ m}} = 349.9 \text{ N}$$

As F_V = 72 kgf = 706.3 N, then

$$\tan \theta = \frac{F_C}{F_V} = \frac{349.9 \text{ N}}{706.3 \text{ N}} = 0.4953$$
$$\theta = 26.3°$$

If the cyclist wanted to cycle at the same speed around a tighter curve, i.e. a smaller radius of curvature, the centripetal force and lean angle would both increase. For example, if the radius of curvature is 27 m, F_C = 479.5 N and α = 34.2° (Fig. 3.43b).

In these examples, it is assumed that the road is horizontal and that, therefore, the centripetal force is the result of friction between the wheels and the road. In this situation, the maximum speed that can be achieved (for a given radius of curvature) is limited by the maximum friction that can be created (maximum friction = $\mu.W$ where μ is the coefficient of friction and W = normal reaction force = weight of cyclist and bike; Eq. 2.1). However, when riding on a banked curve, the need for friction can be significantly reduced or even eliminated. For example, Figure 3.43c shows the cyclist in Figure 3.43a riding at the same speed with the same radius of curvature on a banked curve with a slope that corresponds to the lean angle. Figure 3.43d shows the corresponding situation to that in Figure 3.43b. In these situations, centripetal force is provided by the horizontal component of the ground reaction without the need for friction. Consequently, if the angle of the slope is appropriate for the maximum speed likely to be achieved, friction is not a limiting factor. Velodromes (indoor cycling tracks) and indoor running tracks are banked for this reason. The slope of a velodrome ranges from approximately 15° on the straights to approximately

45° on the bends. The slopes of indoor running tracks range from 0° on the straights to approximately 15° on the bends (Wikipedia 2005).

CENTRIPETAL FORCE IN RUNNING AROUND A CURVED TRACK

As in cycling around a bend, a runner running around a bend leans toward the centre of curvature so that the horizontal component of the ground reaction force creates centripetal force. In cycling, the wheels are continuously in contact with the track so that the change of direction is fairly continuous. Furthermore, there is very little vertical motion of the combined centre of gravity of the cyclist and bike. However, in running, contact with the track is intermittent (each step consists of a ground contact phase and a flight phase) such that change of direction of the runner (in the transverse plane) only occurs during the ground contact phases. During the flight phase of each step, the centre of gravity of the runner moves in a straight line in the transverse plane and up and down in the median plane.

In a standard 400 m running track, each straight is 85 m and each bend is 115 m on the kerb. Consequently, the radius of each bend on the kerb is 36.6 m. The current men's world record for 200 m is 19.32 s (Michael Johnson, USA, mass = 79 kg, height = 1.85 m) which represents an average velocity of 10.35 m/s. To maintain this average speed around the bend in lane 1 (radius of curvature approximately 36.6 m), a male sprinter of mass 79 kg would need to maintain an average centripetal force F_C of 231.2 N, equivalent to 0.3 times his body weight (BW), i.e.

$$F_C = \frac{m.v^2}{r} = \frac{79 \text{ kg} \times (10.35 \text{ m/s})^2}{36.6 \text{ m}}$$
$$= 231.2 \text{ N} = 23.57 \text{ kgf} = 0.30 \text{ BW}$$

As the average magnitude of the vertical component of the ground reaction force F_V (over the total race time, i.e. the sum of ground contact time and flight time) is body weight, it follows from Equation 3.19 that the sprinter

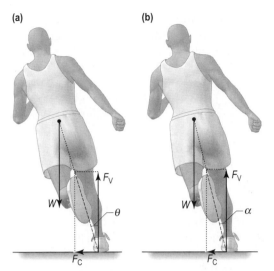

Fig. 3.44   Rear view free body diagram of a sprinter running around a left hand bend of a horizontal track with linear velocity 10.35 m/s (23.15 mph). (a) Radius of curvature = 36.6 m (lane 1), θ = 16.7°. (b) Radius of curvature = 45.1 m (lane 8), α = 13.6°. W = weight of sprinter; F_C = horizontal component of the ground reaction force = centripetal force; F_V = vertical component of the ground reaction force = W

would need to lean toward the centre of curvature at an angle θ of 16.7° (Fig. 3.44a):

$$\tan \theta = \frac{F_C}{F_V} = \frac{0.3 \text{ BW}}{1.0 \text{ BW}} = 0.3$$
$$\theta = 16.7°$$

The lane width in an outdoor track is approximately 1.22 m. Consequently the radius of curvature in lane 8 is approximately 45.1 m (36.6 m in lane 1 plus 7 × 1.22 m). To maintain an average speed of 10.35 m/s in lane 8 the sprinter would need to maintain an average centripetal force of 0.242 BW, which would require a lean angle of 13.6° (Fig. 3.44b).

In the above examples, the average values for F_V and F_C are based on continuous contact with the track. However, in maximum speed sprinting, approximately 55% of the time is spent in flight, i.e. only about 45% of the time is spent in contact with the track (Weyland et al 2000). Consequently, the average magnitude of F_V

would be approximately 2.2 BW (100/45 = 2.2) and the corresponding average magnitude of F_C in the above lane 1 example would be 0.66 BW (2.2 × 0.3 BW = 0.66 BW). Therefore, the average magnitude of the resultant ground reaction force during each period of ground contact would be approximately 2.3 BW rather than 1.04 BW with continuous contact. Since the ratio F_C/F_V would remain the same, so would the lean angle (16.7°).

Centripetal force is the force acting on a body that causes it to move on a curved path. Centrifugal force is the reaction exerted by a rotating object to the centripetal force; it is due to the inertia of the object, which resists a change in direction.

CONCENTRIC FORCE, ECCENTRIC FORCE AND COUPLE

In the earlier sections on moments of force and levers, most of the examples involved rotation or the tendency to rotate about a fixed axis. For example, a seesaw can only rotate about the horizontal axis through the fulcrum and a door can only rotate about the vertical axis through its hinges. When an object is free to rotate within a particular plane, i.e. not constrained to rotate about any particular axis and a force acts on the object that causes or tends to cause the object to rotate, the rotation will occur about an axis that passes through the centre of gravity of the object. For example, Figure 3.45a shows an overhead view of a curling stone resting on a perfectly flat horizontal ice rink. The stone is acted on by a horizontal force F, which is concentric, i.e. the line of action of F passes through the centre of gravity of the stone. A concentric force produces or tends to produce rectilinear translation. Assuming that the friction between the stone and the ice is negligible, the only horizontal force acting on the stone is the concentric force F. Consequently, the stone will experience or tend to experience rectilinear translation, i.e. it will tend to move in a straight line in the direction of F (Fig. 3.45a and b). In a vertical jump, i.e. when the purpose of the movement is simply to

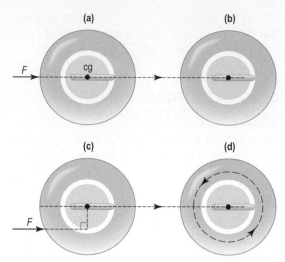

Fig. 3.45 Overhead view of a curling stone. (a) Concentric force. (c) Eccentric force. cg = centre of gravity of the stone

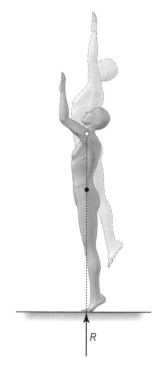

Fig. 3.46 Concentric ground reaction force R in a vertical jump without rotation or horizontal movement

lift the centre of gravity as high as possible off the ground without rotation or horizontal movement, the ground reaction force will be concentric (Fig. 3.46).

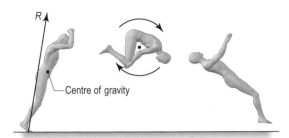

Fig. 3.47   Eccentric ground reaction force *R* during take-off in a forward somersault

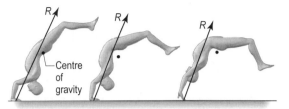

Fig. 3.48   Eccentric ground reaction force *R* during push-off in a headspring

In Figure 3.45c the horizontal force *F* is eccentric, i.e. its line of action does not pass through the centre of gravity of the stone. An eccentric force produces or tends to produce simultaneous rectilinear translation and rotation of an object about an axis that passes through the centre of gravity of the object and is perpendicular to the eccentric force. Consequently, in response to the eccentric force *F* the stone will experience or tend to experience simultaneous rectilinear translation and rotation about the vertical axis passing through its centre of gravity (Fig. 3.45c and d).

Most movements in sport that involve rotation of the whole body during flight are preceded by a ground contact phase prior to take-off in which the ground reaction force is eccentric to the performer's centre of gravity. For example, Figure 3.47 shows a gymnast performing a front somersault following a run-up. Prior to take-off, the line of action of the ground reaction force *R* passes behind the gymnast's centre of gravity. The effect of the eccentric ground reaction force will be to simultaneously move the centre of gravity in the direction of *R* (mainly upward, but also slightly forward in Figure 3.47) and help to generate forward rotation of the body about the mediolateral axis through the centre of gravity.

Similarly, in the final stages of a headspring, the line of action of the ground reaction force (the thrust resulting from arm extension) passes behind the centre of gravity of the body, resulting in translation of the centre of gravity (upward and forward) and the generation of forward rotation of the body (Fig. 3.48).

Another example of the effect of an eccentric force can be seen in the flight of a rugby ball

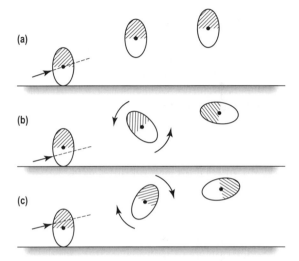

Fig. 3.49   Effect of the line of action of the kicking force on the movement of a rugby ball. (a) Concentric force. (b) Eccentric force resulting in backward rotation. (c) Eccentric force resulting in forward rotation

(Fig. 3.49). If the ball is kicked such that the line of action of the kicking force passes through the centre of gravity of the ball, i.e. a concentric force, then the ball will move through the air without rotation (Fig. 3.49a). However, if the line of action of the kicking force passes directly below the centre of gravity of the ball, i.e. an eccentric force, the ball will rotate backward about the mediolateral axis through the centre of gravity of the ball as it moves through the air (Fig. 3.49b). Similarly, if the line of action of the kicking force passes directly above the centre of gravity of the ball, the ball will rotate forward about the mediolateral axis through the centre of gravity of the ball as it moves through the air (Fig. 3.49c).

Figure 3.50 shows an overhead view of a child's roundabout, which is designed to rotate

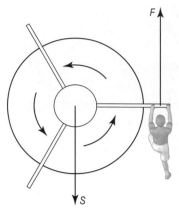

Fig. 3.50 Overhead view of a child's roundabout. F = eccentric force exerted on one of the handrails; S = horizontal force, equal and opposite to F, exerted by the vertical support on the roundabout. F and S form a couple resulting in rotation with no translation

about a fixed vertical axis through its point of support. In response to an eccentric horizontal force F applied to one of the handrails of the roundabout, the vertical support exerts an equal and opposite force S on the roundabout. The tendency of F and S to translate the roundabout (F upward and S downward with respect to Figure 3.50) cancel each other out, but the turning effect of F rotates the roundabout, i.e. the roundabout rotates, but does not translate. The force system produced by F and S is called a couple, i.e. a system of two parallel, equal and opposite forces, one concentric and one eccentric (as in Figure 3.50) or both eccentric, that tend to rotate an object in the same direction about a particular axis. A couple produces or tends to produce rotation without translation. Rotation of any object about a fixed axis is the result of a couple. The magnitude of a couple is the product of one of the forces and the perpendicular distance between the two forces. The larger the couple, the greater the angular acceleration and, therefore, the greater the angular velocity.

The systems of forces that result in translation, rotation or simultaneous translation and rotation may be summarized as follows. Consider an object that is free to translate and rotate within a particular plane, i.e. not constrained to translate

in any particular direction or constrained to rotate about any particular axis:

- *Concentric force system.* If the line of action of the resultant force acting on the object is parallel to the plane of movement and acts through the centre of gravity of the object, the object will experience or tend to experience rectilinear translation, but will not rotate. This is a concentric force system

- *Eccentric force system.* If the line of action of the resultant force acting on the object is parallel to the plane of movement but does not act through the centre of gravity of the object, the object will experience or tend to experience simultaneous rectilinear translation and rotation about an axis perpendicular to the plane of movement that passes through the centre of gravity of the object. This is an eccentric force system

- *Couple.* If the resultant of the forces acting on the object rotate or tend to rotate the object about an axis that does not move (translate) in the plane of movement, the force system is a couple.

ROTATION AND NEWTON'S FIRST LAW OF MOTION

From the previous section, an object at rest will only begin to rotate about a particular axis when the resultant force acting on the object is an eccentric force or couple. Newton's laws of motion apply to linear motion and angular motion. With regard to angular motion, the first law of motion may be expressed as follows:

The resultant moment acting on a body at rest or rotating about a particular axis with constant angular velocity (assuming no change in the shape of the object while rotating) is zero and the body will remain at rest or continue to rotate with constant angular velocity unless acted upon by an unbalanced eccentric force or couple.

For example, consider a bicycle turned upside down so that it rests on its handle bars and saddle (Fig. 3.51a). Each wheel will remain at rest

(a)

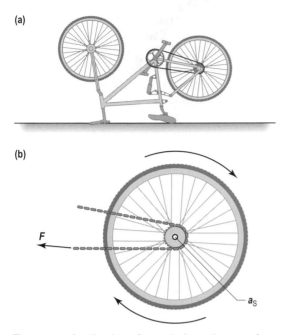

(b)

F

a_S

Fig. 3.51 Application of an unbalanced eccentric force to the rear wheel of a bicycle by the chain as a result of rotation of the pedals. F = force exerted by the chain; a_S = axis through the spindle of the wheel

until an eccentric force or couple is applied to it with respect to the horizontal axis a_S through the spindle of the wheel. When the pedals are turned clockwise with respect to Figure 3.51a, the chain will exert an eccentric force on the rear wheel such that the wheel will start to rotate in a clockwise direction about a_S (Fig. 3.51b). When the pedals are brought to rest (provided that the wheel is not a fixed wheel that rotates clockwise and anticlockwise in direct response to corresponding rotation of the pedals), the wheel will continue to rotate even though there is no couple or eccentric force acting on it. Furthermore, the wheel is likely to rotate for some considerable time unless a counter-rotation eccentric force, in the form of a brake, is applied to the wheel. If a brake is not applied to the wheel, the duration of rotation of the wheel will depend entirely on the amount of friction between the wheel and its spindle. The friction exerts a counter-rotation couple on the wheel and eventually brings it to rest; the greater the friction, the sooner the wheel

is brought to rest. If the friction could be eliminated, the wheel would continue to rotate for ever with constant angular velocity. In movements such as somersaults (Fig. 3.47), in which the human body rotates freely in space during the flight phase of the movement, the rotation of the body will take place about an axis that passes through the centre of gravity of the body. Furthermore, the angular velocity of the body about the axis of rotation will remain constant provided that the orientation of the body segments to each other does not change. The rotation of the body in such movements is ultimately reduced to zero by the action of the ground reaction force on landing (which exerts an unbalanced counter-rotation eccentric force).

MOMENT OF INERTIA

The resistance of an object to an attempt to change its linear motion (resistance to start moving if it is at rest and resistance to change its speed and/or direction if it is moving) is referred to as its inertia. The inertia of an object is directly proportional to its mass; the larger the mass, the greater the inertia. The resistance of an object to an attempt to change its angular motion (resistance to start rotating about a particular axis if it is at rest and resistance to change its angular speed and/or direction if it is rotating) is referred to as its moment of inertia. The moment of inertia of an object about a particular axis depends not only on the mass of the object but also on the distribution of the mass of the object about the axis of rotation. The closer the mass of the object to the axis of rotation or the more concentrated the mass of the object around the axis of rotation, the smaller will be the moment of inertia of the object and the easier it will be (the smaller the moment of force) to start the object rotating or keep it rotating if it is already rotating.

Figure 3.52 shows a gymnast swinging about the axis a_B of a high bar. The human body can be considered to consist of any number of separate masses joined together. Consider the motion of a tiny particle of mass m of the gymnast's body. From Equation 3.13, it follows that the linear acceleration a of the mass m is equal to $r.\alpha$

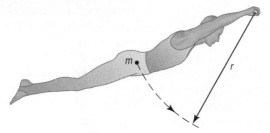

Fig. 3.52   A gymnast swinging about a high bar. r = radius of curvature of particle of mass m

where r = radius of curvature of m about a_B and α = angular acceleration of m about a_B. From Newton's second law of motion, the force F responsible for a is given by

$$F = m.r.\alpha$$

The moment of F about a_B is $F.r$, i.e.

$$F.r = m.r^2.\alpha \qquad \text{Eq. 3.20}$$

The total or resultant moment M of all the forces acting on all the particles that comprise the body is given by

$$M = F_1.r_1 + F_2.r_2 + F_3.r_3 + \cdots F_n.r_n \qquad \text{Eq. 3.21}$$

where n is the number of particles that comprise the body.

It follows from Equations 3.20 and 3.21 that

$$M = m_1.r_1^2.\alpha + m_2.r_2^2.\alpha + m_3.r_3^2.\alpha + \cdots m_n.r_n^2.\alpha \qquad \text{Eq. 3.22}$$

$$M = I.\alpha \qquad \text{Eq. 3.23}$$

where

$$I = \sum_{n=1}^{n=n} m_n.r_n^2 = \text{moment of inertia of the body}$$

about the axis of rotation.

In this example, as the axis of rotation is fixed, the resultant moment is a couple.

Equations 3.22 and 3.23 show that the moment of inertia of an object about a particular axis of rotation is obtained by multiplying the mass of each particle of the object by the square of its distance from the axis of rotation and summing for the whole object. In the SI system, the unit of moment of inertia is kilogram metres squared ($kg.m^2$). As the distribution of the mass of an object about a particular axis changes, so

will the distance of some or all of the particles of mass from the axis of rotation. Consequently, the moment of inertia of the object about the axis of rotation will also change. Figure 3.53 shows the effect of changing body position on the moment of inertia of the human body about the principal X, Y and Z axes (Fig. 2.1; Santchi et al 1963).

> The moment of inertia of an object about a particular axis of rotation is the resistance of the object to an attempt to change its angular motion.

MEASUREMENT OF MOMENT OF INERTIA

It is relatively easy to calculate the moment of inertia about a particular axis of a regular-shaped object of uniform density. For example, Figure 3.54a shows a side view of an object of uniform density of length 1 m, square cross-section 0.05 m $\times$ 0.05 m and mass 2 kg. For the purpose of the illustration, the object is considered to consist of 10 pieces of length 0.1 m joined end to end. Since the object is of uniform density, each piece will have the same mass $m = 0.2$ kg and the centre of gravity of each piece will be at its geometric centre. The moment of inertia I_O of the object about an axis (perpendicular to the page) through the end O is given by

$$I_O = \sum_{n=1}^{n=10} m_n.r_n^2 = m_1.r_1^2 + m_2.r_2^2 + m_3.r_3^2 + \cdots + m_{10}.r_{10}^2$$

where $m_1, m_2, \ldots, m_{10}$ are the masses and $r_1, r_2, \ldots r_{10}$ are the distances of the centres of gravity of the masses from the axis through O. Since all the masses are the same, i.e. 0.2 kg, and $r_1 = 0.05$ m, $r_2 = 0.15$ m, $r_3 = 0.25$ m, $r_4 = 0.35$ m, $r_5 = 0.45$ m, $r_6 = 0.55$ m, $r_7 = 0.65$ m, $r_8 = 0.75$ m, $r_9 = 0.85$ m, $r_{10} = 0.95$ m, then

$$\begin{aligned}
I_O &= m((0.05\,\text{m})^2 + (0.15\,\text{m})^2 + (0.25\,\text{m})^2 \\
&\quad + (0.35\,\text{m})^2 + (0.45\,\text{m})^2 + (0.55\,\text{m})^2 \\
&\quad + (0.65\,\text{m})^2 + (0.75\,\text{m})^2 + (0.85\,\text{m})^2 \\
&\quad + (0.95\,\text{m})^2)
\end{aligned}$$

$$I_O = 0.2\,\text{kg} \times 3.325\,\text{m}^2 = 0.665\,\text{kg.m}^2$$

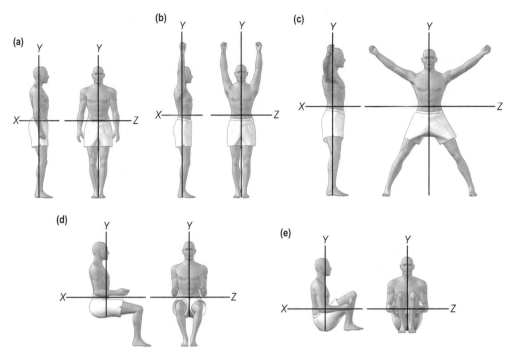

Fig. 3.53   Effect of change in body position on the moment of inertia of the human body about the X, Y and Z axes. (a) Standing. (b) Standing, arms overhead. (c) Star-shape. (d) Sitting. (e) Tucked

	Moment of inertia (kg.m²)			Moment of inertia relative to standing		
	X	Y	Z	X	Y	Z
Standing	13.01	1.28	11.64	1	1	1
Standing, arms overhead	17.20	1.25	15.50	1.32	0.97	1.33
Star-shape	17.07	4.14	12.89	1.31	3.23	1.11
Sitting	6.96	3.79	7.53	0.53	2.96	0.65
Tucked	4.42	2.97	4.30	0.34	2.32	0.37

Parallel axis theorem

In the above example, the axis of rotation was through the end O of the object. For any object, as the axis of rotation (perpendicular to a given plane) moves closer to the centre of gravity of the object, the sum of r^2, where $r_1, r_2, r_3, \ldots, r_n$ are the distances from the axis of rotation of the particles of equal mass that comprise the object, becomes smaller. Consequently, the sum of r^2 and, therefore, the moment of inertia of the object is least when the axis of rotation passes through the centre of gravity of the object. Conversely, the moment of inertia progressively increases with increased distance of the axis of rotation (perpendicular to a given

plane) from the centre of gravity of the object. For parallel axes (within a given plane), the moment of inertia I_A of an object about an axis A that does not pass through the centre of gravity of the object is given by

$$I_A = I_G + m_t.d^2 \qquad \text{Eq. 3.24}$$

where

I_A = moment of inertia of the object about axis A
I_G = moment of inertia of the object about an axis passing through the centre of gravity of the object that is parallel to axis A
m_t = total mass of the object
d = distance from A to the centre of gravity of the object

(a)

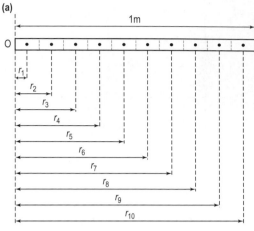

$$I_O = m_1.r_1^2 + m_2.r_2^2 + m_3.r_3^2 \dots + m_{10}.r_{10}^2 = 0.665 \text{ kg.m}^2$$

(b)

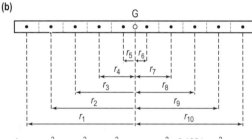

$$I_G = m_1.r_1^2 + m_2.r_2^2 + m_3.r_3^2 \dots + m_{10}.r_{10}^2 = 0.165 \text{ kg.m}^2$$

Fig. 3.54   Side view of an object of uniform density of length 1 m, square cross-section 0.05 m $\times$ 0.05 m and mass 2 kg. (a) Determination of the moment of inertia of the object about an axis (perpendicular to the page) through end O. (b) Determination of the moment of inertia of the object about a parallel axis through the centre of gravity of the object

Equation 3.24 is referred to as the parallel axis theorem. Figure 3.54b shows the same piece of material as in Figure 3.54a. The moment of inertia I_G of the object about the axis passing through its centre of gravity (G), parallel to the axis through O, is given by

$$I_G = \sum_{n=1}^{n=10} m_n.r_n^2 = m_1.r_1^2 + m_2.r_2^2 + m_3.r_3^2 + \dots + m_{10}.r_{10}^2$$

where $m_1, m_2, \dots, m_{10}$ are the masses and $r_1, r_2, \dots, r_{10}$ are the distances of the centres of gravity of the masses from the axis through G. Since all of the masses are the same, i.e. 0.2 kg, and $r_1 = 0.45$ m, $r_2 = 0.35$ m, $r_3 = 0.25$ m, $r_4 = 0.15$ m,

$r_5 = 0.05$ m, $r_6 = 0.05$ m, $r_7 = 0.15$ m, $r_8 = 0.25$ m, $r_9 = 0.35$ m, $r_{10} = 0.45$ m, then

$$\begin{aligned} I_G = m(&(0.45 \text{ m})^2 + (0.35 \text{ m})^2 + (0.25 \text{ m})^2 \\ &+ (0.15 \text{ m})^2 + (0.05 \text{ m})^2 + (0.05 \text{ m})^2 \\ &+ (0.15 \text{ m})^2 + (0.25 \text{ m})^2 + (0.35 \text{ m})^2 \\ &+ (0.45 \text{ m})^2) \end{aligned}$$
$$I_G = 0.2 \text{ kg} \times 0.825 \text{ m}^2 = 0.165 \text{ kg.m}^2$$

According to the parallel axis theorem,

$$I_O = I_G + m_t.d^2$$

where m_t = total mass of the object = 2 kg, d = distance between the parallel axes through O and G = 0.5 m

i.e. $I_O = 0.165 \text{ kg.m}^2 + (2 \text{ kg} \times (0.5 \text{ m})^2)$
     $= 0.165 \text{ kg.m}^2 + 0.5 \text{ kg.m}^2 = 0.665 \text{ kg.m}^2$

As expected, this is the same result for I_O as that obtained by the summation method $(\Sigma m_n.r_n^2)$.

Radius of gyration

When the density of an object is not uniform, like the human body, the summation method cannot be used to determine the moment of inertia of the object. Even if the object could be considered to consist of a number of exactly similar volumes (as in the example in Figure 3.54), it would not be possible to determine the mass of each volume and it could not be assumed that the centre of gravity of each volume was at its geometric centre.

Various methods, summarized by Hay (1974), have been devised to measure the moment of inertia of the human body and body segments. These methods involve complex equipment and are, in general, fairly impractical. Consequently, in most biomechanical analyses of human movement, moments of inertia are estimated from average data on the mass distribution of body segments obtained from cadaver studies.

The mass distribution of an object (of uniform or non-uniform density) about a particular axis is reflected in the radius of gyration of the object about the axis. The moment of inertia I of an object about a particular axis is equivalent to

Table 3.5   Radii of gyration of human body segments about the mediolateral axis through the centre of gravity of the segments, as a proportion of segment length

Segment	Segment endpoints	Radius of gyration
Upper arm	Shoulder joint – Elbow joint	0.322
Forearm	Elbow joint – Wrist	0.303
Forearm and hand	Elbow joint – Wrist	0.468
Hand	Wrist – Knuckle of 2nd finger	0.297
Whole upper limb	Shoulder joint – Wrist	0.368
Thigh	Hip joint – Knee joint	0.323
Shank	Knee joint – Ankle joint	0.302
Shank and foot	Knee joint – Ankle joint	0.416
Foot	Lateral malleolus – Head of 2nd metatarsal	0.475
Whole lower limb	Hip joint – ankle joint	0.326
Trunk, head and neck	Shoulder joint – Hip joint	0.503

Source: adapted from Winter 1990.

that of a mass m_t, equal to the mass of the object, rotating about the axis at a distance k from the axis, where k is the radius gyration, i.e.

$$I = m_t.k^2 \qquad \text{Eq. 3.25}$$

For comparative purposes, the moment of inertia of an object about a particular axis is often expressed in terms of $m_t.k^2$. For a given object, m_t is constant but k, and therefore the moment of inertia of the object, depends upon the distribution of the mass of the object about the axis of rotation. For example, in Figure 3.54a, $I_O = 0.665\,\text{kg.m}^2$ and $m_t = 2\,\text{kg}$. Therefore, from Equation 3.25,

$$k_O = \sqrt{(I_O/m_t)} = 0.5766 \text{ m}$$

where k_O = radius of gyration of m_t about the axis through O. Similarly, in Figure 3.54b,

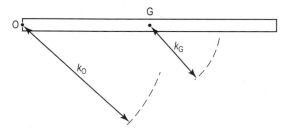

Fig. 3.55   Radius of gyration of the object in Figure 3.54 about the axis through O (k_O) and the parallel axis through G (k_G)

$I_G = 0.165\,\text{kg.m}^2$ and $m_t = 2\,\text{kg}$. Therefore, from Equation 3.25,

$$k_G = \sqrt{(I_G/m_t)} = 0.2872 \text{ m}$$

where k_G = radius of gyration of m_t about the axis through G. k_O and k_G are illustrated in Figure 3.55. k_O is approximately twice the size of k_G ($0.5766/0.2872 = 2.01$). However, since moment of inertia is proportional to the square of the radius of gyration, I_O is approximately four times the size of I_G ($0.665\,\text{kg.m}^2/0.165\,\text{kg.m}^2 = 4.03$).

For objects with the same shape and the same distribution of mass (even if the density is not uniform) but different size, the radius of gyration (with respect to any axis through or on the surface of the object), as a proportion of the length of the segment, is the same. This also applies to the segments of the human body, i.e. corresponding segments of different individuals are very similar in shape and distribution of mass and, therefore, the radii of gyration of corresponding segments, as a proportion of the length of the segments, are very similar. Table 3.5 shows average data, obtained mainly from cadaver studies, for the radii of gyration of body segments as a proportion of segment length about the mediolateral axis through the centre of gravity of the segments (Winter 1990).

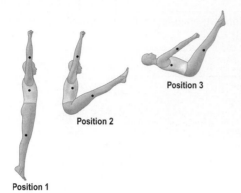

Position 3

Position 2

Position 1

Fig. 3.56 Three positions of a gymnast rotating about a high bar. The dots indicate the centres of gravity of the arm, the leg and the combined trunk, head and neck (see Table 3.6)

DETERMINATION OF THE MOMENT OF INERTIA OF A GYMNAST ABOUT THE AXIS OF A HIGH BAR

Figure 3.56 shows three positions of a gymnast rotating about a high bar. In position 1 the mass of the gymnast is distributed as far away as possible from the axis of rotation. Consequently, the moment of inertia of the gymnast about the axis of rotation will be highest in this position. In position 2, the legs are much closer to the bar than in position 1, such that the moment of inertia of the gymnast about the bar will be smaller in position 2 than in position 1. In position 3, the trunk and legs are much closer to the bar than in positions 1 and 2, such that the moment of inertia of the gymnast about the bar will be smaller in position 3 than in positions 1 and 2.

Table 3.6 shows the stages in the calculation of the moment of inertia of the gymnast about the long axis of the bar in the three positions. The calculations are based on a five-segment model consisting of trunk, head and neck (one segment), right arm, left arm, right leg, left leg. It is assumed that the movement of the gymnast is symmetrical about the median plane such that the movement of the right arm is the same as that of the left arm and the movement of the right leg is the same as that of the left leg. The data on segment mass as a proportion of whole-body mass are taken from Plagenhoef 1983 (Table 3.1). The data on segment length were taken from a video

of the gymnast. The data on radius of gyration are taken from Winter (1990) (Table 3.5) and the data on the distance of the centre of gravity of each segment from the axis of the bar were obtained by applying the centre of gravity locus data of Plagenhoef (1983) (Table 3.1) to the segment length data.

Columns 1–6 of Table 3.6 show the calculation of I_G for each segment, i.e. the moment of inertia of the segment about an axis parallel with the bar through the centre of gravity of the segment. For example, in position 1, I_G for the arm is given by

$$I_G = m.k_G^2 = 4.04\,\text{kg} \times (0.22\,\text{m})^2 = 0.1955\,\text{kg.m}^2$$

where

m = mass of arm (upper arm, forearm and hand) = 4.04 kg
k_G = radius of gyration of the arm about the mediolateral axis through the centre of gravity of the arm = 0.22 m

Columns 7 and 8 show the calculation of $m.d^2$ for the arm in position 1,

i.e. $m.d^2 = 4.04\,\text{kg} \times (0.37\,\text{m})^2 = 0.5531\,\text{kg.m}^2$

where

m = mass of arm = 4.04 kg
d = distance of the centre of gravity of the arm from the axis of the bar = 0.37 m

Column 9 shows the parallel axis theorem calculation of I_O for the arm in position 1, i.e. the moment of inertia of the arm about the axis of the bar:

$$I_O = I_G + m.d^2 = 0.1955\,\text{kg.m}^2 + 0.5531\,\text{kg.m}^2$$
$$= 0.7486\,\text{kg.m}^2$$

Column 10 shows the sum of the moments of inertia of both arms about the axis of the bar in position 1, i.e. 1.4972 kg.m².

Table 3.6 shows that the moment of inertia of the body about the axis of the bar in positions 1, 2 and 3 is approximately 91.2 kg.m², 55.8 kg.m² and 21.4 kg.m² respectively.

ANGULAR MOMENTUM

Just as an object of mass m (kg) moving with linear velocity v (m/s) has linear momentum $m.v$

Table 3.6 Determination of the moment of inertia of a gymnast about the axis of the high bar in three positions (Fig. 3.56)

	1	2	3	4	5	6	7	8	9	10
	Mass (%)	Mass (kg)	Length (m)	k_G (%)	k_G (m)	I_G (kg.m²)	d (m)	$m.d^2$ (kg.m²)	I_0 (kg.m²)	I_0 (kg.m²)
Position 1										
Arm	5.77	4.04	0.60	0.368	0.22	0.1955	0.37	0.5531	0.7486	1.4972
THN	55.1	38.6	0.53	0.503	0.27	2.8118	0.87	29.194	32.005	32.005
Leg	16.7	11.7	0.81	0.326	0.26	0.7896	1.55	28.061	28.851	57.702
Total										91.204
Position 2										
Arm	5.77	4.04	0.60	0.368	0.22	0.1955	0.37	0.5531	0.7486	1.4972
THN	55.1	38.6	0.53	0.503	0.27	2.8118	0.85	27.888	30.699	30.699
Leg	16.7	11.7	0.81	0.326	0.26	0.7896	0.97	11.008	11.798	23.596
Total										55.792
Position 3										
Arm	5.77	4.04	0.60	0.368	0.22	0.1955	0.37	0.5531	0.7486	1.4972
THN	55.1	38.6	0.53	0.503	0.27	2.8118	0.60	13.896	16.708	16.708
Leg	16.7	11.7	0.81	0.326	0.26	0.7896	0.26	0.7896	1.5792	3.1584
Total										21.364

Whole body mass = 70 kg.

Mass (%) = mass of segment as a percentage of whole body mass; Arm = upper arm, forearm and hand; THN = trunk, head and neck; Leg = thigh, shank and foot; Length = length of segment; k_G = radius of gyration of the segment about a mediolateral axis a_G through its centre of gravity as a percentage of segment length; I_G = moment of inertia of the segment about a_G; d = distance between a_G and the axis of the bar; I_0 (column 9) = moment of inertia of the segment about the axis of the bar; I_0 (column 10) = moment of inertia of both arms, both legs and the trunk head and neck about the axis of the bar and the total moment of inertia.

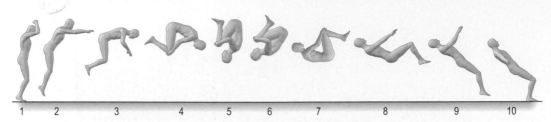

Fig. 3.57 Successive positions of a gymnast during the performance of a front somersault following a run-up

(kg.m/s), an object rotating about a particular axis has angular momentum $I.\omega$ (kg.m^2/s) where I (kg.m^2) is the moment of inertia of the object about the axis and ω (rad/s) is the angular velocity of the object about the axis. Whereas the mass of an object is constant (other than by removing part of the mass or adding more mass), the moment of inertia of a rotating object can be changed by simply redistributing the mass about the axis of rotation. From Newton's first law of motion, the angular momentum of an object about a particular axis of rotation will remain constant until the object is acted upon by an unbalanced eccentric force or couple. Therefore, if the moment of inertia of an object rotating freely about a particular axis is changed, there will be a simultaneous change in the angular velocity of the object so that the angular momentum of the object remains unchanged. This principle is referred to as the conservation of angular momentum and has great significance in movements of the human body that involve rotation during flight.

Figure 3.57 shows the successive positions of a gymnast during the performance of a front somersault following a run-up. During the flight phase (positions 2–9) the gymnast rotates in the median plane about the mediolateral axis a_Z through his centre of gravity. Since there are no unbalanced turning moments acting on the gymnast during flight, the angular momentum of the gymnast about a_Z will be conserved, i.e. remain constant. To land on his feet, the gymnast must complete the forward somersault very quickly. By tucking his body (positions 2–5), the gymnast reduces the moment of inertia of his body about a_Z, which simultaneously results in an increase in his angular velocity about a_Z. Suppose that the moment of

inertia of his body about a_Z in position 5 is half that in position 2. Since his angular momentum about a_Z is the same in both positions, it follows that

$$I_2.\omega_2 = I_5.\omega_5$$

where I_2, I_5 and ω_2, ω_5 are the moments of inertia and angular velocities of the gymnast about a_Z in positions 2 and 5 respectively. As $I_5 = I_2/2$, then

$$I_2.\omega_2 = \frac{I_2}{2}.\omega_5$$

i.e. $\omega_5 = 2\omega_2$

By halving the moment of inertia, the angular velocity is doubled. The increased angular velocity will enable the gymnast to complete the forward somersault in half the time that it would have taken if he had not tucked his body. In the second part of the flight phase (positions 6–9) the gymnast extends his body, which increases his moment of inertia and decreases his angular velocity about a_Z in preparation for landing. Figure 3.58 shows the change in I and ω about a_Z during the flight phase.

> The angular momentum of an object about a particular axis is the product of its moment of inertia and angular velocity about the axis.

Figure 3.59 shows a skater rotating about the vertical axis a_Y through his centre of gravity. If the skater goes into a spin with his arms outstretched at his sides (Fig. 3.59a) and then suddenly brings in his arms close to his sides (Fig. 3.59b), his moment of inertia about a_Y will decrease and his angular velocity about a_Y will

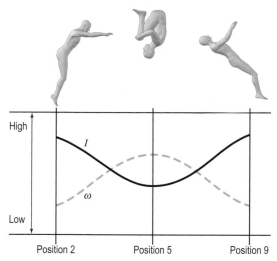

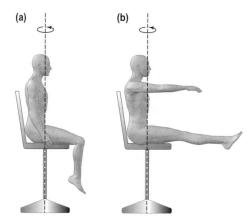

Fig. 3.60 Use of a freely rotating chair to experience the change in angular velocity that accompanies change in moment of inertia in situations where angular momentum is conserved

Fig. 3.58 The relationship between the moment of inertia I and angular velocity ω of a gymnast about the mediolateral axis through his centre of gravity during the flight phase of a front somersault following a run-up (see Fig. 3.57)

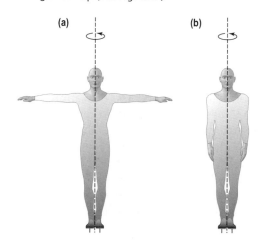

Fig. 3.59 A skater rotating about the vertical axis through his centre of gravity

is conserved can be experienced by using a chair, stool or turntable which is free to rotate about a vertical axis. With the subject and chair rotating as in Figure 3.60a, extending the arms and/or the legs away from the axis of rotation will increase the moment of inertia and decrease angular velocity and vice versa. The effect is more marked if the subject holds a weight in each hand or wears weighted shoes, since the movement of the limbs will result in more marked changes in the moment of inertia of the body about the axis of rotation and, consequently, more marked changes in angular velocity. The angular momentum of subject and chair is not entirely conserved, since there will be a certain amount of friction between the chair and its spindle.

simultaneously increase. In this movement, the skater's angular momentum about a_Y will not be entirely conserved, since the friction between his skates and the ice will exert a small counter-rotation moment such that, if he could rotate for long enough, his angular momentum would eventually be reduced to zero and he would stop spinning.

The change in angular velocity that accompanies a change in moment of inertia of an object in situations where angular momentum

ROTATION AND NEWTON'S SECOND LAW OF MOTION

From Equation 3.23, when a resultant moment M acts on an object about a particular axis of rotation, the angular acceleration α experienced by the object about the axis of rotation will be directly proportional to the magnitude of M and inversely proportional to the moment of inertia I of the object about the axis of rotation, i.e. $\alpha = M/I$. This equation (directly analogous to $a = F/m$; see Eq. 2.14) represents Newton's second law of motion in relation to rotation and may be expressed as follows:

When a moment (resultant moment greater than zero) acts on an object about a particular axis of rotation, the angular acceleration experienced by the object takes place in the direction of the moment and is directly proportional to the magnitude of the moment and inversely proportional to the moment of inertia of the object about the axis of rotation.

If an object has been rotating about a particular axis prior to a change in the resultant moment acting on it, the direction of the change in resultant moment will determine whether the angular momentum of the object is increased or decreased. If the change in resultant moment is in the same direction as the original rotation, the angular momentum of the object will increase; if it is in the opposite direction, it will decrease.

The amount of change in angular momentum of an object about a particular axis of rotation resulting from a change in the resultant moment acting on it depends not only on the direction of the change in resultant moment but also on the duration of the change in resultant moment. From Equations 3.7 and 3.23, it follows that

$$M = \frac{I(\omega_2 - \omega_1)}{t} \qquad \text{Eq. 3.26}$$

where t is the duration of the change in resultant moment and ω_1 and ω_2 are the angular velocities of the object at t_1 and t_2 where $t = t_2 - t_1$.

From Equation 3.26,

$$M.t = I.\omega_2 - I.\omega_1 \qquad \text{Eq. 3.27}$$

Newton's second law of motion in relation to rotation is often expressed in terms of Equation 3.27 (directly analogous to $F.t = m.v - m.u$; see Eq. 2.15) as follows:

When a moment (resultant moment greater than zero) acts on an object about a particular axis of rotation, the change in angular momentum experienced by the object takes place in the direction of the moment and is directly proportional to the magnitude of the moment and the duration of the moment.

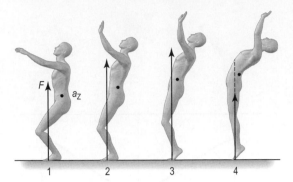

Fig. 3.61 Eccentric ground reaction force *F* prior to take-off in a standing back somersault. The linear impulse of *F* generates linear momentum of the whole-body centre of gravity in the direction of *F* and the angular impulse of *F* about a_Z generates backward angular momentum of the body about a_Z

When the amount of force and size of the moment arm that comprise a particular moment are not specified – as, for example, in describing the turning effect on part of a machine – the term torque is used rather than moment.

From Equation 3.27, it is clear that, to maximize the angular momentum of an object about a particular axis, it is necessary to apply as much moment as possible for as long as possible. The product $M.t$ of the average resultant moment M and duration t of the resultant moment is called the impulse of the resultant moment, i.e. angular impulse. The angular impulse–angular momentum principle is widely used in sports, especially those involving rotation of the whole body such as gymnastics and diving.

Figure 3.61 shows four successive positions of a gymnast prior to take-off during the performance of a standing back somersault. Prior to take-off, the gymnast needs to generate sufficient upward linear momentum and sufficient backward angular momentum about the mediolateral axis a_Z through his centre of gravity in order to perform the somersault and land on his feet. These requirements are met by a vertical eccentric ground reaction force that passes in front of a_Z (Fig. 3.61). Assuming that the gymnast starts the movement from a resting position, then vertical velocity at take-off v (which will determine flight time) and angular

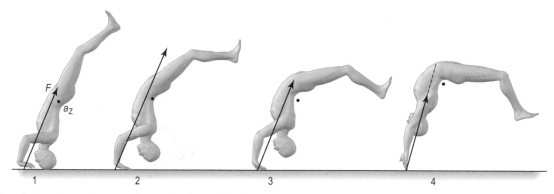

Fig. 3.62   Eccentric ground reaction force *F* during the performance of a headspring. The linear impulse of *F* generates linear momentum of the whole-body centre of gravity in the direction of *F* and the angular impulse of *F* about a_Z generates forward angular momentum of the body about a_Z

momentum at take-off $I.\omega$ (which, together with changes in the moment of inertia about a_Z, will determine the time required to complete the somersault) are given by

$$v = \frac{F.t}{m} \text{ (from Eq. 2.15 where } u = 0)$$

$$I.\omega = M.t \text{ (from Eq. 3.27 where } \omega_1 = 0)$$

where

t = time from the start of movement to take-off
F = average resultant vertical force acting on the gymnast during t
d = average moment arm of F
$M = F.d$ = average moment about a_Z during t (clockwise with respect to Fig. 3.61)
m = mass of the gymnast
I = moment of inertia of the gymnast about a_Z at take-off
ω = angular velocity of the gymnast about a_Z at take-off

F will be largely determined by the strength of the gymnast's leg extensor muscles, t will be determined by the range of motion in the gymnast's hips, knees and ankles and the extent to which this range of motion is utilized and d will be determined by the ability of the gymnast to push vertically downward eccentrically, i.e. with a_Z behind the line of action of F. The line of action of F will determine the extent to which the centre of gravity of the gymnast

moves horizontally during the movement. In a standing back somersault, F would ideally be vertical prior to take-off, resulting in vertical displacement but no horizontal displacement of the centre of gravity.

Figure 3.62 shows four successive positions of a gymnast prior to take-off during the performance of a headspring. In order to land on his feet, the gymnast needs to generate sufficient upward linear momentum and sufficient forward angular momentum about the medio-lateral axis a_Z through his centre of gravity during the push off. These requirements are met by an eccentric ground reaction force F that passes in front of a_Z. The linear impulse of F generates upward linear momentum and the angular impulse of F about a_Z generates forward angular momentum about a_Z. As in the standing back somersault, the line of action of F will determine the extent of horizontal movement of the centre of gravity.

Practical worksheet 6 involves the use of a turntable to determine the moment of inertia and radius of gyration of the human body about a vertical axis while in a seated position.

> To maximize the change in angular momentum of an object about a particular axis of rotation, it is necessary to maximize the angular impulse applied to the object.

TRANSFER OF ANGULAR MOMENTUM

From Equations 3.22 and 3.23,

$$I.\alpha = m_1.r_1^2.\alpha + m_2.r_2^2.\alpha + m_3.r_3^2.\alpha + \cdots + m_n.r_n^2.\alpha$$

Eq. 3.28

where

I = moment if inertia of an object about a particular axis of rotation

α = angular acceleration of the object about the axis of rotation

$m_1, m_2, m_3, \ldots, m_n$ = particles of mass that comprise the object

$r_1, r_2, r_3, \ldots, r_n$ = distances of the particles of mass from the axis of rotation

Since $\alpha = \omega/t$ (Eq. 3.7), it follows from Equation 3.28 that

$$I.\frac{\omega}{t} = m_1.r_1^2.\frac{\omega}{t} + m_2.r_2^2.\frac{\omega}{t} + m_3.r_3^2.\frac{\omega}{t}$$
$$+ \cdots + m_n.r_n^2.\frac{\omega}{t}$$
$$I.\omega = m_1.r_1^2\omega + m_2.r_2^2.\omega + m_3.r_3^2.\omega$$
$$+ \cdots + m_n.r_n^2.\omega$$

$$I.\omega = I_1.\omega + I_2.\omega + I_3.\omega + \cdots + I_n.\omega \qquad \text{Eq. 3.29}$$

where $I_1, I_2, I_3, \ldots, I_n$ are the respective moments of inertia of the particles about the axis of rotation. It follows, therefore, that the angular momentum of the object about the axis of rotation is equal to the sum of the angular momenta of all the individual particles of mass that comprise the object. Consequently, when an object is rotating with constant angular momentum about a particular axis, any change in the angular momentum of one or more parts of the object as a result of internal forces will simultaneously result in a change in the angular momentum of one or more of the other parts of the body so that the angular momentum of the object remains the same.

DEMONSTRATION OF TRANSFER OF ANGULAR MOMENTUM USING A ROTATING TURNTABLE

Figure 3.63 shows a man standing with his arms outstretched at his sides on a turntable that is

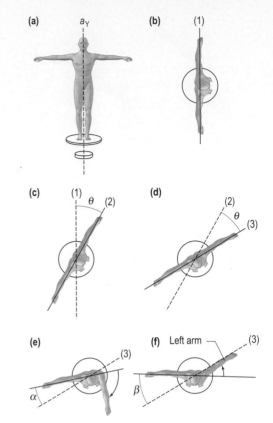

Fig. 3.63 A man standing on a turntable and rotating about the vertical axis a_Y through his centre of gravity with constant angular momentum (subject to friction around the spindle). The time period between (b) and (c), (c) and (d), (d) and (e), and (d) and (f) is the same

free to rotate about a vertical axis a_Y. If the turntable is rotated by an external moment, which is then removed, the system consisting of man and turntable will continue to rotate with constant angular momentum about a_Y (Fig. 3.63b–d). If the man suddenly rotates his left arm relative to the rest of the system, in a horizontal plane and in the direction of rotation of the whole system, the angular velocity of the rest of the system about a_Y will be seen to decrease for the same period of time that the left arm is rotating relative to the rest of the system, i.e. in the same time that it takes the left arm to rotate through 90° about a vertical axis through the left shoulder, the rest of the system rotates through a smaller angle about a_Y than it would have done if the left arm had not rotated relative to the rest of the system (Fig. 3.61d & e, where $\alpha < \theta$). The angular momentum of the whole system about a_Y is equal to the sum of the angular momentum of the left arm about a_Y and the angular momentum of the rest of the system about a_Y. Since rotation of the left arm relative to the rest of the system results in a decrease in the angular momentum of the rest of the system about a_Y, it follows that there must be a simultaneous increase in the angular momentum of the left arm about a_Y so that the angular momentum of the whole system about a_Y is conserved. In effect, rotation of the left arm relative to the rest of the system results in a transfer of angular momentum from the rest of the system to the left arm for as long as the left arm is moving relative to the rest of the system.

If the left arm is rotated relative to the rest of the system in the direction of rotation of the whole system, then angular momentum will be transferred from the rest of the system to the left arm. However, if the left arm is rotated in the opposite direction to that of the whole system, angular momentum will be transferred from the left arm to the rest of the system; the angular velocity of the rest of the system about a_Y will be seen to increase during the same period that the left arm is rotating relative to the rest of the system (Fig. 3.63d & f where $\beta > \theta$).

It is evident that, for a body such as the human body that is comprised of a number of segments that can move relative to each other, angular momentum can be transferred from one segment to another by the action of internal forces exerted between the segments. The angular momentum of any particular segment can be increased/decreased by increasing/decreasing the angular velocity of the segment relative to the axis of rotation of the whole system. This phenomenon is referred to as the principle of transfer of angular momentum. The principle may be demonstrated by using a turntable that is free to rotate about a vertical axis a_Y and a bicycle wheel that has a handle attached to each end of its spindle in line with the spindle so that the wheel can rotate independently of the handles. A person stands on the turntable and holds the wheel, with its

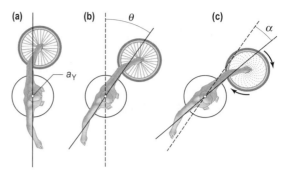

Fig. 3.64   A person standing on a turntable, holding a wheel that is free to rotate about its spindle and the whole system of turntable, person and wheel rotating about a vertical axis a_Y with constant angular momentum (subject to friction around the spindle). The time period between (a) and (b) and (b) and (c) is the same

spindle vertical, in one hand as shown in Figure 3.64. If the turntable is then rotated by an external moment, which is subsequently removed, the whole system (turntable, person and wheel) will continue to rotate about a_Y with constant angular momentum (Fig. 3.64a & b). If the person then rotates the wheel about its spindle in the direction of rotation of the whole system, the angular velocity and, therefore, the angular momentum of the rest of the system, i.e. the turntable and person, will decrease (Fig. 3.64b & c where $\alpha < \theta$). Since the angular momentum of the whole system about a_Y is conserved, the angular momentum lost by the turntable and person is gained by the wheel; by rotating the wheel in the direction of rotation of the whole system, angular momentum is transferred from the turntable and person to the wheel. If the person then stops the wheel rotating by touching the wheel against his/her chest and holds the wheel in its original position, the whole system will rotate about a_Y with the same angular velocity as at the start of the experiment, i.e. after removal of the external moment. Therefore, by stopping the wheel rotating, angular momentum is transferred back from the wheel to the rest of the system. The angular momentum of the system about a_Y will not be entirely conserved because of friction around the spindle.

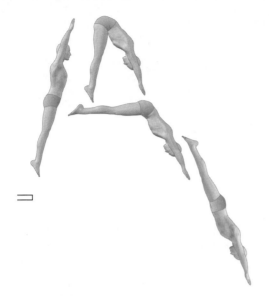

Fig. 3.65 A forward pike dive

TRANSFER OF ANGULAR MOMENTUM IN A FORWARD PIKE DIVE

The principle of transfer of angular momentum is of great significance in many sports. Figure 3.65 shows four successive positions of a diver performing a forward pike dive. The diver leaves the board with a certain amount of upward linear momentum and forward angular momentum about the mediolateral axis a_Z through his centre of gravity. The upward linear momentum and forward angular momentum of the diver are the result of the impulse (linear and angular) of the ground reaction force prior to take-off. Just after take-off, the diver flexes his hips and achieves the pike position shown in Figure 3.65b. The piking action increases the angular velocity and, therefore, the angular momentum of the upper body (trunk, head and arms) about a_Z, which results in a simultaneous decrease in the angular velocity and angular momentum of the legs about a_Z, since the angular momentum of the whole body about a_Z is conserved. If the piking action is carried out very quickly, i.e. the angular velocity of the upper body is rapidly increased, the angular velocity of the legs may be reduced to zero or the direction of rotation of the legs may even be reversed, as shown in Figure 3.65b (compare position of the legs in Figure

3.65a & b). In the last part of the pike dive, the diver needs to straighten out his body in preparation for entry into the water. This is achieved by extension of the hips, which increases the angular velocity and angular momentum of the legs about a_Z and simultaneously decreases the angular velocity and angular momentum of the upper body about a_Z, since the angular momentum of the whole body about a_Z is conserved (Fig. 3.65b–d). In the time that it takes for the position of the body to change from that in Figure 3.65b to that in Figure 3.65d, the legs rotate approximately 150° about a_Z and the upper body rotates approximately 20°.

TRANSFER OF ANGULAR MOMENTUM IN LONG JUMP

The hitch-kick technique of long jumping involves transfer of angular momentum in order to control forward rotation during flight. At take-off, the jumper would like to maximize vertical velocity v_V (to maximize flight time t) and horizontal velocity v_H (to maximize jump distance d where $d = v_H.t$). However, v_V and v_H are not independent of each other, i.e. it is not possible to maximize both at the same time (see trajectory of a long jumper in Ch. 2). Maximal performance (jump distance) involves a compromise between v_V and v_H.

v_H is almost entirely due to the run-up, but v_V is entirely due to the impulse of the vertical component of the ground reaction force acting on the jumper during the thrust from the board. Consequently, in order to generate vertical velocity at take-off, the jumper pushes down on the board, which results in the ground reaction force passing behind the jumper's centre of gravity prior to take-off (Fig. 3.66a). The near-vertical eccentric ground reaction force generates not only upward linear momentum but also forward angular momentum of the body, which is conserved about the mediolateral axis a_Z through the jumper's centre of gravity during the flight phase of the jump. If the forward angular momentum is not controlled during flight, the jumper is likely to rotate forward and land face down (Fig. 3.67). In order to control the angular momentum, i.e. to prevent forward

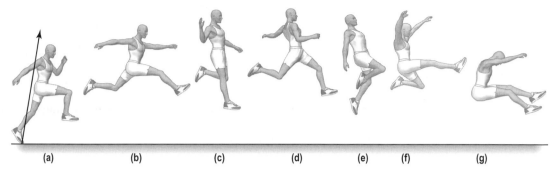

Fig. 3.66 The hitch-kick technique of long jumping

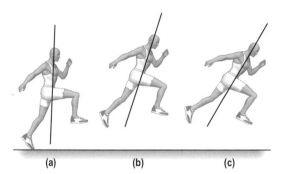

Fig. 3.67 Forward rotation in long jumping. If the forward angular momentum is not controlled during flight, the jumper is likely to rotate forward and land face down

rotation of the body as a whole, the angular momentum of the trunk, head and neck can be transferred to the arms and legs by increasing the angular velocity of the arms and legs relative to a_Z. This is achieved by forward rotation of the arms about the shoulders and similar rotation of the legs about the hips (Fig. 3.66b–f). These actions, referred to as hitch-kick, enable the jumper to keep the trunk upright during flight or even reverse the direction of rotation of the trunk if the action of the arms and legs is sufficiently vigorous (Fig. 3.66d & e). In preparation for landing, the arms and legs are brought to rest in front of the trunk, which transfers angular momentum back from the arms and legs to the trunk, head and neck. Consequently, the trunk, head and neck rotate forward prior to landing, which increases the chance of rotating over the feet rather than falling back in the sand (Fig. 3.66g). The hitch-kick technique enables the jumper to make full use of the ground reaction

force in generating vertical velocity at take-off and also facilitates an effective landing.

TRANSFER OF ANGULAR MOMENTUM IN A STANDING BACK SOMERSAULT

Figure 3.68 shows a gymnast performing a standing back somersault. The movement is initiated by hip flexion and shoulder extension into a position from which a powerful upward thrust can be made (position 1 in Fig. 3.68). The arms are then swung rapidly forward (shoulder flexion; clockwise rotation of the arms with respect to Fig. 3.68) such that much of the backward angular momentum of the body at take-off is contained in the arms (position 11). After take-off, rotation of the body takes place about the mediolateral axis through the gymnast's centre of gravity. Just after take-off, the angular velocity and, therefore, the angular momentum of the arms is rapidly reduced to zero, which is maintained for most of the flight phase (positions 13–22). Therefore, during this period, the angular momentum of the arms is transferred to the rest of the body since the angular momentum of the whole body is conserved during flight.

In a study of platform diving, Hamill et al (1986) showed that in a backward single somersault dive, which is similar to a standing back somersault, about half of the backward angular momentum of the body at take-off is contained in the arms. In both movements, the magnitude and direction of the ground reaction force will vary prior to take-off, but the end result, in terms of linear and angular momentum

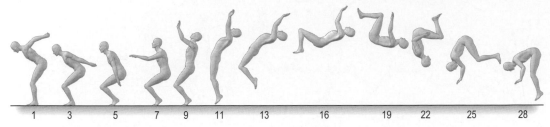

Fig. 3.68   Successive positions of a gymnast during the performance of a standing back somersault

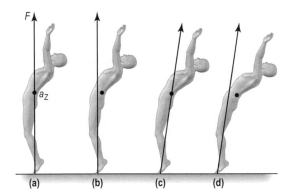

Fig. 3.69   Four variations in the line of action of the ground reaction force at take-off in a standing back somersault. a_Z = mediolateral axis through the gymnast's centre of gravity

of the body at take-off, will depend upon the impulse of the resultant force and impulse of the resultant moment acting on the body.

Figure 3.69 shows four possible positions of a gymnast at take-off in a standing back somersault, together with the line of action of the ground reaction force F in relation to the mediolateral axis a_Z through the centre of gravity of the gymnast in each position. If it is assumed that the line of action of F in each position is typical of the whole of the upward thrust, it will be interesting to consider the effects of F in the different types of action. In Figure 3.69a the line of action of F is vertical and passes through a_Z. This action will produce upward linear momentum, but no backward angular momentum, i.e. the gymnast would jump upward without backward rotation. In Figure 3.69b, the line of action of F is vertical and passes in front of a_Z. This action will produce upward linear momentum and backward angular momentum, i.e. the gymnast would jump upward and rotate backward

during flight. In both situations (Fig. 3.69a & b) the ground reaction force is vertical and therefore the centre of gravity will move vertically (up and down) throughout the whole movement, i.e. the centre of gravity will not move horizontally. If the orientation of the body was the same at take-off and landing, the feet would land in the same place from which they left the ground. In Figure 3.69c the line of action of F passes through a_Z and is inclined with respect to the vertical. This action will produce linear momentum in the direction of F, but no backward angular momentum, i.e. the gymnast's centre of gravity will move up and down (vertically) and backward (horizontally) during flight. In Figure 3.69d the line of action of F passes in front of a_Z and is inclined with respect to the vertical. This action will produce linear momentum in the direction of F, similar to that in Figure 3.69c, and backward angular momentum.

> The angular momentum of a body is conserved during flight, but angular momentum can be transferred between body segments by internal (muscle) forces.

ROTATION AND NEWTON'S THIRD LAW OF MOTION

From Newton's first law of motion, when an object is rotating about a particular axis with constant angular momentum, the resultant moment acting on the object is zero. Internal forces may alter the moment of inertia of the object about the axis of rotation, but angular momentum will be conserved. When internal forces change the moment of inertia of an object about a particular axis, there is a simultaneous change in the angular momentum of each part of the object. For example, in the pike dive shown in Figure 3.65, the pike is achieved by flexion of the hips, which simultaneously increases the angular momentum of the upper body and decreases the angular momentum of the legs about the mediolateral axis a_Z through the centre of gravity so that angular momentum is conserved. When the hip flexors contract to produce the pike position, they pull equally on both of their attachments, the upper body and the legs. Therefore, the angular impulse of the hip flexors on the upper body is exactly the same in magnitude but opposite in direction to that exerted on the legs, so that the angular momentum of the body about the mediolateral axis a_H through the hip joints is unchanged, i.e. it remains zero. To straighten his body in preparation for entry into the water, the diver extends his hips. The hip extensor muscles pull equally on both their attachments, the upper body and the legs. Therefore, the angular impulse of the hip extensors on the upper body is equal in magnitude but opposite in direction to that exerted on the legs, so that the angular momentum of the body about a_H is unchanged, i.e. it remains zero. The action of the hip extensors also results in an increase in the angular momentum of the legs about a_Z and a simultaneous decrease in the angular momentum of the upper body about a_Z so that angular momentum about a_Z is conserved. The above example illustrates that, when an object is rotating about a particular axis with constant angular momentum, such as in the flight phase of a jump, dive or somersault, the angular momentum of the body about any joint axis will be zero.

In a pike dive, the actions of the hip flexors in piking the body and the hip extensors in straightening the body by rotating the upper body and legs in opposite directions are examples of the operation of Newton's third law of motion in relation to rotation. The law may be expressed as follows:

When an object A exerts a moment on another object B, there will be an equal and opposite moment exerted by object B on object A.

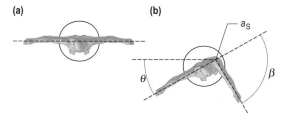

Fig. 3.70 Overhead view of a man standing on a turntable that is free to rotate about a vertical axis through its spindle. a_S = vertical axis through the left shoulder joint

The law may be demonstrated by using a turntable that is free to rotate about a vertical axis through its point of support. A man stands on the turntable, perfectly still, with his arms outstretched at his sides (Fig. 3.70a). If the man flexes his left shoulder such that his left arm is rotated with respect to the rest of the system of man and turntable through an angle β in a horizontal plane about the local vertical axis a_S through his left shoulder joint, the rest of the system will be seen to rotate about a_S in the opposite direction through an angle θ (Fig. 3.70b). Since the angular impulse exerted by the shoulder flexors on the left arm is equal and opposite to that exerted on the rest of the system, the angular momentum of the system about a_S remains unchanged, i.e. zero. In Figure 3.70b,

$$I_A.\omega_A = I_R.\omega_R$$

where

I_A = moment of inertia of the left arm about a_S
ω_A = angular velocity of the left arm about a_S
I_R = moment of inertia of the rest of the system about a_S
ω_R = angular velocity of the rest of the system about a_S

As $\omega_A = \beta/t$ and $\omega_R = \theta/t$, where t = duration of the angular impulse of the shoulder flexors, it follows that

$$I_A.\beta = I_R.\theta$$

Therefore,

$$\theta = \frac{I_A.\beta}{I_R}$$

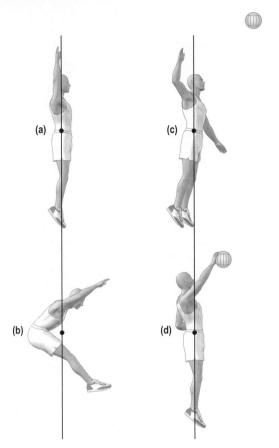

Fig. 3.71 A pike jump (a–b) and a volleyball spike (c–d)

If, for example, $I_A/I_R = \frac{1}{3}$ and $\beta = 90°$, then $\theta = 30°$.

The reaction of the rest of the body to rotation of one part of the body is not always discernible, especially when the larger part is in contact with the ground. In such cases, the reaction of the larger part may be prevented from occurring by friction between the larger part and the ground. The effect of Newton's third law is most clearly seen in movements that occur during flight when the body has little, if any, angular momentum, e.g. in a pike jump (Fig. 3.71a & b) and spiking a volleyball (Fig. 3.71c & d).

SOMERSAULTING AND TWISTING

In a number of sports, including gymnastics, diving, trampolining and freestyle skiing, the main feature of the movements is twisting somersaults during flight, i.e. movements that involve simultaneous rotation of the body about the mediolateral axis a_Z and vertical axis a_Y through the centre of gravity of the body (Fig. 2.4). Rotation about a_Z is referred to as somersaulting and rotation about a_Y is referred to as twisting. Twisting can be produced in three ways: contact twist, counter-rotation twist, tilt twist (Frohlich 1979, 1980, Yeadon 1993a, b, c, d). Contact twist generates angular momentum about a_Y prior to take-off that is conserved during flight and, consequently, results in constant rotation about a_Y during flight. Counter-rotation twist and tilt twist only occur during flight and, in contrast to contact twist, can be initiated and stopped by the performer. Counter-rotation twist is produced as a reaction to rotation of the body or part of the body about a_Y in a manner that facilitates twist but does not change the angular momentum of the body about a_Y. Tilt twist is produced by partitioning existing somersault angular momentum into somersault and twist components by tilting the a_Y axis of the body away from the vertical by asymmetric movements of the arms, chest or hips.

CONTACT TWIST

Contact twist is generated prior to take-off by a pushing/pulling action with the feet and/or hands against the floor/apparatus in such a way that the forces acting on the feet/hands exert a turning moment (in the form of a couple or two eccentric forces) on the body in the required direction of rotation around a_Y. For example, most people of average physical fitness will be able to demonstrate contact twist by jumping vertically and rotating a certain amount about a_Y before landing. This is achieved by a jumping action involving simultaneous whole-body extension along a_Y and torsion of the body around a_Y, i.e. as the body extends upward, the body is forcibly rotated, involving a vigorous upward and lateral swing of both arms, around a_Y in the required direction (Fig. 3.72). If torsion about a_Y occurred during flight, with no angular momentum about a_Y, rotation of the upper body in one direction about a_Y would result in

(a)

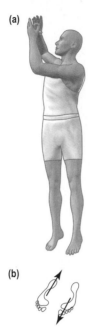

(b)

Fig. 3.72 Contact twist during take-off from the floor. (a) Contact twist to the gymnast's right involving a vigorous upward and lateral swing of the arms. (b) Horizontal components of the ground reaction forces acting on the feet

the lower body rotating in the opposite direction in order to conserve zero angular momentum (similar to the situations in Figures 3.70 and 3.71a & b). However, friction between the feet and the support surface (the horizontal components of the ground reaction forces acting on the feet) normally prevents movement of the feet and simultaneously exerts a turning moment on the body about a_Y. Consequently, the body takes off with angular momentum about a_Y that is conserved during flight. Contact twist is a source of angular momentum about a_Y in all sports that involve twisting somersaults (Frohlich 1979, 1980, Yeadon 1997).

COUNTER-ROTATION TWIST

There are two forms of counter-rotation twist: two-axes twist and hula twist. Both forms are based on the ability of the body to twist about a_Y even though the body has no angular momentum about a_Y.

Two-axes twist

The most frequently cited example of the two-axes twist or 'cat-twist' form of counter-rotation twist is that of the falling cat (McDonald 1960). If a cat is held upside down by its legs about 0.5 m above the floor and then released, it will rotate 180° about its head-to-toe axis a_j in about 0.12 s to land safely on its feet after its 0.30 s fall (Frohlich 1979). This is achieved by a combination of flexion and extension of the trunk with alternate rotation of the upper part of the body (head, neck, upper part of the trunk and front legs) and lower part of the body (lower part of the trunk and back legs). Flexion and extension of the trunk results in the upper body portion a_U of a_j being at an angle to that of the lower part a_L. Consequently, in flexion and extension, the moment of inertia of the upper body about a_U is less than the moment of inertia of the lower body about a_U and the moment of inertia of the lower body about a_L is less than the moment of inertia of the upper body about a_L; the greater the angle between a_U and a_L, the greater the difference in moment of inertia of the upper and lower body about a_U and a_L. Consequently, when the upper body rotates about a_U, the simultaneous rotation of the lower body in the opposite direction is relatively small because of its larger moment of inertia. Similarly, when the lower body rotates about a_L, the simultaneous rotation of the upper body in the opposite direction is relatively small because of its larger moment of inertia. Coordinated flexion and extension of the trunk and rotation about a_U and a_L enables the cat to complete the 180° twist. The action of 'swivel hips' on a trampoline (seat drop, half twist to seat drop) is an example of two-axes counter-rotation twist in human movement (Fig. 3.73).

Hula twist

In the Hawaiian hula dance and when keeping a hula hoop rotating around the body, the hips are moved in a continuous circular manner that effectively rotates the body about a_Y. If this circular movement of the hips occurred during flight, with no angular momentum about a_Y, the

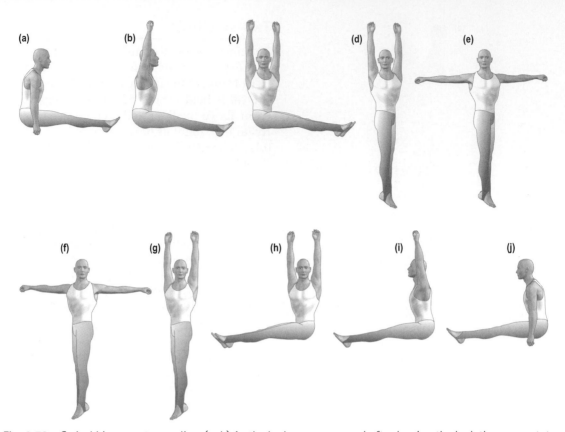

Fig. 3.73 Swivel hips on a trampoline. (a–b) As the body moves upward after leaving the bed, the arms rotate upward in the frontal plane to the overhead position. In (b), the moment of inertia of the upper body (trunk, head, neck and arms) about the vertical axis a_Y through the whole body centre of gravity is much smaller than the moment of inertia of the lower legs about a_Y. (b–c) The upper body rotates about a_Y (shoulders about 90°). The legs hardly move in the opposite direction to their much larger moment of inertia about a_Y in the pike position. (c–d) The body straightens as the upper body and legs rotate in opposite directions about the mediolateral axis a_Z through the whole body centre of gravity; the movement of the upper body is much smaller than that of the legs because of its much greater moment of inertia about a_Z. (d–e) The arms rotate in the frontal plane to the horizontal position, which considerably increases the moment of inertia of the upper body about a_Y. (e–f) The legs rotate (swivel) approximately 180° about a_Y with hardly any reaction from the upper body because of its much larger moment of inertia about a_Y. (f–g) The arms rotate in the frontal plane to the overhead position. (g–h) The body pikes as the upper body and legs rotate in opposite directions about a_Z; the movement of the upper body is much smaller than that of the legs because of its much greater moment of inertia about a_Z. (h–i) The upper body rotates about a_Y to complete the 180° turn with very little reaction from the legs because of their much larger moment of inertia about a_Y in the pike position. (i–j) The arms rotate downward in the frontal plane in preparation for landing

body as a whole would rotate in the opposite direction to that of the hips in order to conserve zero angular momentum about a_Y. This can be demonstrated by a gymnast hanging from a ring that is free to rotate about a_Y. If the gymnast starts to rotate his hips clockwise in a hula manner, he will simultaneously twist anticlockwise (Fig. 3.74). Similarly, if the gymnast starts to rotate his hips anticlockwise in a hula manner, he will simultaneously twist clockwise.

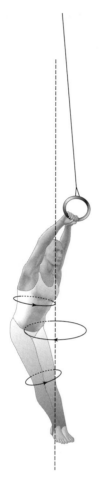

Fig. 3.74 Hula twist in response to rotation of the hips while hanging from a ring

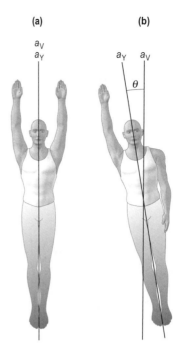

Fig. 3.75 Effect of asymmetric arm action on rotation of the rest of the body during the flight phase of a vertical jump without angular momentum. a_Y = longitudinal axis through the centre of gravity of the gymnast. a_V = vertical axis through the centre of gravity of the gymnast

TILT TWIST

Like linear velocity and linear momentum, angular velocity and angular momentum are vector quantities. At any particular point in time, the angular velocity of an object is the sum of the component angular velocities. For example, when a gymnast is performing a twisting somersault, the angular velocity of the gymnast at any point in time is the resultant of his angular velocities about a_Y (twisting speed) and a_Z (somersaulting speed). Similarly, the angular momentum of the gymnast is the resultant of his angular momentum about a_Y and a_Z. During flight, the total amount of angular momentum of the gymnast will be conserved, but asymmetric

movements of the body can vary the amount of angular momentum and, therefore, angular velocity about a_Y and a_Z. This is the basis of tilt twist.

Figure 3.75 shows a gymnast during the flight phase of a vertical jump in which he has no angular momentum about any axis. If the gymnast rotates his left arm about the anteroposterior axis a_S through his left shoulder from the overhead position in Figure 3.75a to the side position in Figure 3.75b, the rest of his body will simultaneously rotate in the opposite direction about a_S so that zero angular momentum about a_S is conserved. The moment of inertia of the left arm about a_S will be approximately one-20th of the moment of inertia of the rest of the body about a_S so that as the arm rotates about 180°, the rest of the body rotates about 9°. Consequently, the effect of the arm action is to tilt the

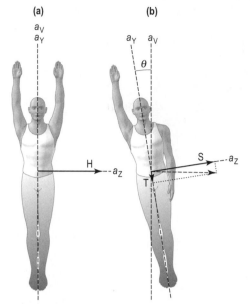

Fig. 3.76 Development of tilt twist by asymmetric arm action during somersaulting. a_Y = longitudinal axis through the centre of gravity of the gymnast. a_Z = mediolateral axis through the centre of gravity of the gymnast; a_V = vertical axis through the centre of gravity of the gymnast; H = angular momentum of the gymnast; S = component of H about a_Z; T = component of H about a_Y

body with respect to the vertical. In the absence of any further movement of body segments, this tilted posture will be maintained till landing. If the same arm action was made while the gymnast was somersaulting forward, he would immediately start twisting to his right while continuing to somersault forward, as described below.

Figure 3.76a shows the front view of a gymnast just after take-off from the floor following a run-up. It is assumed that the gymnast has considerable forward angular momentum about the mediolateral axis a_Z through his centre of gravity, but no angular momentum about the anteroposterior axis a_X or vertical axis a_Y. When showing angular momentum vectors, it is convention that the direction of the arrow indicates clockwise rotation. Consequently, in Figure 3.76a, the angular momentum H of the gymnast is shown as a vector pointing to his left because he is rotating forward about a_Z. If he had been

rotating backward about a_Z, the vector would have pointed to his right.

In the absence of a change in posture, the direction of H will be aligned with a_Z of the gymnast such that he will somersault forward about a_Z with constant angular velocity. However, if the gymnast rotates his left arm in the frontal plane (Fig. 3.76b), his body will tilt with respect to the vertical such that the direction of H will no longer be aligned with a_Z. The tilt will effectively partition H in two components, one along a_Y and one along a_Z, such that the gymnast will immediately start twisting to his right about a_Y as well as somersault forward about a_Z with the total amount of angular momentum being conserved. Furthermore, the gymnast will continue twisting to his right even though there may be no further change in body posture. This source of twist is referred to as tilt twist. Tilt twist can be stopped by the reverse action to that which caused it, i.e. in the above example, reversing the left arm movement. The direction of twist depends upon the direction and amount of tilt. In the above example, anticlockwise rotation of the right arm instead of clockwise rotation of the left arm (with respect to Fig. 3.76) would tilt the body in the opposite direction resulting in tilt twist to the left. In the above example, tilt twist was caused by asymmetric arm action, but any movements that result in left–right asymmetry will result in tilt twist when somersaulting (Yeadon 1993c).

Twist speed depends upon the resultant angular momentum H, the tilt angle and the moments of inertia of the gymnast about a_Y and a_Z while twisting. For example, from Figure 3.76b,

$$T = H.\sin\theta$$
$$S = H.\cos\theta$$

where

θ = tilt angle
T = component of angular momentum about a_Y
S = component of angular momentum about a_Z

Therefore,

$$I_T.\omega_T = H.\sin\theta$$
$$I_S.\omega_S = H.\cos\theta$$

where

I_T = moment of inertia of the gymnast about a_Y
ω_T = angular velocity (twist velocity) of the gymnast about a_Y
I_S = moment of inertia of the gymnast about a_Z
ω_S = angular velocity (somersault velocity) of the gymnast about a_Z

It follows that

$$\frac{I_T.\omega_T}{I_S.\omega_S} = \tan\theta \; (\sin\theta/\cos\theta = \tan\theta)$$

and

$$\omega_T = \frac{I_S.\omega_S.\tan\theta}{I_T}$$

If I_S is 15 times larger than I_T, i.e. $I_S/I_T = 15$ and $\theta = 9°$ ($\tan 9° = 0.158$), then

$$\omega_T = 2.37\omega_S$$

i.e. the body will make 2.37 twists for every somersault.

Elite trampolinists, divers and gymnasts achieve twist speeds of 4–6 twists per somersault (Frohlich 1979, Yeadon 1993c). To maintain counter-rotation twist, the performer needs to continuously change his/her body shape, which tends to restrict the twist speed that can be achieved. High twisting speeds can only be achieved by tilt twisting.

The contribution of contact twist, counter-rotation twist and tilt twist varies between different performers for the same action, but tilt twist appears to be the most important source of twist in multiple twisting somersaults (Yeadon 1993c).

> Twisting can be produced in three ways: contact twist, counter-rotation twist and tilt twist.

REVIEW QUESTIONS

Moment of a force and levers

1. Define the following terms: moment of a force, resultant moment, equilibrium, lever.

2. In Figure 3.3, the seesaw is horizontal and at rest with both boys off the floor. If the centre of gravity of the seesaw coincides with the fulcrum, determine W_B, the weight of boy B, if

   W_A = weight of boy A = 45 kgf

   d_A = moment arm of W_A about the fulcrum
   = 3 m

   d_B = moment arm of W_B about the fulcrum
   = 3.75 m.

3. In Figure 3.10, if S_1 = 10 kgf, S_2 = 42 kgf, W_S = 80 kgf, l = 2.5 m and the height h of the man = 1.8 m, determine (i) the distance d between the vertical plane containing the centre of gravity of the man lying on the board and the parallel plane through knife-edge support A and (ii) d as a percentage of h.

4. In Figure 3.14, if E = 20 kgf, d_E = 25 cm and d_R = 7 cm, calculate R if the nail does not move.

5. In Figure 3.15, calculate the minimum force required to lift the lid further if R = 40 kgf, d_R = 7 cm and d_E = 25 cm.

6. In Figure 3.34c–e, calculate the force (A_1, A_2, A_3 respectively) that the arms have to exert against the support surface in order to raise the body if d_A = 1.45 m, d_{W1} = 0.35 m, d_{W2} = 0.79 m, d_{W3} = 0.99 m and W = 70 kgf.

7. In Figure 3.19, if W = 5 kgf, d_W = 2.5 cm, d_F = 7.5 cm and F, J and W are all vertical forces, calculate F and J.

8. In Figure 3.20, if W = 5 kgf, d_W = 4.5 cm, d_F = 7.5 cm and the line of action of F is 45° with respect to the horizontal, calculate the magnitude of F and the magnitude and direction of J.

9. In Figure 3.23, if W = 60 kgf, d_W = 12 cm, d_A = 7 cm and the line of action of A is 80° with respect to the horizontal, calculate the magnitude of A and the magnitude and direction of J.

10. In Figure 3.25, if $W = 4.5$ kgf, $d_L = 4$ cm, $d = 20$ cm, the line of action of L is 17° with respect to the long axis of the shank (as shown in Fig. 3.25b) and the long axis of the shank is at an angle of 30° with respect to the horizontal, calculate the magnitude of L and the magnitude and direction of T.

11. Figure 3Q.1a shows a gymnast performing a crucifix on the rings. Figure 3Q.1b shows a free body diagram of the right upper limb of the gymnast. Calculate the magnitude and direction of the shoulder joint reaction force S if

  $R =$ force exerted by the ring on the right hand $= 35.54$ kgf

  $A =$ weight of the right upper limb $= 3.5$ kgf (total body weight $= 70$ kgf)

$P =$ force exerted by the pectoralis major muscle

$L =$ force exerted by the latissimus dorsi muscle $= 2P$ (force exerted is twice that of pectoralis major)

$H =$ point of application of R; $G =$ point of application of A; $I =$ point of application of P and L; $J =$ point of application of S

H, G, I and J all lie on the same horizontal line

The line of action of R with respect to the horizontal $= 80°$; the line of action of P with respect to the horizontal $= 20°$; the line of action of L with respect to the horizontal $= 55°$

$d_1 =$ distance between I and $J = 10$ cm

$d_2 =$ distance between G and $J = 29$ cm

$d_3 =$ distance between H and $J = 60$ cm.

(a)

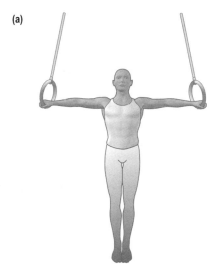

(b)

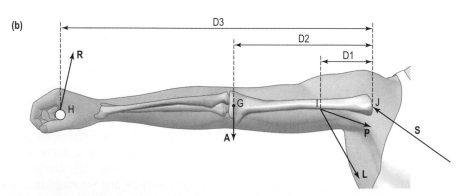

Fig. 3Q.1   (a) A gymnast performing a crucifix on the rings. (b) A free body diagram of the right upper limb of the gymnast

Segmental analysis

12. Figure 3Q.2 shows the outline of a male pole vaulter clearing the bar superimposed onto a centimetre grid. x and y axes are shown on the grid with origin O. The following points are marked on the vaulter's body: top of the head, shoulder joint, wrist joint, hip joint, ankle joint. Assume that the position of the right arm is the same as that of the left arm with respect to the x-y plane and that the position of the right leg is the same as that of the left leg with respect to the x-y plane. Use a five segment model (combined trunk, head and neck, right upper limb, left upper limb, right lower limb, left lower limb) and the segmental data from Plagenhoef et al (1983) in Table 3.1 to determine the x and y coordinates of the

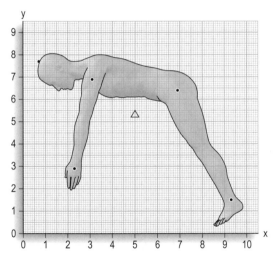

Fig. 3Q.2 A pole vaulter clearing the bar. The x, y coordinates of the top of the head (0.7, 7.7), left shoulder (3.1, 6.9), left wrist (2.3, 2.9), left hip joint (6.9, 6.4) and left ankle joint (9.3, 1.5) are marked

centre of gravity of the vaulter with respect to O. It is not necessary to use the vaulter's mass in the calculations (mass of segments can be incorporated as proportions of total mass), but in order to calculate moments in N.cm, a nominal body mass of 70 kg should be used.

Angular displacement, angular velocity and angular acceleration

13. Define angular displacement, angular velocity, angular acceleration, tangential acceleration, radial acceleration, centripetal force, centrifugal force.

14. In Figure 3.39a, if position A is the reference position, i.e. 0°, and positions B, C, D, E and F are 60°, 125°, 180°, 240° and 305° clockwise from A, determine
    i. the angular displacement θ_C of the gymnast at position C with respect to A and the angular displacement θ_E of the gymnast at position E with respect to A in degrees and radians
    ii. the average angular velocity ω in °/s and rad/s of the gymnast between positions B and D if the time between positions B and D is 0.3 s
    iii. the average angular acceleration α in °/s^2 and rad/s^2 between positions B and D if the time between positions B and D is 0.3 s and ω_B and ω_D are 3.1 rad/s and 5.5 rad/s respectively
    iv. the linear velocity of the centre of gravity of the gymnast at positions B and D if the distance between the bar and the gymnast's centre of gravity is 1 m in both positions and ω_B and ω_D are 3.1 rad/s and 5.5 rad/s respectively
    v. the linear acceleration of the centre of gravity of the gymnast at positions B and D if the distance between the bar and the gymnast's centre of gravity is 1 m in both positions and α_B and α_D are 7.1 rad/s^2 and 9.3 rad/s^2 respectively.

15. In Figure 3.42, if the mass of the thrower = 100 kg, mass of the hammer = 7.26 kg, linear velocity of the hammer = 27.5 m/s and the radius of curvature of the hammer = 1.78 m, calculate the centripetal force F_C on the hammer and the radius of curvature of the thrower r_T.

16. In Figure 3.43, if the mass of the cyclist and bike $m_C = 70$ kg and the radius of curvature of

the cyclist and bike $r_C = 35\,\text{m}$, calculate the centripetal force F_C on the cyclist and bike and the lean angle θ with respect to the vertical required to ride at a speed of 13.5 m/s.

Angular impulse and angular momentum

17. List the metric units and their abbreviations for the following variables:

Variable	Units	Unit abbreviation
Moment of a force		
Time		
Angular impulse		
Moment of inertia		
Angular velocity		
Angular momentum		

18. Use the data from the solution to question 12 to calculate the moment of inertia of the pole vaulter about the mediolateral axis a_G through his centre of gravity. Use the same five segment model, the segmental data from Plagenhoef et al (1983) in Table 3.1, and the radius of gyration data from Winter 1990 in Table 3.5. Total mass of vaulter = 70 kg. 1 cm on the figure $\equiv 0.132\,\text{m}$.

19. In Figure 3.57, if the angular momentum of the gymnast about the mediolateral axis a_Z through his centre of gravity just after take-off is 65 kg.m²/s and his moment of inertia I_Z about a_Z in positions 2 and 5 is 15 kg.m² and 5 kg.m² respectively, calculate the angular velocity of the gymnast about a_Z in positions 2 and 5.

References

Braune W, Fischer O 1889 Cited in Hay 1973

Chow J W 1999 Knee joint forces during isokinetic knee extensions: a case study. Clinical Biomechanics 14: 329–338

Clauser C, McConnville C, Young J 1969 Weight, volume and centre of mass segments of the human body. AMRL-TR-69–70. Wright-Patterson Air Force Base, Ohio

Dapena J 1984 The pattern of hammer speed during a hammer throw and influence of gravity on its fluctuations. Journal of Biomechanics 17: 553–559

Dempster W 1955 Space requirements of the seated operator. WADC Technical Report 55–159. Wright-Patterson Air Force Base, Ohio

Dempster W T 1965 Mechanisms of shoulder movement. Archives of Physical Medicine and Rehabilitation 46: 49–70

Dyson G 1977 The mechanics of athletics. Hodder & Stoughton, London

Frohlich C 1979 Do springboard divers violate angular momentum conservation? American Journal of Physics 47: 583–592

Frohlich C 1980 The physics of somersaulting and twisting. Scientific American 242(3): 112–118, 120

Hamill J, Ricard M D, Golden D M 1986 Angular momentum in multiple rotation nontwisting platform dives. International Journal of Sport Biomechanics 2: 78–87

Hanavan E P 1964 A mathematical model of the human body. AMRL Technical Report 64–102, Wright-Patterson Air Force base, Ohio

Harless E 1860 Cited in Hay 1973

Hatze H 1980 A mathematical model for the computational determination of parameter values of anthropomorphic segments. Journal of Biomechanics 13: 833–843

Hay J G 1973 The center of gravity of the human body. In Kinesiology III. American Alliance for Health, Physical Education and Recreation, Washington DC, p 20–44

Hay J G 1974 Moment of inertia of the human body. In Kinesiology IV. American Alliance for Health, Physical Education and Recreation, Washington DC, p 43–52

Lees A, Fowler, N, Derby, D 1993 A biomechanical analysis of the last stride, touch-down and take-off characteristics of the women's long jump. Journal of Sports Sciences 11: 303–314

Lieber R L 1992 Skeletal muscle structure and function. Williams & Wilkins, Baltimore

Linthorne N P, Guzman M S, Bridgett L A 2005 Optimal take-off angle in the long jump. Journal of Sports Sciences 23: 703–712

McDonald D 1960 How does a cat fall on its feet? New Scientist 7: 1647–1649

Ninio F 1993 Acceleration in uniform circular motion. American Journal of Physics 61: 1052

Plagenhoef S, Evans F G, Abdelnour T 1983 Anatomical data for analysing human motion. Research Quarterly for Exercise and Sport 54: 169–178

Santchi W R, Du Bois J, Omoto C 1963 Moments of inertia and centers of gravity of the living human body. AMRL Technical Documentary Report 63–36, Wright-Patterson Air Force Base, Ohio

Sprigings E J, Burko D B, Watson G, Laverty W H 1987 An evaluation of three segmental methods used to predict the location of the total body CG for human airborne movements. Journal of Human Movement Studies 13: 57–68

Van Eijden T M G J, De Boer W, Weijs W A 1985 The orientation of the distal part of the quadriceps femoris muscle as a function of the knee flexion-extension angle. Journal of Biomechanics 18: 803–809

Wallace D A, Salem G J, Salinas R, Powers C M 2002 Patellofemoral joint kinetics while squatting with and without an external load. Journal of Orthopaedic and Sports Physical Therapy 32: 141–148

Watkins J 1999 Structure and function of the musculoskeletal system. Human Kinetics, Champaign, IL

Weyland P G, Strenlight D B, Bellizza M J et al 2000 Faster top running speeds are achieved with greater ground reaction forces not more rapid leg movements. Journal of Applied Physiology 89: 1991–1999

Whitsett C E 1963 Some dynamic response characteristics of weightless man. AMRL Technical Report 63–18, Wright-Patterson Air Force base, Ohio

Wikipedia 2005 Velodrome. Available online at: http://en.wikipedia.org/wiki/Velodrome. Accessed 6 Dec 2005

Winter D A 1990 Biomechanics and motor control of human movement. John Wiley, New York

Yeadon M R 1990 The simulation of aerial movement. II. A mathematical inertia model of the human body. Journal of Biomechanics 23: 67–74

Yeadon M R 1993a The biomechanics of twisting somersaults part I: rigid body motions. Journal of Sports Sciences 11: 187–198

Yeadon M R 1993b The biomechanics of twisting somersaults part II: contact twist. Journal of Sports Sciences 11: 199–208

Yeadon M R 1993c The biomechanics of twisting somersaults part III: aerial twist. Journal of Sports Sciences 11: 209–218

Yeadon M R 1993d The biomechanics of twisting somersaults part IV: partitioning performances using the tilt angle. Journal of Sports Sciences 11: 219–225

Yeadon M R 1997 The biomechanics of the human in flight. American Journal of Sports Medicine 25: 575–580

Chapter 4

Work, energy and power

There are a number of different forms of energy, including heat, light, sound, electricity, chemical energy and various forms of mechanical energy. The total amount of energy in the universe is constant; it cannot be created or destroyed, it can only be transformed from one form to another. All interactions in nature are the result of transformation of energy from one form to another. For example, the combustion of oil, gas or coal produces heat, which can be used to produce electricity, which can be used to produce heat in a toaster, heat and light in a light bulb, heat, light and sound in a television or mechanical energy in the form of movement in a model train. Living organisms consume nutrients in order to produce chemical energy to maintain all of the life processes. The majority of the energy produced from nutrients is used to produce mechanical energy in the form of movement of the body segments. Transformation of energy into mechanical energy is referred to as work. All forms of energy are equivalent in their capacity to do work, i.e. bring about the transfer of energy from one body to another through the action of a force or forces that deform and/or change the position and/or speed of movement of the bodies. Power is the rate of transformation of energy from one form to another. Mechanical power is the rate at which energy is transformed in the form of work. The purpose of this chapter is to describe the relationships between work, mechanical energy and mechanical power in human movement.

WORK OF A FORCE

Newton's second law of motion expresses the relationship between impulse and momentum. With regard to linear motion,

$$F.t = m.v - m.u$$
Eq. 2.15

where

F = resultant force (greater than zero) acting on an object of mass m

t = duration of the resultant force

u = velocity of the object at the start of force application

v = velocity of the object at the end of force application

If F is a constant force, resulting in constant acceleration, the average velocity v_a of the object during the period t is given by

$$v_a = \frac{u + v}{2}$$
Eq. 2.21

If $u = 0$, then

$$F.t = m.v$$
Eq. 4.1

and

$$v_a = \frac{v}{2}$$
Eq. 4.2

If d is the distance moved by the object during the period t, then

$$v_a = \frac{d}{t}$$
Eq. 4.3

It follows from Equations 4.2 and 4.3 that

$$t = \frac{2d}{v}$$
Eq. 4.4

By substitution of t from Equation 4.4 into Equation 4.1,

$$F.d = \frac{m.v^2}{2}$$
Eq. 4.5

The quantity $F.d$ is the work done by the force on the mass m. A force does work when it moves its point of application in the direction of the force and the amount of work done is defined as the product of the force and the distance moved by the point of application of the force. The quantity $m.v^2/2$ is the change in translational (linear) kinetic energy of the mass m resulting from the work done on it. The translational kinetic energy of an object is the energy possessed by the object due to its linear motion. An object of mass m moving with linear velocity v has translational kinetic energy equal to $m.v^2/2$. A stationary object has no translational kinetic energy, as $v = 0$. Energy is the capacity to do work. A body can do work if it has energy. There are a number of different forms of energy, including heat, light, sound, electricity, chemical energy and various forms of mechanical energy. Translational kinetic energy is a form of mechanical energy and work is the transformation of any form of energy into mechanical energy. Equation 4.5 is referred to as the work–energy equation in relation to the work of a force; it expresses the relationship between the work done on an object by a force and the resulting change in the translational kinetic energy of the object. As will be described shortly, the moment of a force can also do work.

When a body A does work on another body B, energy is transferred from A to B. In doing so, body B is moved and/or its type of movement is changed, i.e. it experiences acceleration or deceleration, usually combined with deformation. Figure 4.1 shows the movement of a soccer ball from the instant of contact with

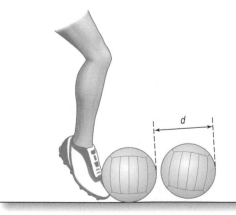

Fig. 4.1 Distance d moved by a soccer ball while in contact with the kicker's foot when kicked from rest

the kicker's foot to the instant of separation of foot and ball. If the ball is at rest before the kick, the velocity of the ball after the kick can be determined by applying Equation 4.5. For example, if

$F = 607.5\,N$ = the average force exerted on the ball during the kick

$d = 0.27\,m$ = contact distance (distance moved by the ball in the direction of F while in contact with the kicker's foot)

$m = 0.45\,kg$ = the mass of the ball

then the work done W on the ball by the kicker is given by

$$W = F.d = 607.5\,N \times 0.27\,m = 164\,J$$

In the SI system, the unit of work is the joule (J) (after James Joule 1818–1889). One joule is the work done by a force of 1 newton (N) when it moves its point of application a distance of 1 metre (m) in the direction of the force. The units of work, energy and moment of a force consist of the same combination of base units, $kg.m^2/s^2$. To distinguish these quantities, the unit for work and energy is the joule (J) and the unit for moment of a force is the newton metre (N.m). From Equation 4.5, the velocity v of the ball after the kick is given by

$$v = \sqrt{(2F.d/m)} = 27.0\,m/s\;(60.4\,mph)$$

> All interactions in nature are the result of transformation of energy from one form to another. Transformation of energy into mechanical energy is referred to as work. In the SI system, the unit of work is the joule.

POWER

Power is work rate, i.e. the rate of doing work. In the SI system, the unit of power is the watt (W). One watt (after James Watt 1736–1819) is a work rate of $1\,J/s$. Power can be measured over a period of time, referred to as average power, or instantaneously, referred to as instantaneous power.

Average power

In the above example of kicking a soccer ball, the contact time t between the kicker's foot and the ball can be determined by applying Newton's second law of motion,

i.e. $F.t = m.v$ Eq. 4.1

$$t = \frac{m.v}{F} = \frac{0.45\,kg \times 27.0\,m/s}{607.5\,N} = 0.02\,s$$

As the kicker does 164 J of work on the ball in 0.02 s, then the average power P_a of the kick, i.e. the average rate at which the kicker transfers energy to the ball in the form of work, is given by

$$P_a = \frac{W}{t} = \frac{164\,J}{0.02\,s} = 8200\,W = 8.2\,kW$$
$$(1\,kW = 1\,kilowatt = 1000\,W)$$

A soccer player kicking a stationary ball is similar, in terms of energy transfer, to a hammer hitting a nail (Fig. 4.2). As the hammer contacts the nail, the hammer has a certain amount of translational kinetic energy due to the work done on it by the person swinging it. As the hammer is rapidly brought to rest, its translational kinetic energy is equally rapidly transferred to the nail in the form of work, which drives the nail a distance d into the wood. Some of the energy of the hammer may be dissipated as heat and sound. If it is assumed that all

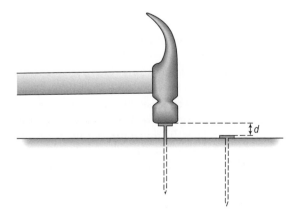

Fig. 4.2   Impact of a hammer on a nail. d = distance that the nail is driven into the wood by the impact

the translational kinetic energy of the hammer is transferred to the nail in the form of work and if

$m = 0.45\,\mathrm{kg}$ = the mass of the hammer
$v = 1.8\,\mathrm{m/s}$ = the velocity of the hammer on impact with the nail
$d = 0.01\,\mathrm{m}$

then, from Equation 4.5, the average force F exerted by the hammer on the nail is given by

$$F = \frac{m.v^2}{2d} = \frac{0.45\,\mathrm{kg} \times (1.8\,\mathrm{m/s})^2}{0.02\,\mathrm{m}}$$
$$= 72.9\,\mathrm{N} = 7.43\,\mathrm{kgf}$$

The duration of the impact t can be determined from Newton's second law of motion, i.e. $F.t = m.v - m.u$, where $F = -72.9\,\mathrm{N}$, $u = 1.8\,\mathrm{m/s}$ and $v = 0$:

$$t = \frac{-(0.45\,\mathrm{kg} \times 1.8\,\mathrm{m/s})}{-72.9\,\mathrm{N}} = 0.011\,\mathrm{s}$$

The average power of the hammer strike on the nail is given by

$$P_a = \frac{W}{t} = \frac{F.d}{t} = \frac{72.9 \times 0.01\,\mathrm{m}}{0.011\,\mathrm{s}} = 66.3\,\mathrm{W}$$

Instantaneous power

Figure 4.3 shows the force–time graph and corresponding velocity–time graph and instantaneous power–time graph of the force exerted by the kicker on the soccer ball in the above example. The corresponding data are shown in Table 4.1. The area between the force–time graph and the time axis represents the impulse of the force; the velocity of the ball increases as the impulse increases. The instantaneous power P_i of the kick, i.e. the instantaneous rate at which the kicker transfers energy to the ball in the form of work, is given by

$$P_i = F_i.v_i$$

where F_i and v_i are the force and velocity of the ball at the instant of time t_i. For example, when

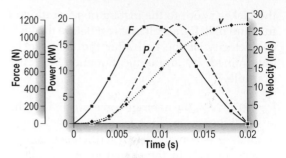

Fig. 4.3   Force–time, velocity–time and instantaneous power–time graphs pertaining to a soccer ball that is kicked from a resting position (see data in Table 4.1). F = force; v = velocity; P = power

Table 4.1   Force–time, velocity–time and instantaneous power–time data pertaining to a soccer ball that is kicked from a resting position (Fig. 4.3)

Time (s)	Force (N)	Velocity (m/s)	Instantaneous power (kW)
0	0	0	0
0.002	200	0.41	0.082
0.004	520	1.99	1.035
0.006	910	5.15	4.686
0.008	1130	9.77	11.040
0.010	1130	14.79	16.713
0.012	970	19.59	19.002
0.014	670	23.24	15.571
0.016	380	25.55	9.709
0.018	150	26.68	4.002
0.020	0	26.99	0

$t_i = 0.01\,\mathrm{s}$, $F_i = 1130\,\mathrm{N}$ and $v_i = 14.79\,\mathrm{m/s}$. Consequently, P_i is given by

$$P_i = 1130\,\mathrm{N} \times 14.79\,\mathrm{m/s} = 16\,712.7\,\mathrm{W}$$
$$= 16.713\,\mathrm{kW}$$

Peak instantaneous power, in the region of 19 kW, occurs at approximately $t_i = 0.012\,\mathrm{s}$ (Table 4.1 and Fig. 4.2).

Transformation of relatively small amounts of energy can have a considerable effect when the transformation involves sufficient power. For example, exposure of a piece of steel to a beam of light for 10 seconds has no visible effect on the steel. However, if the same amount of light is discharged in 1 picosecond (1 millionth of 1 millionth of a second $= 10^{-12}$ s) it will burn a hole in the steel (Frost 1967). This is the basis of laser technology.

> Power is the rate of transformation of energy from one form to another. Mechanical power is the rate at which energy is transformed in the form of work. In the SI system, the unit of power is the watt.

CONSERVATION OF ENERGY

In the above example of a hammer striking a nail, the work done by the hammer would be clearly evident in the distance that the nail was driven into the wood. Similarly, in the example of kicking a soccer ball, the work done by the kicker on the ball would be clearly apparent in the velocity of the ball as it flew away from the kicker's foot. However, most energy transfers are less dramatic and involve relatively small amounts of energy in relation to the mass of the objects upon which the work is done. Figure 4.4a shows a free body diagram of a box resting on the floor. Figure 4.4b shows a free body diagram of the box when a man pushes on the box with a horizontal force S. In order to slide the box across the floor, it is necessary to overcome the friction between the box and the floor. If the weight of the box $B = 30$ kgf and the coefficient of sliding friction between the box and the floor $= 0.45$, then the friction F which resists sliding is given by

$$F = \mu.R = 0.45 \times 294.3 \, \text{N} = 132.4 \, \text{N}$$

where $R =$ the normal reaction force $= B = 294.3$ N (30 kg $\times$ 9.81 N).

Consequently, in order to slide the box across the floor, it is necessary to do work on the box equivalent to the work done by friction on the box in the opposite direction. For example, in order to slide the box a distance $d = 3.5$ m, work W must be done on the box equivalent to $F.d$,

i.e. $W = F.d = 132.4 \, \text{N} \times 3.5 \, \text{m} = 463.4 \, \text{J}$

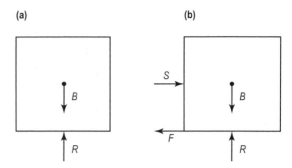

Fig. 4.4 (a) A free body diagram of a box resting on a level floor. (b) A free body diagram of the box when it is pushed from one side by a horizontal force S. $B =$ weight of the box; $R =$ ground reaction force exerted on the box; $F =$ friction between the box and the floor

The speed generated in the box will depend upon the work rate. A relatively low work rate will produce a relatively low speed, resulting in steady movement. A high work rate (a powerful thrust) is likely to generate sufficient translational kinetic energy in the box for it to slide, albeit briefly, in the absence of S. Whether the work rate is low or high, the work done on the box will be quickly dissipated as heat because of the friction, i.e. as energy is transferred to the box in the form of work, the box immediately transfers the energy to itself and the floor in the form of heat, which is reflected in an increase in the temperature of the bottom of the box and the floor. The transfer of energy from work to translational kinetic energy to heat is an illustration of the conservation of energy, i.e. the continual transfer of energy from one form to another while the total amount of energy remains the same.

The principle of conservation of energy was established in the mid 19th century, largely through the work of James Joule and Hermann von Helmholtz (1821–1894) (Brancazio 1984). It originated from the observations that friction produces heat and heat can be used to do work, as in, for example, a steam engine (heat boils the water, which produces steam, which drives the engine). Joule carried out experiments in which he measured the amount of heat generated by electricity, chemical reactions, work in various forms and friction. He discovered that work and heat are equivalent, i.e. a specific amount of work produces an equivalent amount of heat in terms of the amount of energy transformed. It was later discovered that all forms of energy are equivalent. Helmholtz is generally credited with the formulation of the principle of conservation of energy in its most general form, i.e. the total amount of energy (all forms) in a closed system is constant. A closed system is a system that is completely isolated from its surroundings. The earth is not a closed system, since it receives most of its energy from the sun, but the universe as a whole is considered to be a closed system (Brancazio 1984).

THERMODYNAMICS

Thermodynamics is the branch of physics concerning the nature of heat and its association with other forms of energy. The first law of thermodynamics incorporates the principle of conservation of energy, i.e. the total amount of energy in a closed system is constant; energy cannot be created or destroyed, it can only be converted from one form to another. In the above example of sliding a box across the floor, the work done on the box was transformed to translational kinetic energy of the box and then to heat almost immediately. The heat gained by the floor and box would then be dissipated in the form of an increase in the temperature of the surrounding air. Consequently, the total amount of energy transformed in the action of pushing the box across the floor is still in the system but it is present as heat rather than as chemical energy in the muscles of the man just prior to doing the work. The energy transformed to heat is no longer available to do work even though it is still part of the total amount of energy in the system. This is the basis of the second law of thermodynamics, i.e. in any transformation of energy there is always entropy, i.e. energy that is transformed into forms that cannot be recovered to do work.

Heat energy

In the SI system, the unit of heat is the calorie (cal) which is defined as the energy required to raise the temperature of 1 g (gram) of water by 1°C. 1 cal = 4.186 J. 1 cal is equivalent to the work done in lifting a weight of 4.186 N (0.43 kgf) vertically a distance of 1 m. It is also equivalent to pushing a mass of 1 kg a distance of 1 m across a level surface with coefficient of friction = 0.4367.

POTENTIAL ENERGY

Figure 4.5 shows a drawn bow. In drawing the bow, the archer does work on the bow by pulling on the arrow, which in turn pulls on the bowstring. As the bow is drawn, the work done on the bow is stored in the bow, which deforms like a spring; the greater the deformation of the bow, the greater the amount of energy that is stored in it. The amount of work done by the archer on the bow is $F.d$ where F is the average force exerted on the bowstring and d is the distance that the bow is drawn back. When the arrow is released, the bow recoils and the stored energy is transformed into work on the arrow

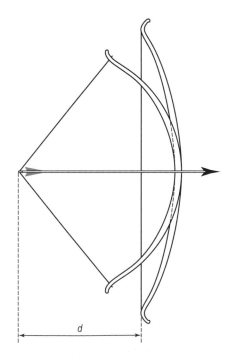

Fig. 4.5   Storage of strain energy in a bow. d = distance that the bow is drawn

via the string. The arrow separates from the bow-string with translational kinetic energy equivalent to the work done on it, i.e. the energy stored in the drawn bow. The energy stored in a drawn bow is referred to as strain energy. Many materials store strain energy in response to loading, for example, a stretched elastic band, a trampoline, a springboard in diving, a beat board in vaulting and a pole in pole vaulting. Strain energy is a form of potential energy, i.e. stored energy that, given appropriate conditions, may be used to do work.

Human movement is brought about by coordinated actions of the skeletal muscles. The muscles do work in moving the body segments. In doing work, the muscles transform chemical energy stored in the muscles into kinetic energy of the moving body segments. The stored energy in the muscles is potential energy in the form of complex chemical substances (chiefly adenosine triphosphate and creatine phosphate). When a muscle contracts isometrically (no change in length) it expends energy but does no work. When a muscle contracts concentrically (shortens) it does work by pulling its skeletal attachments closer together. When a muscle contracts eccentrically (lengthens) it expends energy in creating muscle tension but, in contrast to a concentric contraction, work is done on the muscle–tendon unit, i.e. it lengthens and as it does so the elastic components of the muscle–tendon unit absorb energy in the form of strain energy. For example, when landing from a jump or vault in gymnastics, the kinetic energy of the body is transformed into strain energy in the support surface and strain energy in the muscle–tendon units of the muscles that control the hip, knee and ankle joints by eccentric contraction of these muscles. When the purpose of the landing is to bring the body to rest, the strain energy in the muscle–tendon units is dissipated as heat in the muscle–tendon units and subsequently in the rest of the body and the surrounding air. However, if the landing is part of a rebound, some of the strain energy in the muscle–tendon units may be utilized in the subsequent movement in the form of work (additional to that produced by concentric action of the muscles) resulting from recoil of the elastic components of the muscle–tendon units. The use of this strain energy depends largely on the speed of change-over from eccentric to concentric muscle contraction. Generally, the faster the changeover the smaller the proportion of strain energy dissipated as heat and, consequently, the greater the proportion available to contribute to the subsequent movement (Gregor 1993).

GRAVITATIONAL POTENTIAL ENERGY

If an object is held above ground level and then released, it will fall to the ground because of the force of its own weight. The work done on an object by the force of its own weight W when it falls a distance h is given by $W.h$. Consequently, when an object of weight W is held a distance h above ground level it possesses potential energy equivalent to $W.h$, which may be transformed into kinetic energy if it is allowed to fall. This form of potential energy, usually denoted $m.g.h$ (where $W = m.g$), is called gravitational potential energy because it is due to the effect of gravity: the greater the height of an object above the ground (or some other reference position), the greater its gravitational potential energy.

Figure 4.6a shows a rubber ball held at rest at a height h_1 above the floor, where the floor is the reference level ($h = 0$) for the measurement of gravitational potential energy. While it is held at rest, the ball has no translational kinetic energy, but its gravitational potential energy will be $m.g.h_1$. If the ball is allowed to fall, its gravitational potential energy will be transformed into translational kinetic energy, i.e. its gravitational potential energy will decrease and its translational kinetic energy will increase. When the ball hits the floor, its gravitational potential energy will be zero and its translational kinetic energy will be equal to $m.v^2/2$ where, from Equation 4.5,

$$m.g.h_1 = m.v^2/2$$
$$v = \sqrt{(2g.h_1)}$$

If $h_1 = 1$ m, then

$$v = \sqrt{(2 \times 9.81 \, \text{m/s}^2 \times 1 \, \text{m})} = 4.43 \, \text{m/s}$$

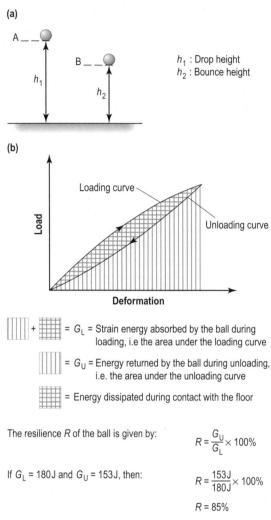

Fig. 4.6   Load–deformation characteristics of a bouncing rubber ball

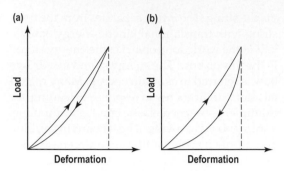

Fig. 4.7   Load–deformation characteristics of material with high resilience (a) and low resilience (b)

HYSTERESIS, RESILIENCE AND DAMPING

In the above example, the ball strikes the floor with translational kinetic energy equivalent to the gravitational potential energy it possessed at release. During contact with the floor the ball will undergo a loading phase in which it is compressed and the translational kinetic energy of the ball is transformed into strain energy in the compressed ball. Following the loading phase the ball undergoes an unloading phase, in which it recoils and the strain energy is released

as translational kinetic energy in the form of the upward bounce of the ball. However, the ball will not bounce as high as the point from which it was dropped. This situation is shown in Figure 4.6a, where h_1 is the drop height and h_2 is the bounce height. Since the ball is at rest at A and B, some of the energy of the ball was dissipated during contact with the floor in the form of, for example, heat and sound. The amount of energy dissipated is reflected in the load deformation curves of the ball during loading and unloading (Fig. 4.6b).

The amount of strain energy absorbed by the ball during loading, the area under the loading curve, is greater than the amount of energy returned during unloading, the area under the unloading curve. The loop described by the loading and unloading curves is the hysteresis loop (from the Greek word *husteros* meaning later or delayed). The area of the hysteresis loop represents the energy dissipated. All materials exhibit hysteresis to a certain extent. The extent of hysteresis in a material is reflected in the resilience of the material, which is defined as the amount of energy returned during unloading as a percentage of the amount of energy absorbed during loading. In accordance with the second law of thermodynamics, there are no 100% resilient materials.

Figure 4.7a shows the load–deformation characteristics of highly resilient material such as ligament and tendon, and Figure 4.7b shows the load–deformation characteristics of low-resilience material, such as some forms of vinyl acetate foam. Damping refers to a low level of

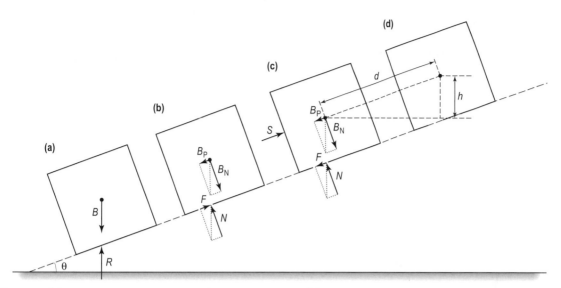

Fig. 4.8   (a) A free body diagram of a box resting on a slope. (b) A free body diagram of the box resting on the slope with the weight of the box B and reaction force R resolved into their components perpendicular (B_N, N) and parallel (B_P, F) to the slope. (c) A free body diagram of the box when it is being pushed up the slope. (d) The vertical displacement of the box after it has been pushed up the slope a distance d

resilience; a damping material returns very little energy during unloading compared to the amount of energy that it absorbs during loading. Damping materials are employed in situations where energy needs to be dissipated rather than returned. For example, the matting used in high jump and pole vault landing areas has low resilience, i.e. good damping properties. Similarly, for protection during transportation, fragile goods are usually packed in materials with good damping properties.

WORK DONE IN PUSHING A BOX UP A SLOPE

Figure 4.8a shows a free body diagram of a box resting on a slope of 20° with respect to the horizontal. There are two forces acting on the box, the weight of the box B and the equal and opposite ground reaction force R. In Figure 4.8b, B and R have been replaced by their components perpendicular and parallel to the slope. The component of B perpendicular to the slope B_N is equal and opposite to the normal reaction force N (component of R perpendicular to the slope). The component of B parallel to the slope B_P is

equal and opposite to the friction force F (component of R parallel to the slope). If the angle of the slope is constant and the surface of the slope is even, N will be constant in magnitude and direction. Consequently, the magnitude of F will be constant ($= \mu.N$). However, the direction of F will depend upon the movement of the box across the slope. F will always act on the box in the opposite direction to the movement of the box or opposite to the direction in which the box tends to move. In Figure 4.8b the box is at rest but tending to slide down the slope as a result of B_P. Consequently, in this situation, F acts on the box up the slope and is equal in magnitude to B_P. However, if someone pushes the box up the slope, F will act on the box down the slope for the period of time that the box is moving up the slope or tending to move up the slope.

Figure 4.8c shows a free body diagram of the box when it is being pushed up the slope by someone applying a force S. In order to push the box up the slope, the person pushing the box must overcome F and B_P, which both oppose the movement of the box up the slope. The work done by S in pushing the box up the slope is the sum of the work done against F (the work done by F on the box) and the increase in the gravitational potential energy of the box as it moves up the slope. For example, if the box moves a distance d up the slope (Figure 4.8c and d), the work done W by S is given by

$$W = S.d = F.d + m.g.h$$

where m = mass of the box and h = vertical displacement of the box as it moves a distance d up the slope. If $m = 30\,kgf$, $\mu = 0.45$, $\theta = 20°$, $d = 3.5\,m$, then

$$N = B.\cos 20° = 30\,kgf \times 9.81\,m/s^2 \times 0.9397$$
$$= 276.55\,N$$
$$F = \mu.N = 0.45 \times 276.55\,N = 124.45\,N$$
$$h = d.\sin 20° = 3.5\,m \times 0.3420 = 1.197\,m$$
$$W = (124.45\,N \times 3.5\,m) + (30\,kg \times 9.81\,m/s^2 \times 1.197\,m)$$
$$= 435.57\,J + 352.28\,J = 787.85\,J$$

Since $W = S.d$, then the average magnitude of S is given by

$$S = \frac{787.85\,J}{3.5\,m} = 225.1\,N$$

The first law of thermodynamics incorporates the principle of conservation of energy, i.e. the total amount of energy in a closed system is constant; energy cannot be created or destroyed, it can only be converted from one form to another.

WORK OF THE MOMENT OF A FORCE

Newton's second law of motion in relation to angular motion expresses the relationship between angular impulse and angular momentum,

i.e. $M.t = I.\omega_2 - I.\omega_1$ Eq. 3.27

where

M = resultant moment of force (greater than zero) acting on an object which has a moment of inertia I about a particular axis

t = duration of the resultant moment

ω_1 = angular velocity of the object at the start of the application of the resultant moment

ω_2 = angular velocity of the object at the end of the application of the resultant moment

If M is a constant moment, resulting in constant angular acceleration, the average angular velocity ω_a of the object during the period t is given by

$$\omega_a = \frac{\omega + \omega_2}{2}$$

If $\omega_1 = 0$, then

$$M.t = I.\omega \text{ (where } \omega = \omega_2) \qquad \text{Eq. 4.6}$$

and

$$\omega_a = \frac{\omega}{2} \qquad \text{Eq. 4.7}$$

If θ is the angular distance in radians moved by the object during the period t, then

$$\omega_a = \frac{\theta}{t} \qquad \text{Eq. 4.8}$$

It follows from Equations 4.7 and 4.8 that

$$t = \frac{2\theta}{\omega} \qquad \text{Eq. 4.9}$$

By substitution of t from Equation 4.9 into Equation 4.6,

$$M.\frac{2\theta}{\omega} = I.\omega$$

$$M.\theta = \frac{1.\omega^2}{2} \qquad \text{Eq. 4.10}$$

The quantity $M.\theta$ is the work done by the moment of force on the object. As the unit of M is newton metres and the unit of θ is radians, the unit of $M.\theta$ is joules, the same as the unit of work done by a force. The work done by the moment of a force is the product of the moment and the angular distance in radians moved by the object during the impulse of the moment.

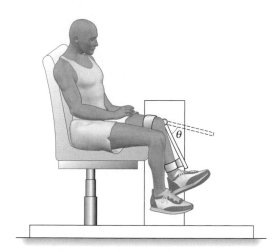

Fig. 4.9   A football player performing a knee extension exercise on a dynamometer. $\theta = 50°$

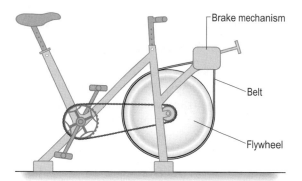

Figure 4.10   A friction-braked cycle ergometer. The friction between the belt and the flywheel can be adjusted by the brake mechanism

The quantity $I.\omega^2/2$ is the change in rotational (angular) kinetic energy of the object resulting from the work done on it by the moment of force. The rotational kinetic energy of an object is the energy possessed by the object due to its angular motion. An object with moment of inertia I and angular velocity ω about a particular axis has rotational kinetic energy equal to $I.\omega^2/2$. A stationary object has no rotational kinetic energy, as $\omega = 0$. Equation 4.10 is referred to as the work–energy equation in relation to the work of the moment of a force; it expresses the relationship between the work done on an object by the moment of a force and the resulting change in the rotational kinetic energy of the object.

Figure 4.9 shows a football player performing a knee extension training exercise on a dynamometer. In this type of dynamometer the resistance exerted by the lever arm matches the force exerted by the trainer. If the player exerts a constant force of 140 N perpendicular to the lever arm of the dynamometer at a distance of 0.25 m from the axis of the lever arm and in extending the knee rotates the lever through 50°, the work done by the player on the dynamometer is given by

$$M.\theta = (140\,\text{N} \times 0.25\,\text{m}) \times 0.8725\,\text{rad}$$
$$(50° = 50 \times 0.017\,45\,\text{rad} = 0.8725\,\text{rad})$$
$$= 35\,\text{N.m} \times 0.8725\,\text{rad} = 30.5\,\text{J}$$

In this exercise, the work done by the trainer on the dynamometer is equivalent to the work done by the friction (or electromagnetic brake) around the axis of the lever arm on the dynamometer in the opposite direction. Consequently, the work done by the trainer on the dynamometer is immediately dissipated as heat within the machine.

Figure 4.10 shows an exercise cycle. Clockwise rotation of the pedals results in clockwise rotation of the flywheel. If the flywheel is a solid mass, the moment of inertia of the flywheel I about its spindle $= m.r^2/2$ where $m =$ mass of the flywheel and $r =$ radius of the flywheel. If $m = 7\,\text{kg}$ and $r = 0.3\,\text{m}$, then $I = 0.315\,\text{kg.m}^2$. If a trainer exerts a constant moment of 0.75 N.m via the pedals for 5 revolutions of the pedals (with no friction between the belt and flywheel), the work done by the trainer on the flywheel is given by

$$M.\theta = 0.75\,\text{N.m} \times (5\,\text{rev} \times 2\pi\,\text{rad/rev})$$
$$(1\,\text{rev} = 2\pi\,\text{rad} = 6.28\,\text{rad})$$
$$= 0.75\,\text{N.m} \times 31.4\,\text{rad} = 23.55\,\text{J}$$

The work done on the flywheel is equivalent to the increase in rotational kinetic energy of the flywheel, i.e., from Equation 4.10,

$$\frac{I.\omega^2}{2} = 23.55\,\text{J}$$
$$\omega = \sqrt{(47.1\,\text{J}/0.315\,\text{kg/m}^2)} = 12.2\,\text{rad/s}$$

CONSERVATION OF MECHANICAL ENERGY

At any particular instant in time, the total mechanical energy of an object is the sum of its kinetic energy (translational and rotational) and its gravitational potential energy (Winter 1979). Transformation of mechanical energy from one form to another within an object is a common occurrence. For example, in a falling object there will be a continuous transformation of gravitational potential energy to translational kinetic energy; as the height of the object and, therefore, its gravitational potential energy decreases, there will be a corresponding increase in its translational kinetic energy. Figure 4.11 shows the transformation of gravitational potential energy to translational kinetic energy of a 1 kg ball after being dropped from a height of 20 m in the absence of air resistance. In this situation, the loss in gravitational potential energy would be equal to the gain in translational kinetic energy so that the total amount of mechanical energy of the ball would be conserved, i.e. remain constant. This concept is referred to as the conservation of mechanical energy.

When an object is acted on by a resultant force that changes the proportions of the different forms of mechanical energy of the object but does not change the total amount of mechanical energy of the object, the resultant force acting on the object is referred to as a conservative force. There are no conservative force systems in nature since the movement of objects is always resisted to a certain extent by friction and/or fluid (air, water) resistance. However, there are a number of situations that approximate to the action of a conservative force system, such as the effect of weight on a falling object. Whereas weight is constant, air resistance will increase as the velocity of the falling object increases (Eq. 2.24). Air resistance will dissipate the energy of a falling object by transforming some of its energy into an increase in the kinetic energy of the layer of air in contact with the falling object.

Another situation that closely approximates a conservative force system is the movement of a pendulum. If a pendulum is stopped from swinging, it will hang vertically; this is the equilibrium position of the pendulum (Fig. 4.12a). If

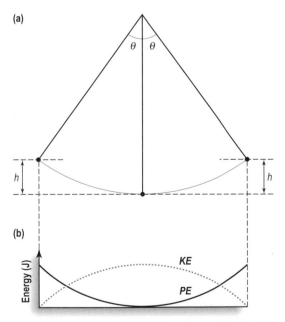

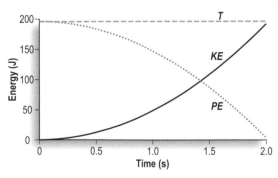

Fig. 4.11 Transformation of gravitational potential energy *PE* to translational kinetic energy *KE* of a 1 kg ball that is dropped from a height of 20 m. In the absence of air resistance, the total mechanical energy *T* of the ball, i.e. the sum of *PE* and *KE*, would remain constant during the fall

Fig. 4.12 The movement of a pendulum. (a) In the absence of friction around the axis of rotation and air resistance, the total mechanical energy of the pendulum would be conserved. (b) Transformation of gravitational potential energy *PE* and translational kinetic energy *KE* of the pendulum during each swing

the equilibrium position is the reference position for the measurement of gravitational potential energy ($h = 0$), then the pendulum will possess no mechanical energy in the equilibrium position. If the pendulum is rotated through an angle θ with respect to the vertical and held at rest, the work done on the pendulum will be equivalent to the gain in gravitational potential energy, i.e. $m.g.h$. If the pendulum is then released, it will oscillate about the equilibrium position for some considerable time and display a continuous transformation of mechanical energy from gravitational potential energy to translational kinetic energy in the downswings and from translational kinetic energy to gravitational potential energy in the upswings (Fig. 4.12b). In the absence of friction around its axis of rotation and air resistance, it would oscillate for ever and the total mechanical energy would be conserved. However, there will always be a certain amount of friction around its axis and air resistance. The friction around the axis will dissipate the energy of the pendulum in the form of heat and air resistance will dissipate the energy of the pendulum in the form of an increase in the kinetic energy of the layer of air in contact with the pendulum.

CONSERVATION OF MECHANICAL ENERGY IN A GYMNAST ROTATING ABOUT A HIGH BAR

The rotation of a gymnast around a high bar is similar to that of a pendulum in terms of transformation of mechanical energy. Figure 4.13 shows a gymnast swinging from rest in a clockwise direction from A through B. If B is the reference position for the measurement of gravitational potential energy ($h = 0$), then the mechanical energy of the gymnast at A and B is given by

Gravitational potential energy at A $= 2\,m.g.h$

Translational kinetic energy at A $= 0$

Rotational kinetic energy at A $= 0$

Total mechanical energy at A $= 2\,m.g.h$

$$\text{Eq. 4.11}$$

Gravitational potential energy at B $= 0$

Translational kinetic energy at B $= m.v^2/2$

Rotational kinetic energy at B $= I.\omega^2/2$

Total mechanical energy at B

$$= m.v^2/2 + I.\omega^2/2 \qquad \text{Eq. 4.12}$$

where m = mass of the gymnast, h = distance between the bar and the centre of gravity of the gymnast, v = linear velocity of the gymnast at B, ω = angular velocity of the gymnast about the bar at B, I = moment of inertia of the gymnast about the bar. From Equations 4.11 and 4.12,

$$2\,m.g.h = m.v^2/2 + I.\omega^2/2 \qquad \text{Eq. 4.13}$$

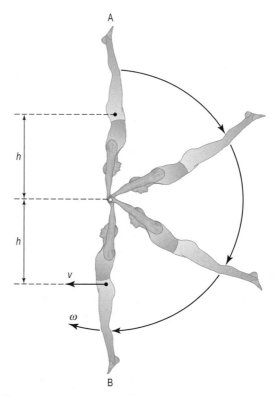

Fig. 4.13   A gymnast swinging around a high bar from a position of rest directly above the bar. h = distance between the bar and the centre of gravity of the gymnast; v = linear velocity of the gymnast at B, ω = angular velocity of the gymnast about the bar at B

As $v = h.\omega$ (Eq. 3.12), substitution for v in Equation 4.13 gives

$$2\,m.g.h = m.(h.\omega)^2/2 + I.\omega^2/2$$
$$4\,m.g.h = \omega^2(m.h^2 + I)$$

$$\omega^2 = \frac{4m.g.h}{m.h^2 + I} \qquad \text{Eq. 4.14}$$

If $m = 70\,kg$, $h = 0.9\,m$ and $I = 90\,kg.m^2$, then from Equation 4.14

$$\omega^2 = \frac{4 \times 70\,kg \times 9.81\,m/s^2 \times 0.9\,m}{(70\,kg \times 0.81\,m^2) + 90\,kg.m^2}$$
$$= 16.86\,rad^2/s^2$$
$$\omega = 4.105\,rad/s$$

As $v = h.\omega$, then $v = 0.9\,m \times 4.105\,rad/s = 3.694\,m/s$.

The total mechanical energy of the gymnast at $A = 2\,m.g.h = 1236\,J$. The total mechanical energy of the gymnast at $B = m.v^2/2 + I.\omega^2/2 = 477.59\,J + 758.29\,J = 1236\,J$. Consequently, in rotating about the bar from A to B the composition of the mechanical energy of the gymnast changes from 100% gravitational potential energy at B (1236 J) to 38.6% translational kinetic energy (477.59 J) and 61.4% rotational kinetic energy (758.29 J) at B. The mechanical energy of the gymnast would not be completely conserved because of friction between the gymnast's hands and the bar.

CONSERVATION OF MECHANICAL ENERGY IN POLE VAULTING

In the pole vault, the vaulter produces translational kinetic energy in the run-up. During the period between take-off and maximum pole bend, much of this translational kinetic energy is transformed into gravitational potential energy (as the centre of gravity of the vaulter rises), rotational kinetic energy (as the body swings about the hand grip) and strain energy in the pole (Figure 4.14a–c). Some of the strain energy in the pole will be dissipated as heat but most of it will be available to do work in lifting the vaulter during the period between maximum pole bend and maximum height (Fig. 4.14c–d). During the

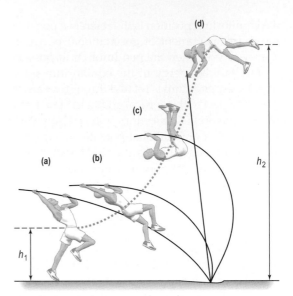

Fig. 4.14   The movement of a pole vaulter. (a) Take-off. (b) Forward swing between take-off and maximum pole bend. (c) Maximum pole bend. (d) Maximum height. h_1 = height of the vaulter's centre of gravity at take-off; h_2 = height of the vaulter's centre of gravity at maximum height

same period (while the pole is straightening), the vaulter normally pushes down on the pole in order to lift his body. Consequently, whereas some mechanical energy is lost as heat, a certain amount of new mechanical energy is added to the system of pole and vaulter in the form of work done by the vaulter in pushing down on the pole. It is difficult to measure the mechanical energy dissipated as heat and gained by muscular effort, but some insight into the loss and gain can be made by considering the mechanical energy of the vaulter at take-off and maximum height.

At take-off, the total mechanical energy E_T of the system of vaulter and pole is equal to the sum of the gravitational potential energy and translational kinetic energy of the vaulter (assuming negligible energy in the pole and negligible rotational kinetic energy of the vaulter),

i.e. $E_T = m.g.h_1 + m.v_1^2/2$ \qquad Eq. 4.15

where h_1 = height of the vaulter's centre of gravity above the ground at take-off and v_1 = linear velocity of the vaulter at take-off (Fig. 4.14). At maximum height, the total mechanical energy E_M of the vaulter is equal to the sum of his gravitational potential energy and translational kinetic energy (assuming negligible rotational kinetic energy),

i.e. $E_M = m.g.h_2 + m.v_2^2/2$ Eq. 4.16

where h_2 = height of the vaulter's centre of gravity above the ground and v_2 = linear velocity of the vaulter = small amount of forward horizontal velocity required to ensure that the vaulter continues to move forward rather than coming to rest over the bar. Consequently, if all the mechanical energy available at take-off is transformed into mechanical energy at maximum height (assuming no losses due to heat and no gains due to muscular effort), then, from Equations 4.15 and 4.16,

$$m.g.h_1 + m.v_1^2/2 = m.g.h_2 + m.v_2^2/2$$

$$h_2 - h_1 = (v_1^2 - v_2^2)/2g$$

The term $(v_1^2 - v_2^2)/2g$ represents the theoretical gain in height between take-off and maximum height for given values of v_1 and v_2. When the theoretical gain is less than the actual gain, this indicates that the work done by the vaulter during the period when the pole is straightening (Fig. 4.14c–d) is greater than the energy losses during the vault; this would be regarded by the coach as good technique. For example, if $h_1 = 1.18$ m, $h_2 = 5.58$ m, $v_1 = 9.3$ m/s and $v_2 = 1.5$ m/s (data from Bogdanis & Yeadon 1994), then the theoretical gain in height = $(v_1^2 - v_2^2)/2g = 4.29$ m. However, the actual gain in height is $h_2 - h_1 = 4.4$ m.

> There are no conservative force systems in nature since the movement of objects is always resisted to a certain extent by friction and/or fluid resistance.

INTERNAL AND EXTERNAL WORK

All human movement is the result of work done by the muscles, i.e. the muscles transform chemical energy stored in the muscles into mechanical work in the form of movement (changes in gravitational potential energy and kinetic energy) of the body segments. The work done by the muscles can be divided into two components, internal work and external work (Winter 1979). Internal work W_I is the work done in changing the kinetic energy of the body segments. External work W_E is the work done against external forces. W_E consists of two components, the work done in changing gravitational potential energy W_{Eg} (weight is an external force) and the work done against other external forces W_{Eo}.

W_{Eo} is comprised of three main types of work: changes in the gravitational potential energy of other objects (e.g. lifting and lowering a box); changes in the kinetic energy of other objects (e.g. throwing and catching a ball, accelerating the flywheel of a cycle ergometer); and work done against friction (e.g. pushing a box across a floor, pedalling a cycle ergometer against the friction brake mechanism, turning a screw). Consequently, the total work done W_T by the human body and the corresponding average power output P_a during any particular period of time t are given by

$W_T = W_I + W_{Eg} + W_{Eo}$ Eq. 4.17

$P_a = W_T/t$ Eq. 4.18

Equation 4.18 should be used to determine the average power output of the human body over a particular period of time. In order to do so, it is necessary to measure all three components of work in Equation 4.17. However, W_I is rarely measured and W_{Eg} and W_{Eo} are usually only partially measured. For example, the cycle ergometer is frequently used to measure human power output (Abbott & Wilson 1995). In pedalling a friction-braked cycle ergometer, W_{Eg} is likely to be negligible (assuming that the person remains seated on the saddle) so that W_T may be considered to consist of $W_I + W_{Eo}$. W_{Eo} consists of the work done in accelerating the flywheel W_F (fluctuations in the angular velocity of the flywheel will be associated with intermittent periods of acceleration) and the work done against the friction-brake mechanism W_K. However, of the three components of work, W_I, W_F and W_K, only W_K is usually measured. Measurement of power output on a rowing ergometer is usually subject to the same limitations.

Stair climbing (Margaria et al 1966) and running up a slope (Kyle & Caiozzo 1985) have been used for many years to measure human power output. In both activities, $W_T = W_I + W_{Eg}$, but only W_{Eg} is usually measured. Practical worksheet 7 involves the measurement of external power output in stair climbing and running up a slope.

MEASUREMENT OF INTERNAL WORK AND WORK DONE IN CHANGING GRAVITATIONAL POTENTIAL ENERGY

In walking, $W_T = W_I + W_{Eg}$. Figure 4.15a–e shows one stride of a man walking at 1.3 m/s (2.9 mph). The time interval between the pictures is approximately 0.25 s. Figure 4.15f and g shows the thigh, shank and foot segments of the right leg in Figure 4.15d (just after toe-off) and Figure 4.15e (just before heel-strike) and the corresponding linear velocity v of the centre of gravity of each segment, the angular velocity ω of each segment about the mediolateral axis through its centre of gravity and the height h of the centre of gravity of each segment above the level floor. The mechanical energy of each segment in each position is the sum of its gravitational potential energy, translational kinetic energy and rotational kinetic energy. For example, the mechanical energy of the thigh segment in Figure 4.15d = 49.68 J (Table 4.2),

i.e. $E_{thigh} = m.g.h + m.v^2/2 + I.\omega^2/2$
$$= 38.23\,J + 10.97\,J + 0.48\,J$$
$$= 49.68\,J$$

The mechanical energy of each leg in each position is the sum of the mechanical energy of thigh, shank and foot segments. For example, the mechanical energy of the leg in Figure 4.15d = 75.51 J (Table 4.2),

i.e. $E_{leg} = E_{thigh} + E_{shank} + E_{foot}$
$$= 49.68\,J + 20.26\,J + 5.57\,J = 75.51\,J$$

Similarly, the mechanical energy of the right leg in Figure 4.15e = 61.95 J (Table 4.2). Consequently, there is a net decrease of 13.56 J in the mechanical energy of the right leg between the positions shown in Figure 4.15d and e.

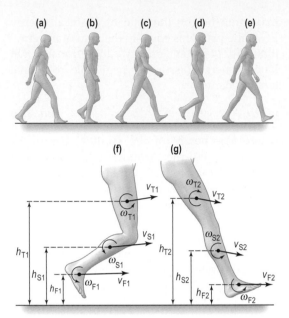

Fig. 4.15 (a–e) One stride of a man walking at 1.3 m/s, (f–g) Thigh, shank and foot segments of the right leg in (d) and (e) showing the height h of the centre of gravity of each segment above the floor, the linear velocity v of the centre of gravity of each segment and the angular velocity ω of each segment about the mediolateral axis through its centre of gravity (see data in Table 4.2)

For a multisegmental linked system like the human body, the total mechanical energy $E(t)$ is given by

$$E(t) = \sum_{i=1}^{n} GPE(i,t) + \sum_{i=1}^{n} TKE(i,t)$$
$$+ \sum_{i=1}^{n} RKE(i,t) \qquad \text{Eq. 4.19}$$

where $E(t)$ = total energy of body at time t; $GPE(i,t)$ = gravitational potential energy of the ith segment at time t; $TKE(i,t)$ = translational kinetic energy of the ith segment at time t; $RKE(i,t)$ = rotational kinetic energy of the ith segment at time t; and n = number of segments (Winter 1979). Net concentric muscular activity, referred to as positive work, increases $E(t)$ and net eccentric work, referred to as negative work, decreases $E(t)$. However, both positive and negative work contribute to the metabolic cost of the activity. Consequently, the work done W on

Table 4.2 Determination of the components of mechanical energy of the right leg of a man just after toe-off (Fig. 4.15d) and just before heel-strike (Fig. 4.15e) while walking at 1.3 m/s

Segment	Mass (kg)		L (m)	k_G		k_G (m)		I_G (kg.m^2)
Thigh	5.95		0.314	0.323		0.1014		0.0612
Shank	2.69		0.425	0.302		0.1283		0.0443
Foot	0.81		0.122	0.475		0.0579		0.0027

Just after TO	h (m)	v (m/s)	ω (rad/s)	GPE (J)	TKE (J)	RKE (J)	Total (J)	S%
Thigh	0.655	1.92	3.98	38.23	10.97	0.48	49.68	65.79
Shank	0.370	2.79	1.24	9.76	10.47	0.03	20.26	26.83
Foot	0.180	3.19	2.75	1.43	4.13	0.01	5.57	7.38
Total				49.42	25.57	0.52	75.51	
E%				65.45	33.86	0.69		

Just before HS	h (m)	v (m/s)	ω (rad/s)	GPE (J)	TKE (J)	RKE (J)	Total (J)	S%
Thigh	0.675	1.54	−0.79	39.40	7.06	0.02	49.68	75.03
Shank	0.340	1.69	1.75	8.97	3.84	0.07	20.26	20.79
Foot	0.105	2.07	1.94	0.84	1.74	0.01	5.57	4.18
Total				49.21	12.64	0.10	61.95	
E%				79.44	20.40	0.16		

Whole body mass = 56.7 kg.
Mass = mass of segment (based on segmental percentage data of Plagenhoef et al 1983); L = length of segment; k_G = radius of gyration of the segment about a mediolateral axis a_G through its centre of gravity as a percentage of segment length (from Winter 1990); I_G = moment of inertia of the segment about a_G; h = height of the centre of gravity of the segment above the floor; v = linear velocity of the centre of gravity of the segment; ω = angular velocity of the segment about a_G; GPE = gravitational potential energy of the segment; TKE = translational kinetic energy of the segment; RKE = rotational kinetic energy of the segment; Total = GPE + TKE + RKE; S% = segment energy as a percentage of the total energy of the leg; E% = energy component as percentage of the total energy of the leg.

the body during a particular period of time is the absolute sum of all the positive and negative changes in $E(t)$ during the time period,

i.e. $W = \sum_{i=1}^{n} |\Delta Ec|$ Eq. 4.20

where ΔEc = change (increase or decrease) in $E(t)$ during the ith change, and n = the number of changes.

Figure 4.16 shows the mechanical energy–time graphs of the arms, legs, combined trunk, head and neck and whole body ($E(t)$) during one stride (right heel-strike to right heel-strike) of a man of approximate mass 72 kg walking at approximately 1.5 m/s (3.3 mph) (based on Pierrynowski et al 1980). The time interval between the data points = 0.062 s and the data corresponding to Figure 4.16 is shown in Table 4.3. The average of $E(t)$ = 845.31 J. The range of $E(t)$ = 33.77 J (829.10 J° − 862.87 J), which is only 4.0% of the average. The arms, legs and combined trunk, head and neck contribute an average of approximately 12%, 19% and 70% respectively to $E(t)$. The change in $E(t)$ per time interval is shown in the eighth column of Table 4.3. The absolute changes are shown in the ninth column of Table 4.3. The sum of the absolute changes in $E(t)$ corresponds to the sum of W_I and W_{Eg} during the single stride (Eq. 4.20), i.e. W = 106.72 J. Since the stride time = 0.99 s, the mechanical work rate = 107.8 W.

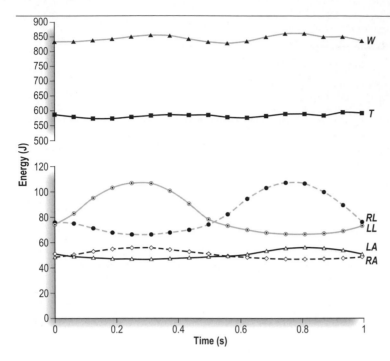

Fig. 4.16 Mechanical energy–time graphs of the arms, legs, combined trunk, head and neck and whole body during one stride (heel-strike to heel-strike of the same leg) of a man walking at approximately 1.5 m/s (adapted from Pierrynowski et al 1980; see data in Table 4.3). *LA* = left arm; *RA* = right arm, *LL* = left leg; *RL* = right leg; *T* = trunk, head and neck; *W* = whole body

Table 4.3 Determination of the total mechanical energy of the human body and work done during a single stride of a man walking at 1.5 m/s on a treadmill (see Fig. 4.16)

Time (s)	Right arm (J)	Left arm (J)	Right leg (J)	Left leg (J)	THN (J)	$E(t)$ (J)	ΔE (J)	Abs ΔE (J)
0	47.57	50.37	75.56	73.69	586.57	833.77	0	0
0.062	49.81	48.51	74.63	82.09	579.10	834.14	0.373	0.373
0.124	52.24	47.57	70.89	94.22	573.51	838.43	4.291	4.291
0.186	54.10	46.64	67.16	102.61	572.57	843.10	4.664	4.664
0.248	55.04	46.27	65.67	106.34	578.17	851.49	8.395	8.395
0.310	55.04	46.27	65.67	106.34	582.84	856.16	4.664	4.664
0.372	53.73	46.64	67.16	100.75	585.63	853.92	−2.239	2.239
0.434	52.24	47.20	69.03	90.48	584.70	843.66	−10.261	10.261
0.496	50.37	48.13	73.13	78.17	584.70	834.51	−9.142	9.142
0.558	48.51	48.51	81.16	72.76	578.17	829.10	−5.410	5.410
0.620	47.57	49.81	93.28	69.22	575.37	835.26	6.157	6.157
0.682	46.64	52.24	102.05	67.16	581.90	850.00	14.739	14.739
0.744	46.27	54.48	106.34	65.86	588.43	861.38	11.381	11.381
0.806	46.08	55.22	106.34	65.86	589.36	862.87	1.492	1.492
0.868	46.08	54.85	99.81	66.23	584.70	851.68	−11.194	11.194
0.930	46.64	53.17	89.55	68.10	594.03	851.49	−0.186	0.186
0.992	47.57	50.37	76.49	71.83	593.10	839.37	−12.127	12.127
Mean	49.74	49.78	81.41	81.28	583.11	845.31		
S%	5.88	5.89	9.93	9.61	68.98			
ΣAbs ΔE								106.72

THN = combined trunk, head and neck; $E(t)$ = total energy at time t; ΔE = change in $E(t)$; Abs ΔE = absolute value of ΔE.
Source: adapted from Pierrynowski et al 1980.

MECHANICAL EFFICIENCY OF THE HUMAN BODY

Mechanical efficiency η is given by

$$\eta = \frac{W}{C} \times 100\%$$

where W = mechanical work done by the body and C = metabolic cost. W is the result of muscular activity (active work) and the utilization of strain energy in the musculoskeletal system (passive work). Consequently,

$$\eta = \frac{\text{active work} + \text{passive work}}{C} \times 100\%$$

Since C reflects active work, a decrease in C indicates a decrease in active work. Consequently, an increase in mechanical efficiency is likely to reflect greater utilization of strain energy.

REVIEW QUESTIONS

1. Define the following terms: work of a force, work of the moment of a force, energy, joule, power, watt, conservation of energy, potential energy, strain energy, entropy, conservative force, conservation of mechanical work, internal work, external work, positive work, negative work.

2. If a soccer ball of mass 0.45 kg is kicked from rest and leaves the kicker's foot with a linear velocity of 25 m/s, calculate (i) the average force exerted on the ball and (ii) the power of the kick if the ball and the kicker's foot were in contact for 0.3 m.

3. If a sledge hammer of mass 2.25 kg has a translational kinetic energy of 7 J at impact with a wall, calculate (i) the average force exerted on the wall if the hammer is brought to rest in 0.03 m and (ii) the power of the impact.

4. If a box of mass 20 kg is at rest on a level floor that has a coefficient of friction with the bottom of the box of 0.4, calculate the work required to push the box a distance of 3 m across the floor.

5. If a box of mass 20 kg is resting on an even 15° slope, calculate (i) the friction between the bottom of the box and the slope if the coefficient of friction = 0.4, (ii) the work required to push the box directly up the slope a distance of 5 m, (iii) the average force, parallel to the slope, required to slide the box steadily up the slope.

6. An iron ball of mass 7.26 kg is dropped from a height of 1.5 m on to the ground. Calculate the average force exerted on the ball by the ground if the ball is brought to rest in (i) 0.04 m and (ii) 0.01 m.

7. If a ball of mass 0.25 kg is dropped from a height of 1.2 m and bounces up 0.8 m, calculate (i) the amount of mechanical energy dissipated during the impact with the ground and (ii) the resilience of the ball.

8. If an arrow of mass 0.015 kg separates from the bowstring with a linear velocity of 60 m/s, calculate (i) the average force exerted on the arrow by the bowstring after release by the archer if the arrow and bowstring are in contact for 0.70 m and (ii) the average force exerted by the target on the arrow if the arrow is brought to rest in 0.04 m (assume no loss of energy during flight).

9. In the most common form of friction-braked cycle ergometer, one revolution of the pedals moves a point on the rim of the flywheel a distance of 6 m. If the friction between the belt and flywheel rim is 2 kgf, calculate the work rate of the cyclist if she pedals at a constant rate of 50 pedal revolutions per minute.

10. At take-off, a pole vaulter of mass 70 kg has a linear velocity of 9.1 m/s and his centre of gravity is 1.1 m above the ground. If the linear velocity of the vaulter at maximum height is 1.0 m/s and all the remaining mechanical energy available at take-off has been transformed into gravitational potential energy at maximum height, calculate (i) the theoretical gain in height and (ii) the theoretical maximum height of the vaulter's centre of gravity. Assume that the mechanical energy in the pole and the rotational kinetic energy of the vaulter at take-off and maximum height are negligible.

References

Abbott A V, Wilson D G 1995 (eds) Human powered vehicles. Human Kinetics, Champaign, IL

Bogdanis G C, Yeadon M R 1994 The biomechanics of pole vaulting. Athletics Coach 28(4): 20–24

Brancazio P J 1984 Sport science: physical laws and optimum performance. Simon & Schuster, New York

Frost H M 1967 An introduction to biomechanics. Charles C Thomas, Springfield, IL

Gregor R J 1993 Skeletal muscle mechanics and movement. In: Grabiner M D (ed.) Current issues in biomechanics. Human Kinetics, Champaign, IL, p 171–211

Kyle C R, Caiozzo V J 1985 A comparison of the effect of external loading upon power output in stair climbing and running up a ramp. European Journal of Applied Physiology 54: 99–103

Margaria R, Aghemo P, Rovelli E 1966 Measurement of muscular power (anaerobic) in man. Journal of Applied Physiology 21: 1662–1664

Pierrynowski M R, Winter D A, Norman R W 1980 Transfers of mechanical energy within the total body and mechanical efficiency during treadmill walking. Ergonomics 23: 147–156

Winter D A 1979 A new definition of mechanical work in human movement. Journal of Applied Physiology 47: 79–83

Chapter 5

Fluid mechanics

Mass exists in three forms, solids, liquids and gases. Structurally, the main difference between solids, liquids and gases is in the strength of their intermolecular bonds. Most substances become less stable (the intermolecular bonds become progressively weaker) with increase in temperature and vice versa, such that a substance may change its state from one form to another. For example, water can exist as a solid (ice), liquid or gas (steam). In general, the stronger the intermolecular bonds, the more stable the structure, the less likely it is to deform in response to load. Whereas the strength of the intermolecular bonds is different in different solids, i.e. in response to load, some solids deform more easily than others, a solid is characterized by a fixed volume and a fixed shape when subjected to no other external force than its own weight. In contrast, a liquid will tend to deform under its own weight and is characterized by a fixed volume and variable shape. In comparison to solids and liquids, the intermolecular bonds in gases are very weak, such that, in response to external pressure, a gas is likely to change not only its shape but also its volume, i.e. gases are characterized by variable volume and variable shape.

Liquids and gases share the characteristic of variable shape, which is reflected in their natural tendency to flow or change shape. A substance that has a natural tendency to flow is called a fluid (Fuchs 1985). Liquids and gases are both fluids. Whenever an object moves through a fluid or a fluid flows over a stationary object, the fluid exerts pressure on the object, which tends to move the object or change the way the object is moving. Fluid mechanics is the study of the forces that act on bodies in fluids and the effects of the forces on the movement of the bodies. Human movement is affected by two fluids, air and water, often simultaneously, as in swimming and sailing. The purpose of this chapter is to describe the fluid mechanics of air and water in relation to the movement of the human body and projectiles.

ATMOSPHERIC PRESSURE

The atmosphere is the layer of gas surrounding any planet or star (Clugston 1998). The earth's atmosphere consists of air, which is a mixture of gases made up largely of nitrogen (about 78%), oxygen (about 21%) and argon (about 1%), with small amounts of other gases, including carbon dioxide. The earth's atmosphere extends upward from the surface of the earth for a distance of approximately 1000 km (620 miles). Like all gases, air has mass and the downward pressure exerted by the atmosphere, referred to as atmospheric pressure, increases with decrease in altitude as a result of the progressive increase in the weight of air above. Consequently, atmospheric pressure is greatest at sea level (zero altitude), i.e. $101\,325\,\text{Pa}$ $(101\,325\,\text{N/m}^2 = 10\,328.7\,\text{kgf/m}^2 = 14.69\,\text{lbf/in}^2)$. Atmospheric pressure at sea level is frequently used as a unit of pressure in meteorology and oceanography, where 1 atm (1 atmosphere) is defined as a pressure of $101\,325\,\text{Pa}$. The progressive increase in atmospheric pressure with decrease in altitude results in a progressive increase in the density of air, which is greatest at sea level ($1.25\,\text{kg/m}^3$) and over half the total mass of the atmosphere is contained within the lowest 5.5 km of the atmosphere. Atmospheric pressure at sea level is equivalent to the pressure exerted by a vertical column of air of height 8263 m, horizontal cross-sectional area $1\,\text{m}^2$ and uniform density $1.25\,\text{kg/m}^3$ (Fig. 5.1). Density is generally reported in terms of mass per unit volume rather than weight per unit volume, i.e. the mass density of air $= 1.25\,\text{kg/m}^3$ and the weight density

of air $= 1.25\,\text{kgf/m}^3 = 12.262\,\text{N/m}^3$. When density is used to determine pressure, density is usually given as weight density because pressure is derived from force.

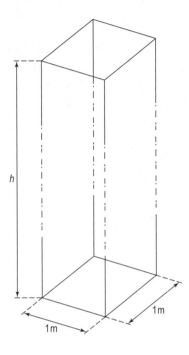

Weight of the column of air $W = V. \rho$ 1
where
V = volume of air
ρ = weight density of the air
  = 1.25 kgf/m^3
  = 12.2625 N/m^3

$V = h.A$ 2
where
h = height of the column
A = horizontal square cross sectional area = 1 m^2

From Equations 1 and 2,
$W = h.A.\rho$ 3

If the pressure on A = 101 325 Pa, then W = 101 325 N

From Equation 3,
101 325 N = h × 1 m^2 × 12.2625 N/m^3
h = 8263 m

Fig. 5.1 The dimensions of a column of air of uniform density exerting a pressure equivalent to atmospheric pressure at sea level.

ARCHIMEDES' PRINCIPLE

The atmospheric pressure at any particular altitude is exerted in all directions. Figure 5.2 shows a side view of the volume of air V (shaded region) of uniform horizontal cross-sectional area A between altitude L_1 and a higher altitude L_2. If P_1 is the upward atmospheric pressure on V at L_1 and P_2 is the downward atmospheric pressure on V at L_2, it follows that

$$P_1 = P_2 + W/A \qquad \text{Eq. 5.1}$$

where W = the weight of V and W/A = the downward pressure exerted by W at L_1. From Equation 5.1,

$$F_1 = F_2 + W \qquad \text{Eq. 5.2}$$

where $F_1 = P_1.A$ = upward force exerted on V at L_1 and $F_2 = P_2.A$ = downward force exerted on V at L_2. From Equation 5.2, $F_1 - F_2 = W$, i.e. V will experience an upward force $B = F_1 - F_2$ that is equal in magnitude to its own weight. If V is replaced by an object of mass m with the same dimensions and, therefore, the same volume as V, the surrounding air will be exactly the same as that previously surrounding the volume of air V. Consequently, the atmospheric pressure at L_1 and L_2 will be the same as that previously acting on the volume of air V and the mass m will experience an upward force that is equal in magnitude to the weight of the displaced air. The force B is referred to as the buoyancy force and buoyancy is a characteristic of all fluids that are within the earth's gravitational field. The equivalence between the magnitude of the buoyancy force and the weight of fluid displaced was discovered by the Greek mathematician Archimedes (c. 287–212 BC) and is expressed in Archimedes' principle, i.e. an object that is partially or completely immersed in a fluid will experience a buoyancy force that is equal to the weight of the fluid displaced.

FLOATING IN AIR

Figure 5.3 shows a child's party balloon floating in the air. The balloon will experience atmospheric pressure over the whole of its surface, which effectively results in four forces: a downward force F_1, an upward force F_2 where $F_1 < F_2$ due to the difference in altitude and a force at each side of equal magnitude F_3. Consequently, the resultant upward force R on the balloon (using the convention of positive upward) is given by

$$R = F_2 - F_1 - W \qquad \text{Eq. 5.3}$$

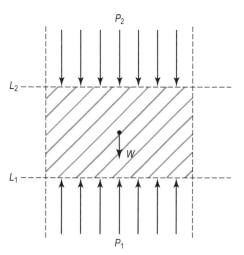

Fig. 5.2 Atmospheric pressure increases with decrease in altitude. P_1 = atmospheric pressure at altitude L_1, P_2 = atmospheric pressure at altitude L_2, W = weight of air between L_1 and L_2

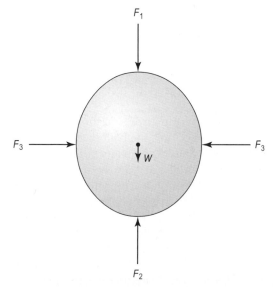

Fig. 5.3 The forces acting on a child's party balloon surrounded by air. F_1, F_2 and F_3 are due to atmospheric pressure, W = the weight of the balloon

where W = weight of the balloon envelope W_E and the weight of air in the balloon W_A. As the buoyancy force $B = F_2 - F_1$ and $W = W_E + W_A$, then from Equation 5.3

$$R = B - W_E - W_A \qquad \text{Eq. 5.4}$$

Consequently, the balloon will float (not move up or down) when $R = 0$, i.e. when $B = W_E + W_A$. When the density of the air inside the balloon is equal to the density of the air outside the balloon, $W_A = B$, i.e. $B < W_E + W_A$ and the balloon would fall to the ground because of the resultant downward force W_E. However, as the density of air decreases with increase in temperature, it should be possible to make the balloon float by filling it with hot air such that $W_A = B - W_E$. For example, if

W_E = 0.5 gf (grams force) = 0.0005 kgf
V = the volume of the inflated balloon = 0.007 24 m³ (the volume of a sphere of radius 0.12 m)
ρ_1 = weight density of the air outside the balloon = 1.25 kgf/m³
$B = V . \rho_1 = 0.007\,24\,\text{m}^3 \times 1.25\,\text{kgf/m}^3 = 0.009\,05\,\text{kgf}$

then the balloon will float if $W_A = B - W_E = 0.009\,05\,\text{kgf} - 0.0005\,\text{kgf} = 0.008\,55\,\text{kgf}$, i.e. if $W_A = V . \rho_2 = 0.008\,55\,\text{kgf}$ where ρ_2 = weight density of the air inside the balloon. Consequently, the balloon will float if

$$\rho_2 = \frac{W_A}{V} = \frac{0.008\,55\,\text{kgf}}{0.007\,24\,\text{m}^3} = 1.18\,\text{kgf/m}^3$$

If the density of the air inside the balloon was less than 1.18 kgf/m³, the balloon would move upward, as B would be greater than $W_E + W_A$. In competitions to see how far a balloon will travel before falling to earth, balloons (like permanent large advertisement balloons) are usually filled with a gas, such as helium, which has a much lower density than air. If the balloon in the above example was filled with helium (weight density $\rho_H = 0.1787\,\text{kgf/m}^3$) instead of hot air, then, from Equation 5.4 the resultant upward force on the balloon would be given by

$$R = B - W_E - W_H = m.a \qquad \text{Eq. 5.5}$$

where

W_H = the weight of helium in the balloon = $V . \rho_H = 0.007\,24\,\text{m}^3 \times 0.1787\,\text{kgf/m}^3 = 0.001\,29\,\text{kgf}$
m = mass of the balloon envelope and helium in the balloon = $m_E + m_H = 0.0005\,\text{kg} + 0.001\,29\,\text{kg} = 0.001\,79\,\text{kg}$
a = acceleration of the balloon

As B and W_E would remain the same as before, it follows from Equation 5.5 that

$$R = 0.009\,05\,\text{kgf} - 0.0005\,\text{kgf} - 0.001\,29\,\text{kgf}$$
$$= 0.007\,26\,\text{kgf} = 0.0712\,\text{N}$$

i.e. $a = \dfrac{R}{m} = \dfrac{0.071\,2\,\text{N}}{0.001\,79\,\text{kg}} = 39.8\,\text{m/s}^2$

Consequently, the balloon would initially accelerate upward at 39.8 m/s².

An object that is partially or completely immersed in a fluid will experience a buoyancy force that is equal to the weight of the fluid displaced.

HYDROSTATIC PRESSURE

The density of air (1.25 kg/m³) is very low compared to that of water (1000 kg/m³) and atmospheric pressure is normally imperceptible. In contrast, the pressure exerted by water on the body, referred to as hydrostatic pressure, is normally clearly noticeable. For example, walking from a beach into the sea will result in a noticeable progressive increase in buoyancy; the greater the degree of immersion, the greater the buoyancy force. Just as atmospheric pressure increases with decrease in altitude, hydrostatic pressure increases with increase in depth. As the density of water is much greater than that of air, hydrostatic pressure increases much more rapidly than atmospheric pressure. For example, 1 atm is equivalent to the pressure exerted by an 8263 m high column of air of horizontal cross-sectional area 1 m² (Fig. 5.1); the same amount of pressure is produced by a 10.3 m high column of water,

i.e. $W = h.A.\rho$

where

W = weight of the column of water = 101 325 N
h = height of the column of water
A = horizontal cross-sectional area of the column = 1 m²
ρ = weight density of water = 1000 kgf/m³ = 9810 N/m³

i.e. $h = \dfrac{W}{A.\rho} = \dfrac{101\,325\,\text{N}}{1\,\text{m}^2 \times 9810\,\text{N/m}^2} = 10.33\,\text{m}$

Consequently, the pressure on a scuba diver at a depth of 10.33 m = 2 atm, i.e. the combined pressure of the atmosphere and the water.

FLOATING IN WATER

From Archimedes' principle, an object will float at the surface of water if the weight of the object W_O is less than the weight of an equal volume of water W_W. The ratio of these two weights is referred to as the specific gravity of the object (a dimensionless number),

i.e. specific gravity of an object $= \dfrac{W_O}{W_W}$ Eq. 5.6

Consequently, an object will float in water if its specific gravity is less than or equal to 1.0. An object with a specific gravity less than 1.0 will be able to float by displacing a volume of water that is less than its own volume, i.e. it will float with part of its mass above the surface of the water (Fig. 5.4a and b). An object with a specific gravity of 1.0 will just float with all its volume immersed (Fig. 5.4c). In Figure 5.4a, the object floats with half of its volume below the surface of the water,

i.e. $W_1 = V_1.\rho_1 = \dfrac{V_1.\rho_W}{2} = \dfrac{W_W}{2}$

where W_1, V_1 and ρ_1 are the weight, volume and density of the object and ρ_W and W_W are the density and weight of the displaced water. As $W_1 = W_W/2$, then

$\dfrac{W_1}{W_W} = 0.5$

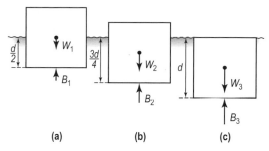

(a)   (b)   (c)

Fig. 5.4   Three cubic objects with the same volume, but different weights (W_1, W_2, W_3) and therefore different specific gravities ($SG_1 = 0.5$, $SG_2 = 0.75$, $SG_3 = 1.0$). B_1, B_2 and B_3 are the buoyancy forces corresponding to W_1, W_2 and W_3

i.e. the specific gravity of the object = 0.5. Similarly, as the object in Figure 5.4b floats with three-quarters of its volume below the surface of the water, its specific gravity = 0.75.

From Equation 5.6, the specific gravity of an object can be expressed as

$\dfrac{W_O}{W_W} = \dfrac{V_O.\rho_O}{V_O.\rho_W} = \dfrac{\rho_O}{\rho_W}$ Eq. 5.7

where W_O, V_O and ρ_O are the weight, volume and density of the object, W_W is the weight of an equal volume of water and ρ_W is the density of water. Consequently, an object will float in water if its density is less than or equal to that of water and it will sink if its density is greater than that of water. The ratio of the density of the object to the density of water, ρ_O/ρ_W (dimensionless number), is referred to as relative density. An object will float in water if its relative density is less than or equal to 1.0 and it will sink if its relative density is greater than 1.0. The specific gravity and relative density of an object have the same value.

The density of water varies depending upon the type and amount of substances that are dissolved in it. The density of fresh water = 1000 kg/m³. The density of sea water is higher than that of fresh water because of its relatively high concentration of salt; the density of sea water ranges between 1020 kg/m³ and 1030 kg/m³ with an average value of 1026 kg/m³ (Pickard & Emery 1995). As the specific gravity of the human body is normally close to 1.0, most people who cannot float in fresh water will be able to float in sea water because of its slightly higher density. Corlett (1980) provides a good illustration of the effect on buoyancy of increasing the salinity of water. A shelled boiled egg will sink if it is placed in a glass of tap water. If salt is gradually dissolved in the water, the density of the water will gradually increase and the egg will soon rise to the surface.

The human body is made up of a number of different tissues, including bone, muscle and fat, that have different specific gravities (Table 5.1). The specific gravity of the whole body depends upon the proportions of the different tissues. These proportions change with age, which in turn changes the specific gravity and therefore the floating ability of the body (Whiting 1963, 1965). In general, non-obese children have a lower specific gravity than non-obese adults because they have a relatively higher proportion of fat (specific gravity = 0.94) and relatively lower proportions of bone (specific gravity = 1.8) and muscle (specific gravity = 1.05) (Malina & Bouchard 1991). Consequently, children tend to float more easily than adults and, for this reason, childhood is a good time to learn to swim (Corlett 1980). Females tend to be more buoyant than males at all ages because of their greater proportion of fat (McArdle et al 1994).

Fully inflating the lungs by a maximal inspiration increases the volume of the body as a whole and, therefore, increases the buoyancy force when floating in water. The increase in buoyancy force is greater than the increase in body weight resulting from the increased volume of air in the lungs. Consequently, the specific gravity of the body will be lower following maximal inspiration and the body will float more easily. Following maximal inspiration, most people will float with at least the face above the surface of the water (Fig. 5.5). However, it is unlikely that two people will be able to float in the same position because of differences in body composition (distribution and proportions of body tissues). The position in which a person can float motionless in water depends upon the points of application of body weight and the buoyancy force. Body weight W acts downward at the whole-body centre of gravity C_G. The buoyancy force B acts upward at the centre of buoyancy C_B, i.e. the centre of gravity of the displaced water. Since the density of the water is uniform and the density of the body is non-uniform, it is unlikely that the C_G and C_B will coincide. In order for the person to float motionless, W and B must be equal in magnitude, opposite in direction and act along the same vertical line. The C_B is usually closer to the head than the

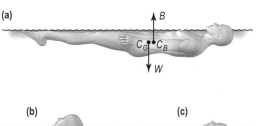

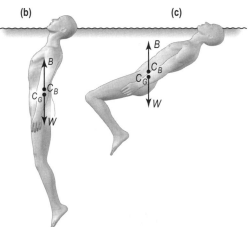

Fig. 5.5   Effect of the position of the centre of gravity C_G and centre of buoyancy C_B on the equilibrium position when floating in water. W = body weight; B = buoyancy force

Table 5.1   Specific gravity of human body tissues and other materials (average values)

Material	Specific gravity
Male adult	0.98
Female adult	0.97
Fat (adipose tissue)	0.94
Muscle	1.05
Bone	1.80
Rubber	0.92
Ice	0.87
Cork	0.21
Expanded polystyrene	0.02

C_G such that, when the body is in a horizontal position, as in Figure 5.5a, W and B form a couple that rotates the body so that the legs sink until an equilibrium position is reached where C_B is directly above C_G (Fig. 5.5b). The distance between C_G and C_B in the position shown in Figure 5.5a is approximately 0.5 cm in adult males and 0.8 cm in adult females (Gagnon & Montpetit 1981). Consequently, a fairly small change in posture is likely to have a significant effect on the magnitude of the W–B couple (by changing the positions of C_G and C_B) and on the orientation of the body in the equilibrium position. For example, most people who normally float in a fairly upright position (Fig. 5.5b) will be able to float in a more horizontal position by flexing the hips and knees (Fig. 5.5c).

> The specific gravity of the whole body depends upon the proportions of the different tissues. These proportions change with age, which in turn changes the specific gravity and therefore the floating ability of the body.

DRAG

When an object moves through a fluid, i.e. when the velocity of the object relative to that of the fluid (referred to as the relative velocity of the object) is greater than zero, the pressure of the fluid on the object exerts a retarding force on the object, which tends to decelerate the object. This retarding force is referred to as drag. Drag has three components, viscous drag, pressure drag and wave drag.

VISCOUS DRAG

A fluid flowing over an object can be considered to consist of layers of fluid called streamlines (Daish 1972). When the relative velocity of the object is low, the streamlines tend to flow fairly smoothly over the object, as in Figure 5.6a. This type of flow is called laminar flow or streamlined flow. Whereas the flow is fairly smooth, the layer of fluid adjacent to the surface of the object, referred to as the boundary layer, sticks to the surface of the object and is dragged along with

the object. As the layer of fluid next to the boundary layer flows over the boundary layer, a certain amount of friction is created between the two layers, which resists the movement of both layers and consequently resists the movement of the object. Similarly, friction is exerted between all of the layers of fluid within a certain distance of the surface of the object but the amount of friction between the layers decreases with distance from the surface of the object. The cumulative effect of the friction between the layers of fluid is a force called viscous drag (also referred to as friction drag and surface drag), which retards the movement of the object. The

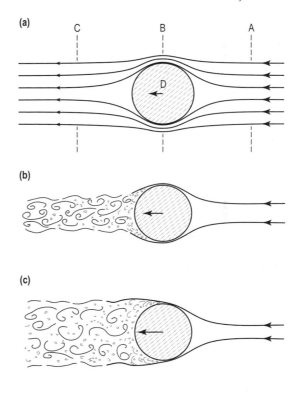

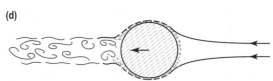

Fig. 5.6 Types of fluid flow over a cylinder.
(a) Laminar or streamlined flow. (b) Partially turbulent flow at moderate relative velocity. (c) Partially turbulent flow at high relative velocity. (d) Fully turbulent flow. D = drag force on the cylinder

magnitude of viscous drag depends upon the viscosity of the fluid, the surface area of the object in contact with the fluid, the relative velocity of the object and the volume of fluid surrounding the object.

The viscosity of a fluid is a measure of the fluid's resistance to flow (how quickly it changes shape in response to external forces) and its stickiness (how strongly it adheres to the surface of the object moving through it). Specifically, it is the resistance of the fluid to shear strain in response to a shear load. Shear stress = viscosity × shear strain rate, i.e. for a given amount of shear stress, the lower the viscosity the greater the shear strain rate. Figure 5.7a shows a flat piece of card separated from a larger flat fixed surface by a layer of fluid. If the area of the card in contact with the fluid is A and a horizontal force F is applied to the card, then the shear stress experienced by the fluid = F/A. The movement of the card is resisted by the viscosity of the fluid; the greater the viscosity, the greater the resistance and the more slowly the card will move. Figure 5.7b shows the displacement of the card in time t. The shear strain experienced by the fluid = d/h where d = the horizontal distance moved by the card in time t in the direction of F and h = thickness of the layer of fluid between the card and the fixed support surface. The shear strain rate experienced by the fluid = $d/(h.t)$ = v/h where $v = d/t$ = average velocity of the card in the direction of F in time t. The term v/h is referred to as the velocity gradient. Shear strain rate and velocity gradient are equivalent. As shear stress = viscosity × shear strain rate, it follows that

$$\frac{F}{A} = \frac{\eta.v}{h}$$

$$F = \frac{\eta.A.v}{h} \qquad \text{Eq. 5.8}$$

where η = the viscosity of the fluid. Equation 5.8 is the general expression for the viscous drag acting on an object moving through a fluid where F = viscous drag, η = the viscosity of the fluid, A = the surface area in contact with the fluid, v = the relative velocity of the object and h = the radius of the tube of fluid around the

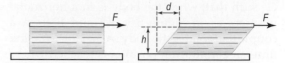

Fig. 5.7 Response of a fluid to shear stress. (a) Start of application of shear stress. (b) Strain on the fluid after time t. F = force exerted on the card; d = horizontal displacement of the card in time t; h = thickness of the layer of fluid

object in which the layers of fluid experience friction. From Equation 5.8, it is clear that viscous drag is directly proportional to η, A and v and inversely proportional to h. The SI unit of viscosity is the poiseuille (Pl) (1 Pl = 1 kg/(m.s) = $1\,\mathrm{kg.m^{-1}.s^{-1}}$), but the poise (P) is more frequently used (1 P = 1 g/(cm.s) = $1\,\mathrm{g.cm^{-1}.s^{-1}}$). 1 P = 0.1 Pl. Both units are named after Jean Louis Poiseuille 1799–1869. The viscosity of fluids decreases with increase in temperature but the viscosity of liquids is always much greater than that of gases (Brancazio 1984). For example, at 20°C the viscosity of water (0.1002 P) is approximately 55 times higher than that of air (0.0018 P). It is difficult to measure viscous drag on the human body during movement since it is difficult to measure the velocity gradient and to separate viscous drag from pressure drag.

PRESSURE DRAG

At low relative velocities the viscosity of a fluid may be sufficient to overcome the inertia of the boundary layer, i.e. the boundary layer adheres to the surface of the object resulting in laminar flow. However, as relative velocity increases, there comes a point where the viscosity of the fluid is no longer able to overcome the inertia of the boundary layer, which becomes detached from the surface of the object, initially toward the rear of the object. The separation of the boundary layer results in a drop in pressure in the region of separation and, in turn, a turbulent wake, which is characterized by disorganized whirls of fluid or eddies (Fig. 5.6b). Since the pressure in the turbulent wake is less than the pressure at the front of the object, a pressure gradient is created, referred to as pressure drag, which retards the movement of the object.

As relative velocity increases, boundary layer separation occurs earlier, i.e. the region around the object where the boundary layer separates from the surface of the object moves progressively forward toward the front of the object. This increases the width of the turbulent wake and, consequently, increases the pressure drag (Fig. 5.6c). At this stage, the flow around the object is described as partially turbulent as there is still a region at the front of the object where the flow is laminar. However, as relative velocity increases further, there comes a point where the whole of the boundary layer becomes turbulent. This results in a decrease in the pressure differential between the front and back of the object and, consequently, a decrease in drag. The decrease in drag is associated with delayed boundary layer separation, which moves back toward the rear of the object, and a reduction in the width of the turbulent wake (Fig. 5.6d). When the whole of the boundary layer becomes turbulent, the flow around the object is described as fully turbulent.

The magnitude of pressure drag depends upon the shape, surface texture, relative velocity and profile area of the object and the density of the fluid. The profile area is the cross-sectional area of the object perpendicular to the direction of movement. Pressure drag is also referred to as profile drag and form drag. Figure 5.8 shows a rod of cross-sectional area A moving in the direction of its long axis through a fluid. If the rod moves a distance d it will displace a mass of fluid $m = A.d.\rho$ where ρ = the density of the fluid. The work done by the rod = $F.d$ where F = average force exerted by the rod on m. The work done by the rod is equal to the change in translational kinetic energy of the mass m, i.e. $F.d = m.v^2/2$ where v = change in velocity of m. As $m = A.d.\rho$ then $F.d = A.d.\rho.v^2/2$, i.e. $F = A.\rho.v^2/2$. From Newton's third law, the rod will experience an equal and opposite force F, i.e. pressure drag, which will retard its movement. Depending upon its shape and surface texture, the movement of the rod will affect the fluid around it as well as in front of it, which, in turn, will affect the magnitude of the pressure drag experienced by the rod. Consequently, pressure drag F is usually expressed as

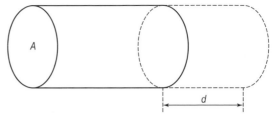

Fig. 5.8 Displacement of a mass of fluid $m = A.d.\rho$ by a rod of cross-sectional area A moving a distance d in the direction of its long axis where ρ = density of the fluid

$$F = C_D.A.\rho.v^2/2 \qquad \text{Eq. 5.9}$$

where C_D = the coefficient of drag, a dimensionless number that reflects the surface texture and shape of the object.

Effect of surface texture and shape on drag

At low to moderate relative velocity, boundary layer separation and, therefore, a marked increase in drag, occurs earlier on rough surfaces than on smooth surfaces. However, pressure drag on objects with smooth surfaces still increases with increase in relative velocity when the flow is partially turbulent. For a given object, pressure drag is lower when the flow is fully turbulent compared to when it is partially turbulent. Consequently, in some situations it may be appropriate to roughen the surface of an object so that fully turbulent flow and, therefore, reduced pressure drag, occur at a lower relative velocity. This is the basis of the fuzzy surface of a tennis ball and the dimples on a golf ball (Brancazio 1984).

Table 5.2 lists the range of drag coefficients for a number of shapes. Streamlined objects tend to have lower drag coefficients than non-streamlined objects. A streamlined object is rounded at the front and tapers to a point at the rear, like an aerofoil, aircraft fuselage or torpedo (Fig. 5.9). In comparison to non-streamlined shapes, streamlined shapes reduce the disruption of fluid flow by reducing the rate of change of direction of the layers of fluid closest to the surface of the object. This delays boundary layer separation (boundary layer separation

Table 5.2 Drag coefficients for various shapes

Shape	Drag coefficient
Aerofoil, torpedo, aircraft fuselage*	0.006–0.12
Airship*	0.02–0.025
Sphere: smooth	0.07–0.1
Bullet*	0.15–0.295
Sphere: rough	0.4–0.5
Sports car*	0.3–0.4
Economy car*	0.4–0.5
Flat plate[†]	1.28–2.0
Freestyle swimmer	0.4–0.5
Bobsleigh[‡]	0.4–0.45
Racing cyclist[‡]	0.8–0.97
Adult male or female[§]	1.0–1.3
Downhill skier in crouch position[‡]	1.0–1.1
Parachutist[‡]	1.0–1.4
Ski-jumper in flight[‡]	1.2–1.3
Motor cyclist[‡]	1.4–1.8

*Flow parallel to the long axis of the structure.
[†]Flow perpendicular to the plane of the plate.
[‡]Flow parallel to direction of movement.
[§]Flow perpendicular to the front of the body when standing upright.
Source: adapted from Wright 2005 and Filippone 2005.

(a)

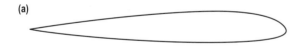

(b)

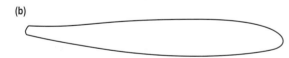

(c)

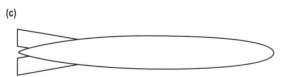

Fig. 5.9 Streamlined shapes. (a) Aerofoil (aircraft wing). (b) Aircraft fuselage. (c) Torpedo

occurs at a higher relative velocity) and, therefore, reduces pressure drag. The degree of streamlining of an object is reflected in the fineness ratio, i.e. the ratio of the length of the object to the diameter of the object with respect to the direction of fluid flow. In general, the higher the fineness ratio, the lower the drag coefficient. For objects of equal volume, total drag is least (other variables held constant) when the fineness ratio is about 4.5 (Alexander 1968). Not surprisingly, the fineness ratio of the fuselages of passenger aircraft tends to be about 4.5, since this is the best compromise between drag, which determines fuel consumption, and volume, which determines the number of passengers.

Drag on a rugby ball

The total drag on an object that is completely immersed in a fluid is the sum of the viscous drag and the pressure drag. Whereas it is relatively easy to measure the total drag, for example, in a wind tunnel, it is difficult to measure the viscous drag and pressure drag components. Equation 5.8 shows that viscous drag is proportional to v and Equation 5.9 shows that pressure drag is proportional to v^2. Consequently, pressure drag tends to increase much more rapidly than viscous drag as relative velocity increases. At the high speeds of movement generated in most sports (of participants and implements such as bats and balls), viscous drag is very small relative to pressure drag, such that pressure drag provides a reasonable estimate of total drag.

The fineness ratio of a rugby ball in flight depends upon the orientation of the ball to the air flow. Changing the orientation of the ball changes the fineness ratio and, consequently, changes the drag coefficient and the profile area. When the long axis of the ball is parallel to the air flow (nose-on), its fineness ratio, drag coefficient and profile area are approximately 1.47, 0.1 and 0.0287 m^2 respectively (Fig. 5.10a). When the short axis of the ball is parallel to the air flow (broadside), its fineness ratio, drag coefficient and profile area are approximately 0.68, 0.6 and 0.0435 m^2 respectively (Fig. 5.10b). Consequently, if $v = 22.35$ m/s (50 mph) and $\rho = 1.25$ kg/m^3, then (from Eq. 5.9) the pressure drag on the ball in the nose-on and broadside orientations is approximately 0.9 N and 8.15 N respectively. Clearly, changing the orientation of the ball has a marked effect on pressure drag.

(a)

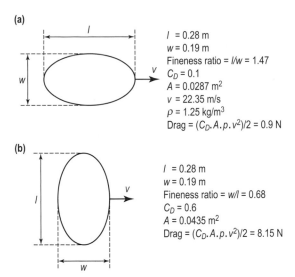

l = 0.28 m
w = 0.19 m
Fineness ratio = l/w = 1.47
C_D = 0.1
A = 0.0287 m^2
v = 22.35 m/s
ρ = 1.25 kg/m^3
Drag = $(C_D.A.\rho.v^2)/2$ = 0.9 N

(b)

l = 0.28 m
w = 0.19 m
Fineness ratio = w/l = 0.68
C_D = 0.6
A = 0.0435 m^2
Drag = $(C_D.A.\rho.v^2)/2$ = 8.15 N

Fig. 5.10   Drag on a rugby ball. (a) Long axis of the ball in the same direction as the velocity of the ball. (b) Long axis of the ball at right angles to the direction of the velocity of the ball. l = long axis of the ball; w = width of the ball

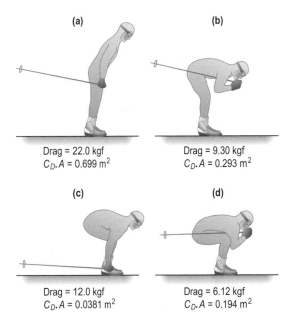

(a)   Drag = 22.0 kgf $C_D.A$ = 0.699 m^2

(b)   Drag = 9.30 kgf $C_D.A$ = 0.293 m^2

(c)   Drag = 12.0 kgf $C_D.A$ = 0.0381 m^2

(d)   Drag = 6.12 kgf $C_D.A$ = 0.194 m^2

Fig. 5.11   Drag on a skier in a wind tunnel

Drag on a skier in a wind tunnel

At the elite level, the time between the medal winners in bobsleigh, luge, skeleton and ski races is usually a fraction of a second. In such events, the difference between the times of the competitors is largely dependent upon differences in drag, which is a combination of air resistance and friction with the slope. Not surprisingly, considerable effort is made to reduce drag as much as possible. Friction drag is largely dependent upon the quality of the turns: the smoother the turns, the lower the friction drag. Air resistance is largely dependent on shape and surface texture. With regard to skiing, smooth, skin-tight clothing tends to reduce drag but changes in shape and profile area are likely to be more important sources of drag. Changes in body shape are necessary to negotiate turns and sudden changes in slope, but downhill skiers try to maintain a compact crouch position, referred to as the egg position, as much as possible, since this position has been shown to minimize drag. Figure 5.11 shows the drag on a skier in four different positions while standing in a wind tunnel with a wind velocity of 22.2 m/s (50 mph). It is clear that the compact crouch position produces the least drag (Fig. 5.11d). It is, perhaps, surprising that dropping the arms outside the lower legs from the compact crouch increases the drag more than extending the legs from the crouch position (Fig. 5.11b, c).

Terminal velocity of a downhill skier

Even though downhill skiers experience both air resistance and friction with the slope, very high speeds can be produced when conditions are favourable, i.e. minimal turns, dry snow and a steep slope (Armenti 1984). An estimate of the maximum velocity that a downhill skier may achieve can be made by consideration of the pressure drag on the skier. There are three forces acting on a downhill skier, body weight W, the ground reaction force S and the drag force D (Fig. 5.12a). D is parallel to the slope. In Figure 5.12b W and S have been replaced by their components parallel and perpendicular to the slope. W_P is the component of W parallel to the slope. The component of W perpendicular to the slope W_N is equal and opposite to the normal reaction force N, which is the component of S perpendicular to the slope. F is the frictional force which is the component of S parallel to the

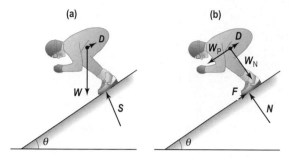

Fig. 5.12 Free body diagram of a downhill skier. W = weight of the skier, clothing and skis; D = drag force; S = ground reaction force; W_P = component of W parallel to the slope; W_N = component of W perpendicular to the slope; F = component of S parallel to the slope; N = component of S perpendicular to the slope

slope. The resultant force R acting on the skier down the slope (positive down) is given by

$$R = W_P - F - D = m.a \qquad \text{Eq. 5.10}$$

where m = mass of skier and skis and a = linear acceleration of the skier. When $R > 0$, the skier will accelerate down the slope. Whereas W_P and F will remain fairly constant, D is proportional to relative velocity, i.e. it increases as relative velocity increases such that terminal (maximal) velocity will occur when $R = 0$ and, therefore, $a = 0$. Consequently, from Equation 5.10, terminal velocity v will occur when $W_P - F - D = 0$, i.e. when

$$W.\sin\theta - \mu.W.\cos\theta - C_D.A.\rho.v^2/2 = 0 \quad \text{Eq. 5.11}$$

where μ = coefficient of friction between the skis and the slope, C_D = coefficient of drag, A = profile area and ρ = density of air. From Equation 5.11,

$$v = \sqrt{\frac{2(W.\sin\theta - \mu.W.\cos\theta)}{C_D.A.\rho}} \qquad \text{Eq. 5.12}$$

Determinations of drag on particular objects are usually made in wind tunnels so that the density of air (ρ) and velocity of air (v) can be held constant. Under these circumstances, drag varies directly with change in shape, which simultaneously changes C_D and A. As it is difficult to measure A, it is usual to report the product $C_D.A$

rather than C_D and A separately. For a downhill skier, $C_D.A$ is approximately 0.25 m² (Wagner & Wood 1996). Consequently, if W = 80 kgf, θ = 35°, μ = 0.04 (dry snow), $C_D.A$ = 0.25 m² and ρ = 1.2 kg/m³, then

$$W.\sin\theta = 80\,\text{kg} \times 9.81\,\text{m/s}^2 \times 0.5736 = 450.1\,\text{N}$$

$$\mu.W.\cos\theta = 0.04 \times 80\,\text{kg} \times 9.81\,\text{m/s}^2 \times 0.8191$$
$$= 25.7\,\text{N}$$

$$C_D.A.\rho = 0.25\,\text{m}^2 \times 1.2\,\text{kg/m}^3 = 0.3\,\text{kg/m}$$

From Equation 5.12

$$v = \sqrt{\frac{2(450.1\,\text{N} - 25.7\,\text{N})}{0.3\,\text{kg/m}}} = \sqrt{2829.3\,\text{m}^2/\text{s}^2}$$
$$= 53.19\,\text{m/s} = 119\,\text{mph}$$

The world record speed for a downhill skier is reported to be 124.23 mph (Armenti 1984).

Terminal velocity of a skydiver

In contrast to a downhill skier, the only source of drag on a skydiver is air resistance. There are two forces acting on a skydiver, body weight W and air resistance D (Fig. 5.13). The resultant force R acting on the skydiver (positive down) is given by

$$R = W - D = m.a \qquad \text{Eq. 5.13}$$

where m = mass of skydiver, clothing and parachute and a = linear acceleration of the skydiver. Terminal velocity v will occur when $R = 0$. Consequently, from Equation 5.13, terminal velocity v will occur when $W - D = 0$, i.e. when

$$W - C_D.A.\rho.v^2/2 = 0 \qquad \text{Eq. 5.14}$$

where C_D = coefficient of drag, A = profile area and ρ = density of air. From Equation 5.14,

$$v = \sqrt{2W/(C_D.A.\rho)} \qquad \text{Eq. 5.15}$$

For a skydiver, $C_D.A$ is approximately 0.56 m² before the parachute opens (Wagner & Wood 1996). Consequently, if W = 80 kgf, $C_D.A$ = 0.56 m² and ρ = 1.2 kg/m³, then, from Equation 5.15,

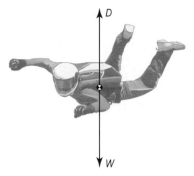

Fig. 5.13   Free body diagram of a skydiver.
W = weight of the skydiver; clothing and parachute;
D = drag force

$$v = \sqrt{\frac{2 \times 80\,\text{kg} \times 9.81\,\text{m/s}^2}{0.56\,\text{m}^2 \times 1.2\,\text{kg/m}^3}}$$

$$v = \sqrt{2335.7\,\text{m}^2/\text{s}^2} = 48.33\,\text{m/s} = 108.1\,\text{mph}$$

Consequently, it is possible for the terminal velocity of a downhill skier to be greater than that of a skydiver. Terminal velocity in the two activities depends largely on the profile area A, which in turn determines C_D. In the above examples, $C_D.A = 0.25\,\text{m}^2$ for the skier and $0.56\,\text{m}^2$ for the skydiver.

After the skydiver opens his/her parachute, C_D and A change considerably. A typical parachute has a diameter of approximately 8.5 m when fully opened. Consequently, A is approximately 57 m². In this situation C_D is approximately 1.42 (Wagner & Wood 1996). Therefore, from Equation 5.15, if $W = 80\,\text{kgf}$, $C_D = 1.42$ and $\rho = 1.2\,\text{kg/m}^3$, the terminal velocity v of the skydiver with parachute fully open is given by

$$v = \sqrt{\frac{2 \times 80\,\text{kg} \times 9.81\,\text{m/s}^2}{1.42\,\text{m}^2 \times 57\,\text{m}^2 \times 1.2\,\text{kg/m}^3}}$$

$$v = \sqrt{16.2\,\text{m}^2/\text{s}^2} = 4.02\,\text{m/s} = 9.0\,\text{mph}$$

Consequently, the terminal velocity of the skydiver with parachute fully open is the same as free-falling a distance of just 0.82 m.

WAVE DRAG

In addition to viscous drag and pressure drag, an object moving through the boundary between two different fluids experiences wave drag. For example, swimming, with part of the body in the water and part of the body out of the water, creates a wave in front of the body. The wave is the result of work done on the water by the body and the amount of work done is directly proportional to the size and speed of the wave. As the body pushes against the wave, the body experiences a force, wave drag, that is equal and opposite to that exerted by the body on the wave. Barthels (1977) likens wave drag to the force exerted by the water against a bridge support in a fast flowing river. As flow velocity increases, so does the size of the wave and the force exerted by the wave against the support. In flood conditions, the support may collapse under the strain.

> Drag has three components, viscous drag, pressure drag and wave drag.

SLIPSTREAMING

As the pressure drag on a runner increases with increase in relative velocity, so does the metabolic cost of overcoming the drag. In sprint events, where the runners run in lanes, the drag experienced by each runner is largely dependent upon his/her speed. Similarly, the drag on the leading runner in a middle- to long-distance event is largely dependent upon his/her speed. However, the drag on the other runners is significantly affected by their positions with respect to each other. As the air pressure on the front of each runner is higher than the pressure in the turbulent wake at his back, a runner can reduce the drag on his body by running in the turbulent wake or 'slipstream' of the runner in front. Whereas the second to last runners all benefit from the slipstream effect between the leading and second runner by a reduction in drag of approximately 4% (assuming that the runners are in single file, one behind the other), place in the line appears to confer no additional benefit (Pugh 1971).

The beneficial effect of slipstreaming increases with increase in relative velocity. For example, the reduction in drag due to streamlining in cycling is approximately 40%, which results in a 33% decrease in energy expenditure (Kyle 1979). Not surprisingly, the members of cyclist teams usually take turns at leading, as this is likely to maximize team performance.

BERNOULLI'S PRINCIPLE

Figure 5.6a shows the streamlines of a fluid flowing smoothly over a cylindrical object. The closer the streamlines to the object, the more they are disrupted as they flow over the object. The greater the disruption, the greater the distance that the particles of fluid in these streamlines have to travel as they pass over the object. As the particles of fluid in these streamlines have to travel a greater distance in the same time as particles of fluid in the undisrupted streamlines, it follows that the speed of the particles of fluid in the disrupted streamlines must be greater than the speed of the particles in the undisrupted streamlines as they flow between the regions of undisrupted flow upstream and downstream of the object, i.e. between regions A and C in Figure 5.6a. In Figure 5.6a, the speed of the particles in the disrupted streamlines increases between regions A and B and decreases between regions B and C. The changes in the speed of the particles of fluid in the disrupted streamlines are due to differences in pressure, i.e. pressure decreases between regions A and B resulting in an increase in speed and the pressure increases between regions B and C resulting in a decrease in speed. The inverse relationship between the pressure in a fluid and its speed is a well established phenomenon referred to as Bernoulli's principle after Daniel Bernoulli (1700–1782), i.e. when a fluid flows over a surface, the pressure exerted by the fluid on the surface is inversely proportional to the speed of flow, i.e. the lower the pressure the higher the speed and vice-versa.

Gardner (1993) describes a good demonstration of Bernoulli's principle. One end of a strip of paper about 20 cm long and 3.5 cm wide (the

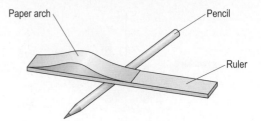

Fig. 5.14   Demonstration of Bernoulli's principle

width of a ruler) is attached to one end of a 30 cm ruler and the other end of the strip of paper is attached to the ruler about 18 cm along the ruler so that the piece of paper forms an arch (Fig. 5.14). The ruler is placed on a round-stemmed pencil lying on a table. The pencil is rotated until the end of the ruler with the paper arch just overbalances the other end. If air is then blown along the ruler from the end that is elevated, the speed of the air flow decreases the pressure above the paper arch so that the ruler tips the other way.

HYDRODYNAMIC LIFT

In accordance with Bernoulli's principle, differences in the speed of flow of fluid over the opposite sides of an object will result in differences in pressure and, therefore, a pressure gradient that will tend to move the object in the direction of the pressure gradient, i.e. from the region of higher pressure to the region of lower pressure. Consequently, whereas all objects moving through fluids experience drag, an object may also simultaneously experience a force at right angles to the drag force if the speed of flow of fluid over the opposite sides of the object is different. This force is referred to as hydrodynamic lift force and its effect is referred to as hydrodynamic lift, where lift is a general term indicating movement or tendency to move in a direction at right angles to the drag force. Hydrodynamic lift can be produced in four ways: asymmetric shape, asymmetric orientation of a regular shape, asymmetric surface texture and spin.

LIFT DUE TO ASYMMETRIC SHAPE

Objects that are specifically designed to produce hydrodynamic lift by asymmetric shape are

(a)

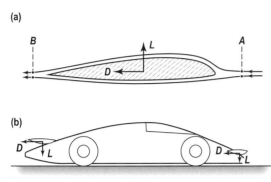

(b)

Fig. 5.15 Drag D and lift L forces on an aerofoil. (a) Cross-section of an aircraft wing. (b) Aerofoils on the front and rear of a sports car

referred to as aerofoils. An aircraft wing is an aerofoil. Figure 5.15a shows the cross-section of an aircraft wing. The distance from the front edge of the wing to the back edge is greater over the upper surface than over the lower surface. Consequently, as each particle of air must move between A and B in Figure 5.15a in the same time, the speed of air flowing over the upper surface must be greater than the speed over the lower surface which, in accordance with Bernoulli's principle, results in a pressure gradient (the pressure on the lower surface is greater than the pressure on the upper surface) tending to lift the wing.

Like pressure drag (Eq. 5.9), the magnitude of the hydrodynamic lift force F_L on an aerofoil depends upon the density of the fluid ρ, the relative velocity v of the aerofoil through the fluid, the profile area A perpendicular to v and a dimensionless coefficient, referred to as the coefficient of lift C_L, reflecting the surface texture and shape of the aerofoil,

i.e. $F_L = C_L.A.\rho.v^2/2$ Eq. 5.16

For example, consider the lift force required for a fighter aircraft to take off. The aircraft will take off if the lift force F_L is greater than the weight of the aircraft W, i.e. if

$$\frac{C_L A.\rho.v^2}{2} > W$$

$$v > \sqrt{\frac{2W}{C_L.A.\rho}}$$ Eq. 5.17

If $C_L = 0.8$, A = wing area = $55.74\,\text{m}^2$, ρ = density of air = $1.25\,\text{kg/m}^3$ and m = mass of the aircraft = $11\,800\,\text{kg}$ (Duke 1999), then the aircraft will take off when

$$v > \sqrt{\frac{2 \times 11\,800\,\text{kg} \times 9.81\,\text{m/s}^2}{0.8 \times 55.74\,\text{m}^2 \times 1.25\,\text{kg/m}^3}}$$

$$v > 65.78\,\text{m/s} = 147.1\,\text{mph}$$

Whereas aerofoils in the form of wings are used to produce upward force in aircraft, aerofoils are fitted to the front and rear of racing cars to produce downward force in order to increase the grip between the tyres and the track. In this situation, the downward pressure differential is created by an aerofoil in which the lower surface is larger than the upper surface, i.e. the reverse of an aircraft wing (Fig. 5.15b).

LIFT DUE TO ASYMMETRIC ORIENTATION

The lift force produced by an aerofoil can be increased to a certain extent by increasing the angle of attack of the aerofoil, i.e. the angle that the axis of the aerofoil makes with respect to the linear velocity of the aerofoil (Fig. 5.16a). As the angle of attack increases from zero, there is an increase in both hydrodynamic lift and drag, with hydrodynamic lift increasing at a faster rate than drag. However, as the angle of attack increases, there comes a point where the increase in drag decreases the linear velocity of the aerofoil so much that hydrodynamic lift cannot be maintained and the aerofoil stalls, i.e. the aerofoil experiences a dramatic decrease in hydrodynamic lift and forward movement (Fig. 5.16b). A typical aerofoil will stall when the angle of attack is approximately 15–20°. In an aircraft, stalling results in an almost vertical, often uncontrollable, fall (Brancazio 1984).

Paddle propulsion

In comparison to lift force, which decreases rapidly after the stall point, drag continues to increase over the 0–90° range if the relative velocity of the object is maintained (Fig. 5.16b). In terms of the type of force created, the action

(a)

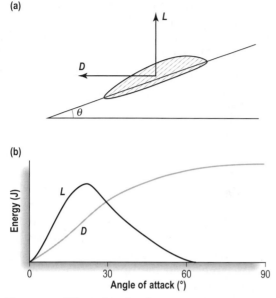

(b)

Fig. 5.16   Effect of angle of attack on the magnitude of the lift L and drag D forces on a typical aerofoil for a given relative velocity. (a) Angle of attack θ. (b) Change in drag and lift force with increase in angle of attack

(a)

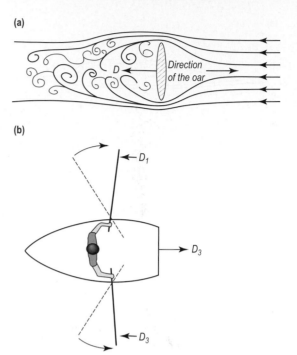

(b)

Fig. 5.17   Paddle propulsion in water. (a) Drag D on an oar blade. (b) Drag forces D_1 and D_2 on the oars and drag D_3 on the boat

of an oar or paddle in producing propulsion in water is similar to an aerofoil with an angle of attack of 90° (Fig. 5.17a). Figure 5.17b shows a person rowing a boat with two oars. As the oar blades sweep downstream through the water, turbulence is created on the upstream side of each blade such that the pressure on the upstream side of each blade is less than the pressure on the downstream side. Consequently, the pressure differential on each blade results in drag, which resists its movement. If the resultant drag force on the oar blades is greater than the drag force on the boat, the boat will be accelerated upstream as the oar blades move downstream. This form of propulsion is called paddle propulsion or drag propulsion (Brown & Counsilman 1971).

Screw propulsion

Even fairly flat symmetrical objects can experience lift force if oriented asymmetrically to the linear velocity of the object. For example, Figure 5.18 shows a boat being propelled forward by one oar operated from a rowlock in the stern. If the oar is moved sideways alternately left and right, i.e. in a direction at right angles to the intended direction of travel, and the oar blade is angled in order to create an angle of attack with respect to the water flow, the movement of the blade will produce hydrodynamic lift force on the blade and the boat will move forward. The movement of the oar blade, referred to as sculling, will also produce drag such that the boat will zigzag as it moves forward. The form of propulsion produced by sculling is similar to that produced by a propeller and is referred to as screw propulsion (Barthels 1977).

The blades of a propeller in a ship cut through the water in a plane at right angles to the intended direction of the ship. As the propeller blades are angled on the propeller shaft, the angle of attack with respect to the water

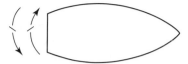

Fig. 5.18 Screw propulsion using a single oar operated from a rowlock in the stern of a rowing boat

creates hydrodynamic lift force on the blades, which pushes the propeller, and therefore the ship, forward. The rotation of the propeller also produces drag on the blades but, as the drag force is evenly distributed around the propeller and acts at right angles to the lift force, it hasno effect on the movement of the ship. Consequently, propulsion in a propeller-driven ship is entirely due to hydrodynamic lift force. In a propeller-driven aircraft, both the forward movement (resulting from the rotation of the propellers) and upward movement (resulting from air flow over the wings) are due to hydrodynamic lift force.

Propulsion in swimming

Prior to the advent of equipment (notably slow-motion cameras) and facilities (notably observation windows) necessary for the detailed analysis of underwater movements, it was assumed that swimmers propelled themselves through the water by pulling the arm or arms straight back through the water, i.e. paddle propulsion. However, slow-motion underwater filming showed that elite swimmers do not pull straight back in any of the swimming strokes, but move the hands in a three-dimensional path involving considerable mediolateral movement. This is illustrated in Figure 5.19a, which shows a typical bottom-view right-hand–body plot of an elite freestyle swimmer, i.e. the path of the right hand in relation to the body as seen from underneath the swimmer. Of even greater significance in terms of coaching was the discovery of how the hand moved in relation to the water, i.e. the hand–water plot, as it is the flow of water over the hands that produces most of the propulsion. Figure 5.19b shows the hand–water plot

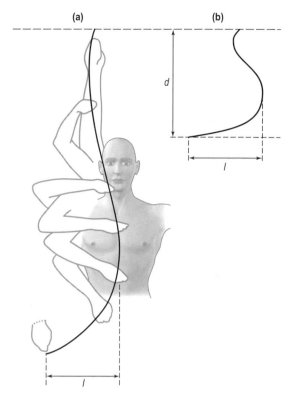

Fig. 5.19 (a) Hand–body plot and (b) corresponding hand–water plot of the movement of the right hand of an elite freestyle swimmer in the propulsion phase of the stroke as seen from underneath the swimmer. d = backward displacement of the hand during the propulsion phase of the stroke; l = range of mediolateral movement of the hand during the propulsion phase of the stroke

corresponding to the hand–body plot in Figure 5.19a. The discovery of three-dimensional hand–water plots led some coaches to suggest that elite swimmers derived some propulsion from hydrodynamic lift force by asymmetric orientation of their hands to the flow of water over them (Brown & Counsilman 1971). It is now generally accepted that elite swimmers use a combination of paddle and screw propulsion (Costill et al 1992, Counsilman & Counsilman 1994).

Figure 5.20a shows a typical bottom-view right-hand–water plot of an elite breaststroke swimmer during the propulsion phase of the stroke. The hand–water plot can be described as

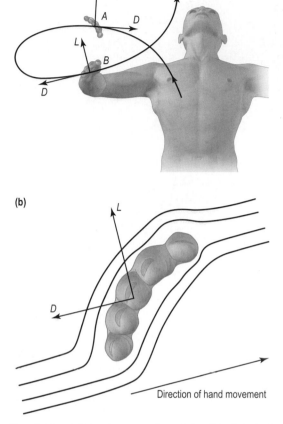

Fig. 5.20 (a) Hand–water plot of the right hand of an elite breaststroke swimmer in the propulsion phase of the stroke as seen from underneath the swimmer. (b) Angle of attack of the hand at point B in the stroke. D = drag; L = lift force

an elongated loop at right angles to the direction of body movement. Throughout the stroke, the plane of the hand maintains an angle of attack with respect to the flow of water, which results in lift force as well as drag on the hand. The hand position is shown at two points A and B in the stroke and the flow of water over the hand in position B and the associated lift force and drag are shown in Figure 5.20b.

When a swimmer's hand produces lift and drag forces, it is the resultant of the two forces that determines the effect of the hand movement on body movement. Ideally, the resultant force acting on each hand in the alternate arm

action events (freestyle and backstroke) and the resultant of the resultant forces acting on both hands in the dual arm action events (butterfly and breaststroke) would act in the intended direction of body movement. It is reasonable to assume that swimmers differ in their ability to (a) produce the most effective combination of paddle and screw propulsion and (b) direct the resultant propulsion force in the intended direction of body movement. However, it would appear that elite swimmers naturally adopt a sculling–pulling (or screw–paddle) action. The main advantage of a sculling–pulling action over a pulling action is reduced backward displacement of the hand relative to the water during the propulsion phase (d in Figure 5.19b). Consequently, stroke length (the distance moved forward by the body per stroke) is increased, which in turn increases the speed of body movement (assuming the same stroke frequency).

Propulsion from a sail

Depending on the number and distribution of sails, sailing boats utilize drag propulsion and screw propulsion. Drag propulsion is used when running with the wind, i.e. sailing with the wind blowing directly from behind. In this situation, the wind creates drag force on the sails, which pushes the boat forward (similar to the drag on an oar in Figure 5.17a). Screw propulsion is used when tacking, i.e. moving obliquely into the wind. In this situation the sails act as aerofoils and experience drag and lift force. Figure 5.21a shows a sailing dinghy with a single sail. The wind produces lift force L and drag D on the sail with resultant S. The tendency of S to move the boat in the direction of S is resisted by the reaction force P exerted by the water on the hull (Fig. 5.21b). The tendency of S_X, the transverse component of S, to move the boat sideways is resisted by P_X, the transverse component of P. P_Y, the posterior component of P is the drag force exerted by the water on the hull. The boat will move forward if S_Y, the anterior component of S, is greater than P_Y.

(a)

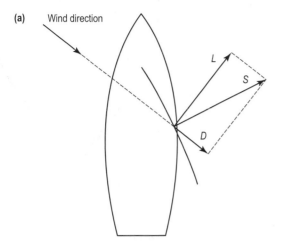

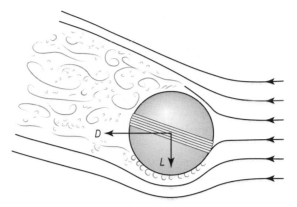

Fig. 5.22 Drag *D* and lift force *L* on a cricket ball released without spin

(b)

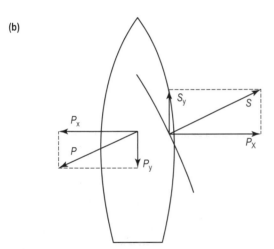

Fig. 5.21 Lift and drag forces on a sail. *L* = lift force on the sail; *D* = drag force on the sail; *S* = resultant of *L* and *D*; *P* = force exerted by the water on the hull in reaction to *S*; P_X and S_X = transverse components of *P* and *S*; P_Y and S_Y = anteroposterior components of *P* and *S*

LIFT DUE TO ASYMMETRIC SURFACE TEXTURE

When shape, orientation, relative velocity and fluid density are constant, surface texture will determine the timing of the transitions between the different types of fluid flow (laminar, partially turbulent, fully turbulent) and therefore the pressure on different parts of the surface of an object. Consequently, differences in surface texture on opposite sides of an object are likely to result in differences in pressure and therefore hydrodynamic lift force, which will tend to move the object sideways as it moves forward. This is the principle underlying the swing of a cricket ball in flight. The surface of a cricket ball consists of two leather hemispheres that are bound together around a solid core by several parallel rows of stitches that constitute the seam. In a new ball, the leather is highly polished and the seam is slightly proud of the rest of the surface. At fast bowling speed, 40 m/s–45 m/s (90 mph–100 mph), the ball can be made to swing by releasing the ball with the seam asymmetric to the linear velocity of the ball. Figure 5.22 shows an overhead view of a cricket ball projected left to right with respect to the figure. On the left side of the ball (upper part of the figure), the air flows over the uninterrupted highly polished surface. At fast bowling speed, this tends to produce partially turbulent flow with boundary layer separation close to the front of the ball and, consequently, considerable turbulence. On the right side of the ball (lower part of the figure), the seam presents a region of roughness to the air flow, which tends to produce fully turbulent flow, delayed boundary layer separation and, consequently, reduced turbulence. The different types of flow on the left and right sides of the ball are associated with differences in pressure (pressure on the left side is higher than that on the right side), which results in hydrodynamic lift force that tends to move the ball sideways from left to right. The combination of simultaneous sideways and forward movement is referred to as swing. The amount and direction of swing will be influenced by any change in the surface of the ball. Cricketers frequently polish one side of the ball and roughen the other side with moisture or grease in order to affect swing.

LIFT DUE TO SPIN

Figure 5.23 shows an overhead view of a ball with uniform surface texture projected left to right with respect to the figure and spinning clockwise about a vertical axis. The left side of the ball (upper part of the figure) is moving in the opposite direction to that of the adjacent streamlines. This results in a significant increase in the friction (relative to when the ball is not spinning) between the boundary layer and the adjacent streamlines. The increased friction results in early boundary layer separation, which is associated with an increase in pressure and a decrease in the speed of flow of air. The right side of the ball (lower part of the figure) is moving in the same direction as the adjacent streamlines. This results in a significant decrease in the friction (relative to when the ball is not spinning) between the boundary layer and the adjacent streamlines. The decreased friction delays boundary layer separation and is associated with a decrease in pressure and an increase in the speed of flow of air. The pressure differential results in hydrodynamic lift force, which tends to move the ball sideways from left to right. The production of hydrodynamic lift as a result of spin is referred to as the Magnus effect after Gustav Magnus (1802–1870).

Swing due to the Magnus effect is an important feature of many ball games, especially at the elite level. The Magnus effect can be used to produce swing in any direction, but topspin and backspin (about a horizontal axis perpendicular to the linear velocity of the ball) and sidespin (about a vertical axis perpendicular to the linear velocity of the ball) are the most common forms. Topspin produces a downward lift force (as in

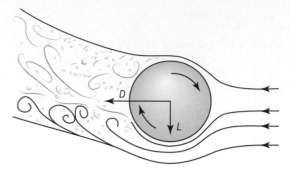

Fig. 5.23   Drag D and lift force L on a ball spinning clockwise

Figure 5.23 if the plane of the figure is assumed to be vertical) and is used in situations where the player wants to hit the ball hard but also keep the ball in court, as in tennis, or on the table, as in table-tennis. Backspin produces an upward lift force and is the key feature of drop-shots in tennis and table-tennis. Backspin is also the major feature of golf shots. The angled face of golf clubs produces considerable backspin of the ball, which, due to lift force, significantly increases the range through the air. Sidespin (as in Fig. 5.23) is also an important feature of golf shots. A shot that is intended to swing left to right (for a right-hander) is referred to as a fade. Similarly, a shot that is intended to swing right to left is referred to as a draw. Recreational golfers are more familiar with unintended shots in these directions, which are referred to as a slice and a hook respectively.

> All objects moving through fluids experience drag and they may simultaneously experience hydrodynamic lift force due to asymmetric shape, asymmetric orientation, asymmetric surface texture, spin or a combination of these influences.

EFFECT OF DRAG AND LIFT FORCE ON BALL FLIGHT

In the absence of air resistance (no drag or lift force), the trajectory of a ball when projected into the air would be a parabola, i.e. the second half of the trajectory (from maximum height to landing) would be a mirror image of the first part of the trajectory (from release to maximum height) and the only force acting on the ball would be its weight (Fig. 5.24a). If projected at the same velocity in air, without spin (and uniform surface texture), the ball would experience two forces, drag and weight, and the drag force would result in reduced range (Fig. 5.24b). If projected at the same velocity with topspin, the ball would experience three forces, drag, lift force and weight. The net effect of the three forces would be a shorter range than when projected without spin (Fig. 5.24c). If projected at the same velocity with backspin, the ball would experience three forces, drag, lift force and weight, but the lift force would

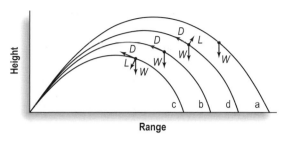

Fig. 5.24   Effect of drag and lift force on the trajectory of ball flight. (a) No air resistance. (b) Air resistance, no spin. (c) Air resistance and topspin. (d) Air resistance and backspin. W = weight of ball; D = drag; L = lift force

be in the opposite direction to that of topspin. The net effect of the three forces would be a longer range than when projected without spin (Fig. 5.24d).

REVIEW QUESTIONS

1. Define the following terms: atmospheric pressure, hydrostatic pressure, fluid, Archimedes' principle, buoyancy force, centre of buoyancy, specific gravity, viscosity, boundary layer, drag, viscous drag, pressure drag, slipstreaming, paddle propulsion, Bernoulli's principle, hydrodynamic lift force, screw propulsion, Magnus effect.

2. When fully inflated, a balloon used to provide overhead views at televised golf tournaments has a volume of 1000 m³. Calculate the maximum load that the balloon can carry in order to be able to float if the weight of the balloon envelope W_E = 50 kgf, the weight density of air outside the balloon ρ_o = 1.25 kgf/m³ and the weight density of hot air inside the balloon ρ_i = 1.10 kg/m³.

3. If the density of sea water ρ_w = 1025 kg/m³, what is the weight of a boat that floats with 1.5 m³ of its hull submerged?

4. In freestyle swimming events each swimmer dives into the water and then glides underwater for a short distance before rising to the surface and starting to swim. During the glide, each swimmer tries to adopt a streamlined position (fully extended body in line with the linear velocity of the swimmer) in order to minimize drag.
   i. Calculate the viscous drag and pressure drag on a swimmer during the glide (assume no change in body position) if the linear velocity of the swimmer v = 3.5 m/s, viscosity of water η = 0.010 02 Pl, density of water ρ = 1000 kg/m³, body surface area A_S = 1.8 m², velocity gradient v/h = 1.75/s, coefficient of drag C_D = 0.2, profile area A_P = 0.06 m².
   ii. Calculate the instantaneous deceleration of the swimmer if the mass of the swimmer m = 70 kg.

5. i. Calculate the viscous drag and pressure drag on a soccer ball moving through the air if the linear velocity of the ball v = 22.35 m/s (50 mph), viscosity of air η = 0.000 18 Pl, density of air ρ = 1.25 kg/m³, surface area of the ball A_S = 0.152 m², velocity gradient v/h = 2/s, coefficient of drag C_D = 0.2, profile area A_P = 0.04 m².
   ii. Calculate the instantaneous deceleration of the ball if the mass of the ball m = 0.45 kg.

6. Calculate the theoretical terminal velocity of a two-man bobsleigh sliding down a consistent slope of 5° with no turns if the combined mass of the bobsleigh and two-man team $m = 390\,kg$, the coefficient of sliding friction between the sleigh and the slope $\mu = 0.03$, coefficient of drag of the sleigh $C_D = 0.45$, profile area of the sleigh $A = 0.413\,m^2$, density of air $\rho = 1.25\,kg/m^3$.

7. Following a free kick in soccer, if the ball moves through the air with sidespin that results in a 0.1% difference in atmospheric pressure on the opposite sides of the ball, calculate the distance that the ball swings sideways during a flight of 1 s if the mass of the ball $m = 0.45\,kg$ and the radius of the ball $r = 0.11\,m$.

References

Alexander R M 1968 Animal mechanics. Sidgwick & Jackson, London

Armenti A 1984 How can a downhill skier move faster than a sky diver? Physics Teacher 22: 109–111

Barthels K 1977 Swimming biomechanics: resistance and propulsion. Swimming Technique 14(3): 66–70

Brancazio P J 1984 Sport science: physical laws and optimum performance. Simon & Schuster, New York

Brown R M, Councilman J E 1971 The role of lift in propelling the swimmer. In Cooper J M (ed) Selected topics in biomechanics. The Athletic Institute, Chicago, IL, p 179–190

Clugston M J 1998 The Penguin dictionary of science. Penguin, Harmondsworth

Counsilman J E, Counsilman B E 1994 The new science of swimming. Prentice-Hall, Englewood Cliffs, NJ

Corlett G 1980 swimming teaching, theory and practice. Kaye & Ward, London

Costill D L, Maglischo E W, Richardson A B 1992 Handbook of sports medicine and science in swimming. Blackwell Science, Oxford

Daish C B 1972 The physics of ball games. English University Press, London

Duke L 1999 Flight testing Newton's laws. Available on line at: http://trc.dfrc.nasa.gov/trc/ntps/index.html 12 November 1999

Filippone A 2005 Aerodynamic database: drag coefficients. Available on line at: http:// aerodyn.org/ Drag/tables.html 19 September 2005

Fuchs V 1985 (ed) Oxford illustrated encyclopedia, vol 1: the physical world. Oxford University Press, Oxford

Gagnon M, Montpetit R 1981 Technological development for the measurement of the center of volume in the human body. Journal of Biomechanics 14: 235–241

Gardner M 1993 Bernoulli's principle. Physics Teacher 31: 304

Kyle C R 1979 Reduction in wind resistance and power output of racing cyclists and runners travelling in groups. Ergonomics 22: 387–397

McArdle W D, Katch F I, Katch V L 1994 Essentials of exercise physiology. Lea & Febiger, Philadelphia, PA

Malina R M, Bouchard C 1991 Growth, maturation, and physical activity. Human Kinetics, Champaign, IL

Pickard G L, Emery W J 1995 Descriptive physical oceanography: an introduction. Butterworth-Heinemann, London

Pugh L G C E 1971 the influence of wind resistance on walking and running and the mechanical efficiency of work against horizontal or vertical forces. Journal of Physiology (London) 213: 255–276

Wagner G, Wood R 1996 Skydiver survives depth plunge. Physics Teacher 34: 543–545

Whiting H T A 1963 Variations in floating ability with age in the male. Research Quarterly 31: 84–91

Whiting H T A 1965 Variations in floating ability with age in the female. Research Quarterly 36: 216–218

Wright J 2005 Shape effects on drag. Available on line at: http://www.grc.nasa.gov/WWW/Wright/airplane/shaped.html 22 September 2005

Chapter 6

Biomechanical analysis of human movement

There are basically two methods of movement analysis, qualitative and quantitative (Hay & Reid 1982). A qualitative analysis is based on observation and results in a more or less subjective evaluation of the performance under consideration. In a quantitative analysis, performance is evaluated fairly objectively on the basis of measurements of the variables that determine performance. The purpose of this chapter is to outline the qualitative and quantitative methods.

QUALITATIVE ANALYSIS

Qualitative analysis is used in the context of teaching and coaching to provide the learner with detailed feedback in order to improve his/her performance and in the context of judging performance in order to differentiate between individuals in competitive sports such as gymnastics, diving and figure skating (Watkins 1987a).

In the context of teaching and coaching, qualitative analysis is a two-stage process, observation and instruction. The observation stage involves observing the performer in order to identify any discrepancies between the expected and actual movement pattern and to diagnose the cause of any discrepancies. The instruction stage involves providing verbal feedback to the performer and formulating appropriate exercises and/or training to improve performance. In the context of judging, qualitative analysis consists only of the observation stage.

Clearly, the ability to observe accurately is of prime importance in teaching and coaching. In order to observe accurately, it is necessary to know what to look for, i.e. the desired response. Knowing the desired response for a particular movement depends upon the knowledge and experience of the observer, in particular, the observer's ability to identify the mechanical requirements of the movement. Without a thorough understanding of the underlying mechanics, instructions to the learner are likely to be of limited value. Poor instructions tend to be of two types:

- Vague instructions such as 'jump higher' or 'run faster' that highlight obvious deficiencies but do not help the learner to improve his/her performance. The learner needs to know how to jump higher or run faster

- Instructions directed at symptoms of faulty technique rather than the causes. For example, in golf, a player who continually tops the ball may be told that her problem is lifting her head. Lifting her head may be a symptom of the problem, but the cause of the problem is lifting the clubhead, which may result, for example, from extending the hips or knees or flexing the elbows just prior to contact with the ball (Norman 1975).

SEQUENTIAL APPROACH

A teacher's or coach's desired response for a particular movement may consist of a mental checklist of the body configurations at different stages during the movement, i.e. a mental picture sequence such as that shown in Figure 6.1. This sequential approach to qualitative analysis of movement tends to focus on what the observer expects to see and is usually based on the technique of elite performers. However, it is possible for a performer to be successful in a sport without necessarily having a very good technique; other factors such as physical conditioning and motivation may compensate for an imperfect technique. A good technique is likely to result in greater consistency of performance and reduced risk of injury. An individual is unlikely to achieve full potential in a sport if s/he can occasionally perform very well but is injured most of the time because of a poor technique that overloads particular muscles or joints. Consequently, the technique of elite performers is not necessarily a good model for formulating

a desired response, especially for the purpose of teaching or coaching children.

Another major disadvantage of the sequential approach is that, while it may be possible to identify faulty technique, there is no systematic basis for diagnosing the cause of the faulty technique. For example, it may be clear that a gymnast's performance of a standing back somersault is poor because he does not achieve sufficient height and, therefore, sufficient flight time. However, the gymnast needs to know how to achieve greater height. Without a systematic basis for diagnosing the cause of faulty technique, instructions tend to be vague and/or directed at symptoms rather than causes.

MECHANICAL APPROACH

To be effective, the desired response needs to be based not only on what the observer expects to see, but also why s/he expects to see it, i.e. an expected movement pattern based on the mechanical requirements of the movement. This is referred to as the mechanical approach to qualitative analysis of movement. In a standing back somersault (Fig. 6.1), there are two main mechanical requirements at take-off: upward linear velocity to provide sufficient flight time and backward angular momentum to ensure sufficient backward rotation to complete the somersault within the flight time. Figure 6.2, referred to as a deterministic model (Hay & Reid 1982), shows these two mechanical requirements in relation to the mechanical and anthropometric factors that determine them.

Upward linear velocity at take-off will be determined by the impulse of the vertical

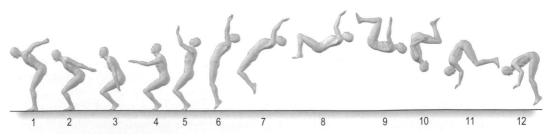

1   2   3   4   5   6   7   8   9   10   11   12

Fig. 6.1   Picture sequence of a standing back somersault

component of the resultant force acting on the gymnast during the propulsion phase. The resultant force is the resultant of the weight of the gymnast and the ground reaction force. The ground reaction force is the result of the forces exerted by the muscles of the arms, legs and trunk during the propulsion phase. The magnitude of the ground reaction force will largely depend upon the strength of the hip and knee extensors and the ankle plantar flexors; the stronger the muscles the greater the potential for developing a large ground reaction force. The duration of the propulsion phase will depend largely on the flexibility of the hips, knees and ankles and the extent to which the flexibility of these joints is utilized; the greater the flexibility and the greater the range of motion the greater the propulsion time. Whereas leg extension will produce most of the upward linear impulse, the arms can also contribute; the faster the upward swing of the arms the greater the ground

reaction force. Consequently, in order to generate upward linear momentum at take-off, the ideal movement pattern should consist of a vigorous vertical thrust involving full extension of the legs together with a vigorous upward swing of the arms culminating in a fully extended body at take-off.

Backward angular velocity during flight will depend upon the amount of angular momentum at take-off and the moment of inertia of the body about the somersault axis a_Z through the centre of gravity of the gymnast during flight; the greater the angular momentum and the smaller the moment of inertia about a_Z, the greater the average angular velocity. The moment of inertia during flight will depend upon the position of the body during flight; the tighter the tuck about a_Z, the smaller the moment of inertia and the greater the angular velocity. Angular momentum at take-off will be determined by the impulse of the moment of

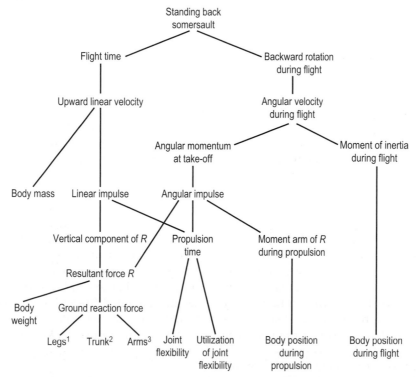

Fig. 6.2   Deterministic model of performance in a standing back somersault
[1] Ground reaction force component due to leg action during propulsion time
[2] Ground reaction force component due to trunk action during propulsion time
[3] Ground reaction force component due to arm action during propulsion time

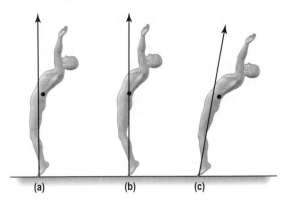

Fig. 6.3 Variation in body position and line of action of the ground reaction force at take-off in a standing back somersault

the resultant force during the propulsion phase which, in turn, will be determined by the resultant force R, the moment arm d of the resultant force about a_Z and propulsion time t. The magnitude and direction of R and the magnitude of d will vary during the propulsion phase, but, for a given propulsion time, the larger the average R and the larger the average d about a_Z, the greater the angular momentum. The magnitude and direction of R will depend largely on the magnitude and direction of the ground reaction force and the moment arm of R will depend upon the position of the body in relation to the ground reaction force. Increasing the moment arm of the ground reaction force about a_Z will tend to reduce the magnitude of the ground reaction force and vice versa, i.e. it is physically impossible to maximize both the ground reaction force and the moment of the ground reaction force (emphasizing one will reduce the other). Consequently, good performance involves a compromise between the generation of upward linear momentum and backward angular momentum. This is achieved by a vertical thrust involving whole body extension and a slight backward lean of the upper body in order to create a moment arm about a_Z (Fig. 6.3a). If the body is too upright during propulsion, the moment arm of the ground reaction about a_Z will be close to zero and result in little or no backward angular momentum (Fig. 6.3b). If the ground reaction force is inclined backward prior to take-off, as

in Figure 6.3c, the body will travel backward during flight and land some distance behind the take-off point.

The basic principles of generating linear and angular momentum, as described in the above example, are the same for all movements. The mechanical approach to qualitative movement analysis is based on the application of these basic principles, whereas the sequential approach is based on memorizing a very large number of largely irrelevant body configurations.

> Qualitative analysis of movement is a two-stage process, observation and instruction. Without a systematic basis for diagnosing the cause of faulty technique, instructions tend to be vague and/or directed at symptoms rather than causes.

QUANTITATIVE ANALYSIS

Whereas qualitative analysis is based on observation, usually in real time, quantitative analysis is based on measurements of the variables that determine performance. There are two types of measurements, direct and indirect (Watkins 1987b). Direct measurements are those that determine the end result of a movement or movement sequence and include time (e.g. running, swimming, cycling, rowing) distance (e.g. jumping, throwing) and score (e.g. target sports such as darts and archery). Indirect measures are used to evaluate the sequence of movements or movement pattern that culminates in a particular end result. Measures in this category are usually obtained indirectly by analysing recordings of various aspects of the movement. For example, stride rate and stride length (obtained from video analysis) and the forces acting on the feet (obtained with the use of a force platform) may be used to evaluate the technique of a runner.

MOVEMENT SEQUENCES

In the context of quantitative analysis, a movement sequence refers to a sequence of discrete movements involving static and dynamic postures that are performed one after the other; the order in which the movements are performed may be chosen beforehand, as in gymnastics, or may be random, as in a game of soccer. Quantitative analysis of a movement sequence involves an analysis of the type, duration and frequency of the discrete movements that comprise the sequence. This kind of information can be used in a variety of ways. For example, in soccer, knowledge of the types of movement exhibited (e.g. jogging, sprinting, jumping) and the duration and frequency of the movements will help the coach to structure specific physical conditioning training programmes for different playing positions. The information on type, duration and frequency of movements can be obtained from video of individual players over several games (Reilly & Thomas 1976). Similarly, in tennis, knowledge of the type of strokes and the success rate of the strokes exhibited by an individual player will help the coach to plan future practice sessions (Morrison et al 1978).

MOVEMENT PATTERNS

In the context of quantitative analysis, a movement pattern refers to the way that the body as a whole moves in relation to its spatial environment (the movement of the whole body centre of gravity) and the way that the body segments move in relation to each other. Quantitative analysis of a movement pattern involves a kinematic and/or kinetic analysis of the movement.

> Quantitative analysis of movement is based on direct measurements that determine the end result and indirect measurements that are used to evaluate the sequence of movements or movement pattern that culminates in the end result.

Kinematic analysis of whole body movement

A kinematic analysis of the movement of the body as a whole in a particular activity would involve a description of the displacement, velocity and acceleration of the whole-body centre of gravity during the movement. The kinematic analysis of a 100 m sprint in Chapter 2 is an example of this type of analysis. Whereas the displacement–time and acceleration–time histories of the movement of the whole body centre of gravity are likely to provide useful information for the teacher or coach, most attention is usually directed at the velocity–time history of the movement of the centre of gravity, especially in sports where time is the determinant of performance. This category includes all sports that are based on the different forms of human locomotion, such as running and swimming. In all these sports, movement is cyclic, i.e. based on repetition of a movement pattern. For example, in swimming, speed of movement V of the body as a whole is the product of stroke length SL (the distance that the centre of gravity moves forward per stroke) and stroke frequency SF (the number of strokes per unit of time), i.e. $V = SL \times SF$.

Figure 6.4 shows the change in speed and the corresponding changes in stroke length and stroke frequency for a swimmer in a 200 m freestyle race. The data used to produce Figure 6.4 were obtained from video analysis. For each 50 m length, the stroking distance d, stroking time t and number of strokes n were recorded and were used to calculate average stroking speed (d/t) average stroke length (d/n) and average stroke frequency (n/t). The average stroking speed V shows a steady decline throughout the race. This decline could have been due to a decline in SL, SF or both. However, it is clear that the decline in V was almost entirely due to a steady decline in SL, with SF staying fairly constant throughout the race. This relationship between V, SL and SF is fairly typical of the performance of elite swimmers in all events and highlights the importance of SL (Counsilman & Counsilman 1994). Craig et al (1985) compared the velocity, stroke length, stroke frequency relationships of swimmers in all events at the 1976 and 1984 US Olympic trials and concluded that improvements in performance between 1976 and 1984 were almost entirely due to increased stroke length.

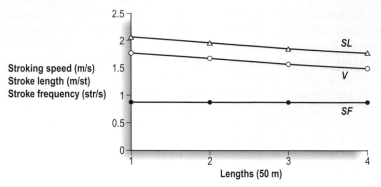

Fig. 6.4   Stroking speed *V*, stroke length *SL* and stroke frequency *SF* of a swimmer in a 200 m freestyle race

Kinematic analysis of the movement of body segments

The most widely used and well documented method of obtaining kinematic information on the movement of body segments is analysis of film or video. The video is projected one frame at a time and the positions of the body segments are recorded in terms of the X and Y coordinates of various points on the body with respect to an appropriate reference origin. Reference distances in the X and Y directions are also recorded so that distances on the image can be converted to actual distances for the purpose of calculating velocity and acceleration data. Other reference points may also be recorded, such as the positions of the reuther board and vaulting horse when analysing the performance of a vault in gymnastics. The points recorded for each frame of video comprise the spatial model and the number of points in the spatial model is determined prior to analysis. The points in the spatial model that define the body segments are usually the main joint centres. The process of recording the X and Y coordinates of the points in the spatial model in computer-based video analysis systems is referred to as digitization. The X–Y coordinate data can be used in a variety of ways, in particular, representation of the movement of the body in the form of a stick figure and the calculation of linear kinematics (e.g. the movement of the whole-body centre of gravity) and angular kinematics (e.g. angular movement of particular body segments).

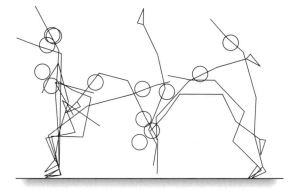

Fig. 6.5   Stick figure sequence of a standing flic-flac on a fixed frame of reference

Stick-figure sequence

Figure 6.5 shows a stick-figure sequence of a standing flic-flac presented on a fixed frame of reference, i.e. with respect to the same origin. This method produces a set of overlapping images that may be difficult to interpret if too many images are presented. This problem can be overcome by presenting the images on a displaced frame of reference, i.e. the images are displaced horizontally by a fixed amount to produce one or more rows of images so that the change in body position between images can be more clearly seen. Figure 6.6 shows the same sequence as in Figure 6.5 presented on a displaced frame of reference.

Angular kinematics

Figure 6.7 shows a stick-figure sequence of a place kick in rugby presented on a displaced frame of reference together with the corresponding hip angle–time and knee angle–time graphs. The graphs show two distinct phases, the backswing of the leg (frames 5–12), which involves simultaneous hip extension and knee flexion, followed by the kicking action (frames 12–22), which involves simultaneous hip flexion and knee extension.

Centre of gravity

Figure 6.8 shows the change in the position of the whole-body centre of gravity during the hand–ground contact phase of the flic-flac shown in Figures 6.5 and 6.6. The vertical displacement of the centre of gravity is minimal and similar to the movement of the axle of a wheel rolling along the ground. This indicates minimal work done in moving the centre of

gravity during the ground contact phase and, therefore, good technique. Poor technique would be characterized by the centre of gravity moving downward during the first part of ground contact (eccentric muscle activity) and upward during the second part of ground contact (concentric muscle activity).

A MODEL OF MOVEMENT ANALYSIS

Kinematic data obtained by the above methods can be combined with the corresponding ground

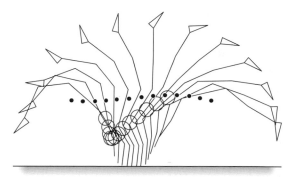

Fig. 6.8   Change in position of the whole-body centre of gravity during the hand–ground contact phase in a standing flic-flac on a displaced frame of reference

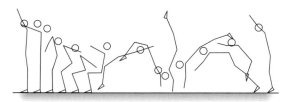

Fig. 6.6   Stick figure sequence of a standing flic-flac on a displaced frame of reference

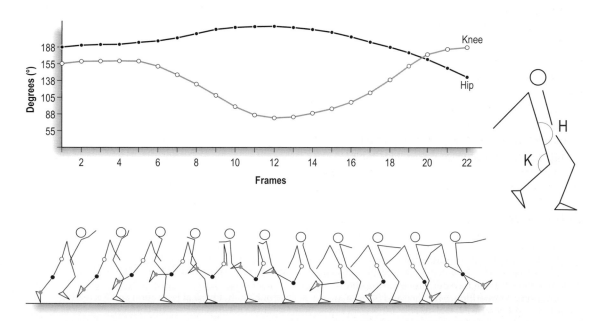

Fig. 6.7   Hip and knee angular displacement–time graphs for the kicking leg in a place kick in rugby

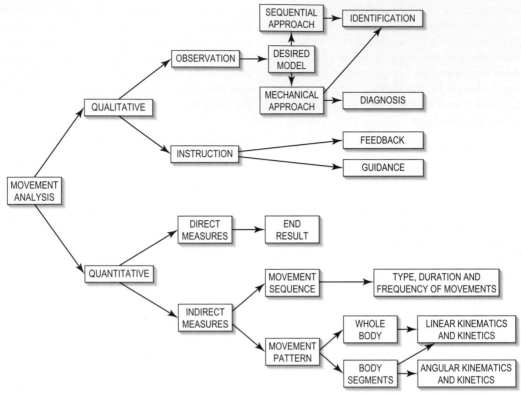

Fig. 6.9 A model of movement analysis

reaction and other external force records to carry out a kinetic analysis of performance, in particular, the muscle moments about the joints that are responsible for the observed kinematics. However, this is beyond the scope of the book. Figure 6.9 summarizes the qualitative and quantitative approaches to movement analysis.

REVIEW QUESTION

1. Define the following terms: qualitative analysis of movement, quantitative analysis of movement, desired response, sequential approach, deterministic model, mechanical approach.

References

Counsilman J E, Counsilman B E 1994 The new science of swimming. Prentice-Hall, Englewood Cliffs, NJ

Craig A B, Skehan P L, Pawelczyk J A et al 1985 Velocity, stroke rate and distance per stroke during elite swimming competition. Medicine and Science in Sports and Exercise 17: 625–634

Hay J G, Reid J G 1982 Anatomy, mechanics and human motion. Prentice-Hall, Englewood Cliffs, NJ

Morrison S, Morgan J C, Heaton D A et al 1978 Tennis: analysing play for coaching. New Zealand Journal of Health, Physical Education and Recreation 11(3): 104–106

Norman R W 1975 Biomechanics for the community coach. Journal of Health, Physical Education and Recreation 46(3): 49–52

Reilly T, Thomas V 1976 A motion analysis of work rate in different positional roles in professional football match play. Journal of Human Movement Studies 2: 87–97

Watkins J 1987a Qualitative movement analysis. British Journal of Physical Education 18: 177–179

Watkins J 1987b Quantitative movement analysis. British Journal of Physical Education 18: 271–275

Practical Worksheet 1

Linear kinematic analysis of a 15 m sprint

Objective

To record the 5 m split times during a 15 m sprint and use the distance–time data to produce the distance–time, speed–time and acceleration–time graphs of the sprint.

Location

Indoor or outdoor area with minimum length of 30 m.

Apparatus and equipment

Four sets of photo cells linked to a timer.

Method

Subject's clothing and footwear
Sports clothing and trainers.

Layout of equipment
The four sets of photo cells are arranged as in Figure PW1.1. Each set of photo cells is placed approximately 3 m apart at each side of the running track. The photo cells are mounted on tripods at a height of about 1 m. One set of photo cells is located at the start, with the other sets located 5 m, 10 m and 15 m from the start line.

Data collection
1. Using a standing start from 1 m behind the start line (so that the first set of photo cells will start the timer as you run between them), perform three maximum effort trials and record the 5 m, 10 m and 15 m times for each trial in Table PW1.1.

2. Plot the distance–time data (distance on the vertical axis and time on the horizontal axis) of your fastest trial on centimetre squared graph paper and draw a smooth curve through the origin and the three data points to produce the distance–time graph. If necessary, extend the

Fig. PW1.1
Location of photo cells (A, B, C, D) for Practical Worksheet 1

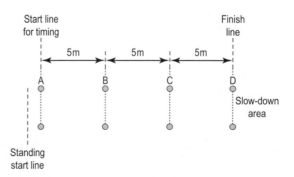

graph beyond the 3 s point on the time axis. It is suggested that a scale of 1 cm on the graph paper = 1 m for the distance axis and a scale of 5 cm on the graph paper = 1 s for the time axis.

3. From the distance–time graph, read the distance at 1, 2 and 3 s after the start and record these data in the second column of Table PW1.2.

4. Calculate and record in the third column of Table PW1.2 the change in distance during each of the three 1 s intervals.

5. Record the average speed in each of the three one-second intervals in the fourth column of Table PW1.2 (same numbers as in column 3).

6. Plot the average speed–time data (column 4 of Table PW1.2) on the same sheet of graph paper, choosing an appropriate scale for speed (vertical axis). It is suggested that a scale of 2 cm on the graph paper = 1 m/s for the speed axis. Since the data represent average speed, plot the data at the midpoints of the corresponding time intervals.

7. Draw a smooth curve through the origin and the three data points to produce the speed–time graph. If necessary, extend the graph beyond the 3 s point on the time axis.

8. From the speed–time graph, read the speed at 1, 2 and 3 s after the start and record these data in the second column of Table PW1.3.

Table PW1.1
5 m, 10 m and 15 m
times (s) in three
maximum effort
trials

Distance (m)	Trial 1	Trial 2	Trial 3
5			
10			
15			

Table PW1.2
Average speed

Time interval (s)	Distance (m)	Change in distance (m)	Average speed (m/s)
1			
2			
3			

Table PW1.3
Average acceleration

Time interval (s)	Speed (m/s)	Change in speed (m/s)	Average acceleration (m/s^2)
1			
2			
3			

9. Calculate and record in the third column of Table PW1.3 the change in speed during each of the three 1 s intervals.

10. Record the average acceleration in each of the three 1 s intervals in the fourth column of Table PW1.3 (same numbers as in column 3).

11. Using the same axis and scale for acceleration as that used for speed, plot the average acceleration–time data (column 4 of Table PW1.3) on the same sheet of graph paper. Since the data represent average acceleration, plot the data at the midpoints of the corresponding time intervals.

12. Draw a smooth curve through the origin and the three data points to produce the acceleration–time graph.

Example results

Example data are shown in Tables PW1.4–PW1.6. The distance–time, speed–time and acceleration–time graphs based on the data in Tables PW1.4–PW1.6 are shown as Figure PW1.2. The speed–time graph indicates that speed continued to increase throughout the trial. This is clearly reflected in the progressive increase in the slope of the distance–time graph over the corresponding period. Whereas speed continued to increase throughout the trial, the slope of the speed–time graph progressively decreased, i.e. acceleration was always positive but decreasing. This is clearly reflected in the acceleration–time graph.

Table PW1.4
5 m, 10 m and 15 m times (s) in three maximum effort trials

Distance (m)	Trial 1	Trial 2	Trial 3
5	1.33	1.35	1.32
10	2.22	2.11	2.12
15	3.25	3.01	2.83

Table PW1.5
Average speed

Time (s)	Distance (m/s)	Change in distance (m/s)	Average speed (m/s)
1	3.45	3.45	3.45
2	9.25	5.80	5.80
3	16.25	7.00	7.00

Table PW1.6
Average acceleration

Time interval (s)	Speed (m/s)	Change in speed (m/s)	Average acceleration (m/s^2)
1	4.875	4.875	4.875
2	6.45	1.575	1.575
3	7.50	1.05	1.05

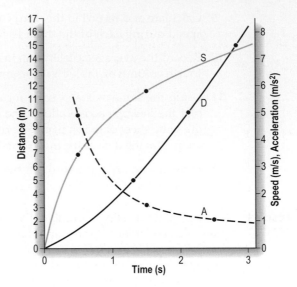

Fig. PW1.2
Distance–time (*D*),
speed–time (*S*) and
acceleration–time (*A*)
graphs based on the
data in Tables
PW1.4–PW1.6

Practical Worksheet 2

The effect of increase in speed on stride length, stride rate and relative stride length

Objective

To obtain stride length, stride rate and relative stride length data for subjects running on a treadmill over a speed range of 1.5–3.5 m/s and to produce the corresponding stride length–speed, stride rate–speed and relative stride length–speed graphs.

Location

Motion analysis laboratory.

Apparatus and equipment

Variable speed treadmill with handrails, stop watches, steel tape.

Method

Subject's clothing and footwear
Sports clothing and trainers.

Data collection
Height of subject
The subject's height is measured (m) with the subject standing upright without shoes and looking straight ahead. The height is recorded in Table PW2.1 (results sheet).

Leg length
1. The subject lies supine with legs straight and together.
2. The subject relaxes legs so that legs rest naturally with feet turned out.
3. The length of each leg is measured with a steel tape; this is the distance between the anterior superior iliac spine and medial malleolus.
4. The subject's average leg length is recorded in Table PW2.1.

Time measurements
1. For each subject, in a single trial, the time for 10 complete stride cycles at speeds of 1.5 m/s, 2.5 m/s and 3.5 m/s is measured and recorded in Table PW2.1.
2. At the start of each trial, the subject stands on the treadmill with hands on the handrails. The speed of the treadmill is gradually increased to 1.5 m/s (moderate walking pace) as the subject accommodates to the increase in speed.
3. After the subject has settled into a natural rhythm at a speed of 1.5 m/s, the time (s) for 10 complete stride cycles is measured using a stop watch (heel strike to heel strike of the same foot). The time for 10 complete stride cycles can be measured by any number of timers with the average

time being recorded in Table PW2.1. (For example, the class can be divided into groups of six people with each member of a group taking turns as subject, treadmill operator and timer).

4. After the time for 10 complete stride cycles at a speed of 1.5 m/s has been measured, the speed of the treadmill is gradually increased to 2.5 m/s (slow jog). After the subject has settled into a natural rhythm at a speed of 2.5 m/s, the time (s) for 10 complete stride cycles is measured and recorded in Table PW2.1.

5. The speed of the treadmill is then gradually increased to 3.5 m/s (moderate running pace) and the time for 10 complete stride cycles is measured as before and recorded in Table PW2.1. The speed of the treadmill is then gradually reduced to zero.

6. After the times for 10 complete stride cycles at all three speeds have been recorded, the stride rate, stride length, relative stride length (height) and relative stride length (leg length) are calculated for each speed as follows:

$$\text{Stride rate (SR)} = \frac{10 \text{ cycles}}{t}$$

where t = time for 10 complete stride cycles.

Example: If t = 9.56 s at a speed of 1.5 m/s, then

$$\text{SR} = \frac{10 \text{ cycles}}{9.56 \text{ s}} = 1.046 \text{ Hz}$$

$$\text{Stride length (SL)} = \frac{\text{Speed}}{\text{SR}}$$

Example: If SR = 1.046 Hz at a speed of 1.5 m/s, then

$$\text{SL} = \frac{1.5 \text{ m/s}}{1.046 \text{ Hz}} = 1.434 \text{ m/stride}$$

$$\text{Relative stride length with respect to height (RH)} = \frac{\text{SL}}{\text{H}}$$

Example: If SL = 1.434 m/stride and H = 1.694 m, then RH = 0.846.

$$\text{Relative stride length with respect to leg length (RL)} = \frac{\text{SL}}{\text{L}}$$

Example: If SL = 1.434 m/stride and L = 0.90 m, then RL = 1.593.

Presentation of results

1. Present a results table showing individual and group (mean and SD) results for the subjects in your group. Show the results for females and males separately, i.e. list the subjects as two groups.

2. Present two sets of graphs of the results:
   i. Group mean results for stride rate and stride length (females and males separately)

Table PW2.1 Individual and group results for height, leg length, stride rate, stride length and relative stride length

Subject	H (m)	L (m)	1.5 m/s					2.5 m/s					3.5 m/s				
			Time (s)	SR (Hz)	SL (m/str)	RSL:H (SL/H)	RSL:L (SL/L)	Time (s)	SR (Hz)	SL (m/str)	RSL:H (SL/H)	RSL:L (SL/L)	Time (s)	SR (Hz)	SL (m/str)	RSL:H (SL/H)	RSL:L (SL/L)
Females																	
1																	
2																	
3																	
4																	
5																	
6																	
Mean																	
SD																	
Males																	
1																	
2																	
3																	
4																	
5																	
6																	
Mean																	
SD																	

H = height; L = average leg length; m/str = metres per stride.

Vertical axis: stride rate (Hz) and stride length (m/stride)

Horizontal axis: speed (m/s).

ii. Group mean results for relative stride length (females and males separately)

Vertical axis: relative stride length

Horizontal axis: speed (m/s).

NB: The unit of relative stride length is 'heights per stride' (length of stride as a proportion of the subject's height) for RH and 'leg lengths per stride' (length of stride as a proportion of the subject's average leg length) for RL.

Example results

Example data (obtained in an actual practical session with students) are shown in Table PW2.2. The corresponding group mean graphs for stride length–speed, stride rate–speed and relative stride length–speed are shown in Figure PW2.1. As in the study by Elliot & Blanksby (1979), Figure PW2.1 shows that (a) the females had a shorter average stride length and a higher average stride rate than the males at each of the three speeds and (b) the average relative stride length (with respect to height and leg length) at each speed was very similar for both groups.

Reference

Elliot B C, Blanksby B A 1979 Optimal stride length considerations for male and female recreational runners. British Journal of Sports Medicine 13: 15–18

Table PW2.2   Individual and group results for height, leg length, stride rate, stride length and relative stride length

Subject	H (m)	L (m)	1.5 m/s Time (s)	SR (Hz)	SL (m/str)	RSL:H (SL/H)	RSL:L (SL/L)	2.5 m/s Time (s)	SR (Hz)	SL (m/str)	RSL:H (SL/H)	RSL:L (SL/L)	3.5 m/s Time (s)	SR (Hz)	SL (m/str)	RSL:H (SL/H)	RSL:L (SL/L)
Females																	
1 Laura	1.652	0.89	10.35	0.97	1.55	0.94	1.74	7.8	1.28	1.95	1.18	2.19	7.1	1.4085	2.49	1.51	2.8
2 Georgina	1.694	0.9	9.56	1.05	1.43	0.84	1.59	7.66	1.31	1.91	1.13	2.12	7.09	1.4104	2.48	1.46	2.76
3 Sam	1.615	0.81	10.4	0.96	1.56	0.97	1.93	7.6	1.32	1.89	1.17	2.33	7.19	1.3908	2.52	1.56	3.11
4 Carly	1.647	0.875	9.46	1.06	1.42	0.86	1.62	6.97	1.43	1.75	1.06	2	6.47	1.5456	2.26	1.37	2.58
5 Sarah	1.681	0.91	10.31	0.97	1.55	0.92	1.7	7.53	1.33	1.88	1.12	2.07	6.69	1.4948	2.34	1.39	2.57
6 Amanda	1.65	0.87	9.5	1.05	1.43	0.87	1.64	7	1.43	1.75	1.06	2.01	6	1.6667	2.1	1.27	2.41
Mean	1.657	0.876	9.93	1.01	1.49	0.9	1.7	7.43	1.35	1.86	1.12	2.12	6.76	1.49	2.37	1.43	2.71
SD	0.03	0.04	0.47	0.05	0.07	0.05	0.12	0.35	0.06	0.08	0.05	0.12	0.46	0.11	0.16	0.1	0.24
Males																	
1 Lewis	1.852	0.96	11.04	0.91	1.65	0.89	1.72	8.13	1.23	2.03	1.1	2.11	7.6	1.3158	2.66	1.44	2.77
2 Neil	1.831	0.955	11	0.91	1.65	0.9	1.73	8.	1.18	2.12	1.16	2.22	8.09	1.2361	2.83	1.55	2.96
3 Andy	1.807	0.85	10.63	0.94	1.6	0.89	1.88	7.84	1.28	1.95	1.08	2.29	7.63	1.3106	2.67	1.48	3.14
4 Rhys	1.688	0.887	10.94	0.91	1.65	0.98	1.86	8.16	1.23	2.03	1.2	2.29	7.47	1.3387	2.61	1.55	2.94
5 Matt	1.885	0.983	10.5	0.95	1.58	0.84	1.61	7.87	1.27	1.97	1.05	2	7.53	1.328	2.64	1.4	2.69
6 Mark	1.806	0.965	10.15	0.99	1.52	0.84	1.58	7.62	1.31	1.91	1.06	1.98	7.15	1.3986	2.5	1.38	2.59
Mean	1.8115	0.9333	10.71	0.94	1.61	0.89	1.73	8.02	1.25	2	1.11	2.15	7.58	1.32	2.65	1.47	2.85
SD	0.07	0.05	0.35	0.03	0.05	0.05	0.12	0.31	0.05	0.07	0.06	0.14	0.3	0.05	0.11	0.07	0.2

H = height; L = average leg length; m/str = metres per stride.

Fig. PW2.1
(a) Group mean results for males (M) and females (F) for stride rate (SR) and stride length (SL). (b) Group mean results for males (M) and females (F) for relative stride length for height (H) and leg length (L).

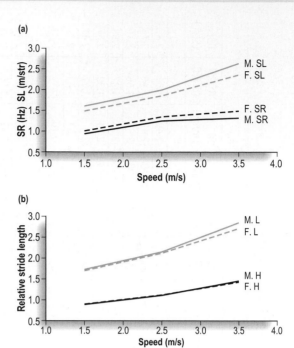

Practical Worksheet **3**

Force–time analysis of ground reaction force in running

Objective

To (i) record the anteroposterior (F_x) and vertical (F_y) components of the ground reaction force acting on a runner during ground contact when running at a moderate pace and (ii) perform a force–time analysis of the F_y–time graph.

Location

Biomechanics laboratory.

Apparatus and equipment

Force platform system.

Method

Subject's clothing and footwear
Sports clothing and trainers.

Data collection
Measurement of subject's mass
1. Subject's mass (kg) is measured with subject standing upright without shoes.
2. Record the mass of the subject in Table PW3.1.
3. Calculate and record the weight (N) of the subject in Table PW3.1.

Record the ground reaction force–time components during contact time of the right foot
1. On signal from the system operator, the subject runs across the force plate at a moderate speed, making sure that only the right foot contacts the force plate.
2. The operator prints the anteroposterior (F_x) and vertical (F_y) force–time components of the ground reaction force acting on the right foot during contact with the force plate. The time of contact of the right foot with the force plate is referred to as contact time.

Analysis of the F_y–time graph
1. From the F_y–time graph, estimate the forces (N) and times (s) corresponding to the variables listed 1–5 in Table PW3.1. Record these forces and times in Table PW3.1.
2. Calculate the forces in units of body weight and record the forces in Table PW3.1.

Table PW3.1
Analysis of the
vertical component
(F_y–time) of the
ground reaction force
acting on the right
foot of a subject
during contact time
in running

Name of subject			
		Mass (kg)	Weight (N)
Mass of subject			
Key points on F_y–time graph	Time (s)	Force (N)	Force (BW)
1. Heel contact (t_1, F_{y1})		0	0
2. Impact force peak IFP (t_2, F_{y2})			
3. End of the passive phase (minimum force following IFP) (t_3, F_{y3})			
4. End of absorption phase (t_4, F_{y4}) (when $F_x = 0$)			
5. Toe-off (t_5, F_{y5})		0	0
	Time (s)	Proportion of contact time (%)	
6. Contact time ($t_5 - t_1$)		100	
7. Time to IFP ($t_2 - t_1$)			
8. Duration of passive phase ($t_3 - t_1$)			
9. Duration of absorption phase ($t_4 - t_1$)			
10. Duration of propulsion phase ($t_5 - t_4$)			
	L_R (N/s)	L_R (BW/s)	
Rate of loading (L_R) during impact ($F_{y2}/(t_2 - t_1)$)			

3. Using the time data in Table PW3.1 for points 1–5, calculate and record the time variables 6–10 in Table PW3.1.
4. Calculate and record in Table PW3.1 the rate of loading (L_R) during impact in N/s and BW/s.

Presentation of results

Your submission should consist of:

1. A labelled figure (using the original print provided by the operator) showing the F_x and F_y force–time graphs.
2. A table showing the results of the analysis of the F_y–time graph, i.e. a completed copy of Table PW3.1.

Example results

An example print of F_x and F_y force–time graphs is shown in Figure PW3.1. The force–time analysis of the F_y–time graph in Figure PW3.1 is shown in Table PW3.2.

Fig. PW3.1
Anteroposterior (F_x)
and vertical (F_y)
components of the
ground reaction force
acting on a runner
during ground contact
when running at
approximately 3.5 m/s

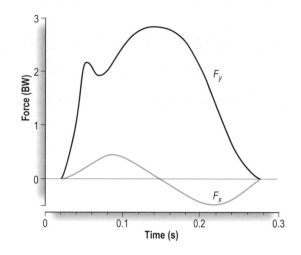

Table PW3.2
Analysis of the
vertical component
(F_y–time) of the
ground reaction force
acting on the right
foot of a subject
during contact time
in running

Name of subject			
	Mass (kg)	Weight (N)	
Mass of subject	75.3	738.7	
Key points on F_y–time graph	Time (s)	Force (N)	Force (BW)
1. Heel contact (t_1, F_{y1})	0.02	0	0
2. Impact force peak IFP (t_2, F_{y2})	0.055	1605.93	2.174
3. End of the passive phase (minimum force following IFP) (t_3, F_{y3})	0.069	1419.0	1.921
4. End of absorption phase (t_4, F_{y4}) (when $F_x = 0$)	0.148	2086.09	2.824
5. Toe-off (t_5, F_{y5})	0.276	0	0
	Time (s)	Proportion of contact time (%)	
6. Contact time ($t_5 - t_1$)	0.256	100	
7. Time to IFP ($t_2 - t_1$)	0.035	13.67	
8. Duration of passive phase ($t_3 - t_1$)	0.049	17.75	
9. Duration of absorption phase ($t_4 - t_1$)	0.128	50.0	
10. Duration of propulsion phase ($t_5 - t_4$)	0.128	50.0	
	L_R (N/s)	L_R (BW/s)	
Rate of loading (L_R) during impact ($F_{y2}/(t_2 - t_1)$)	45 883.4	62.11	

Practical Worksheet 4

Determination of the position of the whole-body centre of gravity by the direct method using a one-dimension reaction board

Objectives
1. To determine the position of the whole-body centre of gravity in the anatomical position.
2. To examine the effect of changes in body shape on the position of the whole-body centre of gravity relative to the anatomical position.

Location
Motion analysis laboratory.

Apparatus and equipment
One-dimension reaction board (approximately $2.5 \times 0.5\,m$) with a centi-metre scale running left to right on one side.
One set of weighing scales.

Method
Subject's clothing
Shorts and shirt.

Data collection
1. Record the height h (cm) without shoes and weight W (kgf) of the subject in Table PW4.1.
2. Record in Table PW4.1 the distance l between the knife-edge supports.
3. Support the reaction board in a horizontal position with knife-edge support B resting on the weighing scales (Fig. PW4.1a).
4. Record in Table PW4.1 the vertical force S_1 (kgf) exerted on the scales, i.e. the vertical support force acting on knife-edge support B.
5. Position 1: anatomical reference position:
   a. Subject lies on the board with arms by sides and soles of feet in the same plane as knife-edge support A (Fig. PW4.1b)
   b. Record in Table PW4.2 the force S_2 on the scales

Table PW4.1
Height and weight of subject, distance between knife-edge supports and initial load on knife-edge support B

Name of subject:	
Weight W (kgf)	
Height h (cm)	
l (cm)	
S_1 (kgf)	

Fig. PW4.1
(a) Reaction board without the subject.
(b) Subject lying on the reaction board in position 1

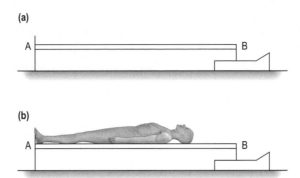

Table PW4.2
Individual results for d in the six positions and change in d in positions 2–6 with respect to position 1

Body position	S_2 (kgf)	d (cm)	d (% of h)	Δd (cm)*	Δd (% of h)
1	0	0			
2					
3					
4					
5					
6					

*Change in d with respect to position 1

    c. Calculate the horizontal distance d (cm) between knife-edge support A and the parallel vertical plane containing the whole-body centre of gravity of the subject using:

$$d = \frac{l(S_2 - S_1)}{W}$$

    Eq. PW4.1

    d. Calculate d as a percentage of h and record the result in Table PW4.2.

6. Position 2: From position 1, fold arms across chest (Fig. PW4.2):
    a. Record S_2 in Table PW4.2
    b. Calculate d (cm) using equation PW4.1 and record the result in Table PW4.2
    c. Calculate d as a percentage of h and record the result in Table PW4.2
    d. Calculate the change in d (Δd, cm) between positions 1 and 2 and record the result in Table PW4.2
    e. Calculate Δd as a percentage of h and record the result in Table PW4.2.

7. Position 3: From position 1, fully abduct both arms (Fig. PW4.2):
    a. Record S_2 in Table PW4.2
    b. Calculate d (cm) using equation PW4.1 and record the result in Table PW4.2
    c. Calculate d as a percentage of h
    d. Calculate Δd between positions 1 and 3 and record the result in Table PW4.2
    e. Calculate Δd as a percentage of h and record the result in Table PW4.2.

Fig. PW4.2
Positions 2, 3, 4, 5 and
6 of the subject

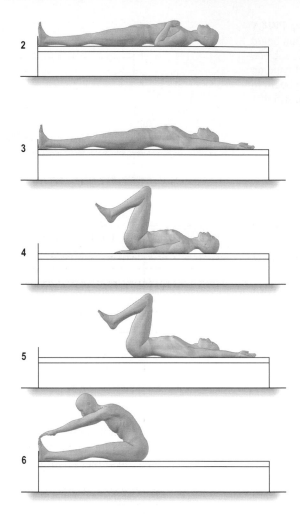

8. Position 4: From position 1, fully flex hips and knees (Fig. PW4.2):
   a. Record S_2 in Table PW4.2
   b. Calculate d (cm) using equation PW4.1 and record the result in Table PW4.2
   c. Calculate d as a percentage of h
   d. Calculate Δd between positions 1 and 4 and record the result in Table PW4.2
   e. Calculate Δd as a percentage of h and record the result in Table PW4.2.
9. Position 5: From position 1, fully abduct both arms and fully flex hips and knees (Fig. PW4.2):
   a. Record S_2 in Table PW4.2
   b. Calculate d (cm) using equation PW4.1 and record the result in Table PW4.2
   c. Calculate d as a percentage of h
   d. Calculate Δd between positions 1 and 5 and record the result in Table PW4.2
   e. Calculate Δd as a percentage of h and record the result in Table PW4.2.

Table PW4.3   Individual and group results for d and change in d with respect to position 1

Subjects	h (cm)	W (kgf)	Position 1		Position 2		Position 3		Position 4		Position 5		Position 6	
			$d\%$	$\Delta d\%$	$d\%$	$\Delta d\%$	$d\%$	$\Delta d\%$	$d\%$	$\Delta d\%$	$d\%$	$\Delta d\%$	$d\%$	$\Delta d\%$
Women														
1														
2														
3														
4														
5														
Mean														
SD														
Men														
1														
2														
3														
4														
5														
Mean														
SD														

$d\% = d$ as a percentage of height h; $\Delta d\% = $ change in d with respect to position 1 as a percentage of h

10. Position 6: From position 1, sit up to touch toes (Fig. PW4.2):
    a. Record S_2 in Table PW4.2
    b. Calculate d (cm) using equation PW4.1 and record the result in Table PW4.2
    c. Calculate d as a percentage of h
    d. Calculate Δd between positions 1 and 6 and record the result in Table PW4.2
    e. Calculate Δd as a percentage of h and record the result in Table PW4.2.

Presentation of results

1. Present your individual results, i.e. completed Tables PW4.1 and PW4.2.
2. Present the completed results, Table PW4.3, for the subjects in your group.

Example results

Example data (obtained from a practical session with students) are shown in Tables PW4.4 and PW4.5. Table PW4.6 also shows group mean results for 10 students (5 women and 5 men). The group mean data (Table PW4.6) show that the change in the position of the whole-body centre of gravity is on average very similar for the men and women subjects even though there is considerable variation in height and weight.

Table PW4.4
Height and weight of subject, distance between knife-edge supports and initial load on knife-edge support B

Name of subject:	Anne
Weight W (kgf)	67.0
Height h (cm)	167.0
l (cm)	244.0
S_1 (kgf)	10.0

Table PW4.5
Individual results for d in the six positions and change in d in positions 2–6 with respect to position 1

Body position	S_2 (kgf)	d (cm)	d (% of h)	Δd (cm)*	Δd (% of h)
1	36.0	94.7	56.7	0	0
2	36.5	96.5	57.8	1.8	1.08
3	37.5	100.1	59.9	5.4	3.23
4	41.5	114.7	68.7	20.0	11.98
5	42.0	116.5	69.8	21.8	13.05
6	29.0	69.2	41.4	−25.5	−15.27

*Change in d with respect to position 1

Table PW4.6   Individual and group results for d and change in d with respect to position 1

Subjects	h (cm)	W (kgf)	Position 1		Position 2		Position 3		Position 4		Position 5		Position 6	
			$d\%$	$\Delta d\%$	$d\%$	$\Delta d\%$	$d\%$	$\Delta d\%$	$d\%$	$\Delta d\%$	$d\%$	$\Delta d\%$	$d\%$	$\Delta d\%$
Women														
1 Anne	167	67	56.7	0	57.8	1.08	59.9	3.23	68.7	11.98	69.7	13.05	51.4	−15.27
2 Sarah	153.4	52	54.8	0	56.1	1.24	58.5	3.71	64.8	9.97	67.3	12.45	39.9	−14.93
3 Dawn	157	52.5	57.8	0	58.9	1.21	61	3.25	68.6	10.83	71	13.23	42.1	−15.63
4 Susan	172	68	53.2	0	54.2	1.04	56.3	3.13	64.7	11.47	66.7	13.56	41.7	−11.47
5 Kylie	167	61	55.6	0	56.6	0.96	59.5	3.89	65.4	9.75	67.3	11.7	41	−14.67
Mean	163.28	60.1	55.62	0	56.72	1.11	59.04	3.44	66.44	10.8	68.4	12.8	41.22	−14.39
SD	7.76	7.65	1.76	0	1.78	0.12	1.77	0.34	2.04	0.95	1.85	0.73	0.84	1.67
Men														
1 Paul	176.5	77	58.3	0	59.2	0.9	62.8	4.49	68.2	9.88	71.8	13.47	45.78	−12.56
2 Richard	181.3	76	61.9	0	62.9	0.88	65.5	3.54	69.1	7.08	72.6	10.62	46	−15.94
3 Bruce	189.4	80.5	59.8	0	60.4	0.63	63.1	3.27	68.9	9.13	72.8	12.98	44.8	−14.94
4 David	171	78	58.7	0	60.2	0.54	62.4	3.72	68.4	9.66	73.6	14.86	43.1	−15.61
5 John	169	68	59.6	0	60.5	0.89	62.2	2.66	68.6	8.99	70.4	10.82	43.3	−16.27
Mean	177.44	75.9	59.66	0	60.64	0.77	63.2	3.54	68.64	8.95	72.24	12.55	44.6	−15.06
SD	1.65	0.94	0.28	0	0.27	0.03	0.27	0.13	0.07	0.22	0.24	0.36	0.27	0.3

$d\%$ = d as a percentage of height h; $\Delta d\%$ = change in d with respect to position 1 as a percentage of h

Practical Worksheet 5

Comparison of the direct and segmental analysis methods of determining the position of the whole–body centre of gravity of the human body

Objective

To compare the direct and segmental analysis methods of determining the transverse plane containing the centre of gravity (CG) of the human body in static equilibrium in the anatomical position using a one-dimension reaction board.

Location

Motion analysis laboratory.

Apparatus and equipment

One-dimension reaction board (approximately $2.5 \times 0.5\,\text{m}$) with a centimetre scale running left to right on one side.
One set of weighing scales.

Method

Subject's clothing

Shorts and a sleeveless top so that the following points on the skin on the *left side of the body* can be easily identified:

- A point on the skin of the left arm at a distance of 3 cm below the tip of the acromion process, i.e. 3 cm to the left of the acromion process when the subject is lying horizontally in the anatomical position. This point will indicate the plane of the left shoulder joint centre when lying on the reaction board

- The tip of the styloid process of the left ulna. This point will indicate the plane of the left wrist when lying on the reaction board

- The tip of the left greater tuberosity. This point will indicate the plane of the left hip joint centre when lying on the reaction board

- The tip of the lateral malleolus of the left fibula. This point will indicate the plane of the left ankle joint centre when lying on the reaction board.

Data collection

1. Record in Table PW5.1 the weight W (kgf) of the subject (shorts, sleeveless top, no shoes).
2. Record in Table PW5.1 the height h (cm) of the subject (no shoes).
3. Support the board in a horizontal position with knife-edge support B resting on the scales (Fig. PW5.1a).
4. Record in Table PW5.1 the distance l (cm) between the two knife-edge supports.

5. Record in Table PW5.1 the vertical force S_1 (kgf) exerted on the scales.
6. Subject lies on the board with arms by sides and soles of feet against the foot block, i.e. with the soles of the feet in the vertical plane containing knife-edge support A (Fig. PW5.1b).
7. Record in Table PW5.1 the vertical force S_2 (kgf) exerted on end B.
8. Using the centimetre scale on the side of the board, record in Table PW5.1 the horizontal distances (cm) between the plane of the soles of the feet (reference zero) and the following points on the left side of the

Table PW5.1
Results

Subject	
W (kgf)	
h (cm)	
l (cm)	
S_1 (kgf)	
S_2 (kgf)	
d_M (cm)	
d_H (cm)	
d_U (cm)	
d_S (cm)	
d_D (cm)	
W_A (kgf)	
W_L (kgf)	
W_{THN} (kgf)	
d_{GA} (cm)	
d_{GL} (cm)	
d_{GTHN} (cm)	
M_C (kgf.cm)	
d_W (cm)	
d (cm)	

Fig. PW5.1
(a) Reaction board without the subject.
(b) Subject lying on the reaction board

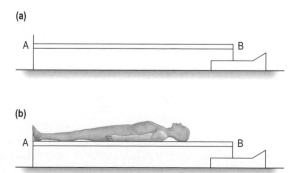

(a)

(b)

body (Fig. PW5.2): lateral malleolus (d_M), greater trochanter (d_H), styloid process of the ulna (d_U), shoulder joint (d_S), vertical plane through the top of the head (d_D).

Data analysis

1. Calculate the horizontal distance d between the plane of the soles of the feet and the plane containing the CG of the body by the direct method using Equation PW5.1 and record the result in Table PW5.1:

$$d \ (cm) = \frac{l(S_2 - S_1)}{W}$$

Eq. PW5.1

2. Calculate the horizontal distance d_W between the plane of the soles of the feet and the plane containing the CG of the body by the indirect method (segmental analysis method):

   i. Calculate the weight (kgf) of each upper limb W_A, the weight of each lower limb W_L and the weight of the combined trunk, head and neck W_{THN}. Record the results in Table PW5.1. Use the Plagenhoef et al (1983) data for segment weight percentages in Table 3.1 for men and Table 3.2 for women, i.e.

Men:	$W_A \ (kgf) = 0.0577 \times W$
	$W_L \ (kgf) = 0.1668 \times W$
	$W_{THN} \ (kgf) = 0.551 \times W$

Women:	$W_A \ (kgf) = 0.0497 \times W$
	$W_L \ (kgf) = 0.1843 \times W$
	$W_{THN} \ (kgf) = 0.532 \times W$

   ii. Calculate the moment arms, about end A of the board, of the centres of gravity of each upper limb (d_{GA}) (assume that the moment arms are the same for the left and right upper limb), each lower limb (d_{GL}) (assume

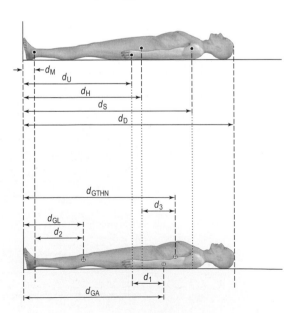

Fig. PW5.2
Location of segmental centres of gravity

that the moment arms are the same for the left and right lower limb) and the combined trunk, head and neck (d_{GTHN}). See Figure PW5.2. Record the results in Table PW5.1. Use the Plagenhoef et al (1983) data for segment centre of gravity loci in Table 3.1 for men and Table 3.2 for women, i.e.

Men:
$$d_{\text{GA}} \text{ (cm)} = d_{\text{U}} + d_1 = d_{\text{U}} + 0.50(d_{\text{S}} - d_{\text{U}})$$
$$d_{\text{GL}} \text{ (cm)} = d_{\text{M}} + d_2 = d_{\text{M}} + 0.564(d_{\text{H}} - d_{\text{M}})$$
$$d_{\text{GTHN}} \text{ (cm)} = d_{\text{H}} + d_3 = d_{\text{H}} + 0.434(d_{\text{D}} - d_{\text{H}})$$

Women:
$$d_{\text{GA}} \text{ (cm)} = d_{\text{U}} + d_1 = d_{\text{U}} + 0.514(d_{\text{S}} - d_{\text{U}})$$
$$d_{\text{GL}} \text{ (cm)} = d_{\text{M}} + d_2 = d_{\text{M}} + 0.580(d_{\text{H}} - d_{\text{M}})$$
$$d_{\text{GTHN}} \text{ (cm)} = d_{\text{H}} + d_3 = d_{\text{H}} + 0.397(d_{\text{D}} - d_{\text{H}})$$

iii. Calculate the combined moment (M_C) about end A of the board of the five segments of the body (two upper limbs, two lower limbs, combined trunk, head and neck). Record the result in Table PW5.1:

$$M_C \text{ (kgf.cm)} = 2(W_A \times d_{\text{GA}}) + 2(W_L \times d_{\text{GL}}) + W_{\text{THN}} \times d_{\text{GTHN}}$$

iv. Calculate the moment arm of total body weight (d_W) about end A by the principle of moments, i.e.

$$d_W \text{ (cm)} = M_C/W$$

Table PW5.2 Individual and group results for d, d_W and $d_W - d$

Subjects	h (cm)	W (kgf)	d (cm)	d* (%)	d_W (cm)	d_W* (%)	$d_W - d$ (cm)	$d_W - d$* (%)
Women								
1								
2								
3								
4								
5								
Mean								
SD								
Men								
1								
2								
3								
4								
5								
Mean								
SD								

* = % of h

v. Compare d with d_W. If the anthropometric data (segmental masses and mass centre loci) used in the calculation of M_C were accurate, then d and d_W should be exactly the same. This is unlikely, since the anthropometric data were estimated from mean data obtained by volumetric analysis. Nevertheless, the anthropometric data are accurate enough for most analyses of human movement.

Presentation of results

1. Present your individual results, i.e. completed Table PW5.1.
2. Present the completed results Table PW5.2 for the subjects in your group.

Example results

Example data (obtained from a practical session with students) are shown in Table PW5.3. Table PW5.4 shows group mean results for 10 students (five women and five men). The group mean data show that the indirect result was greater than the direct result for both the women and the men by an average of 2.4 cm (1.5% of height) and 4.1 cm (2.3% of height) respectively.

Table PW5.3
Results

Subject	Pamela
W (kgf)	57
h (cm)	165.8
l (cm)	198.8
S_1 (kgf)	13
S_2 (kgf)	40.5
d_M (cm)	8
d_H (cm)	86
d_U (cm)	91
d_S (cm)	139
d_D (cm)	168
W_A (kgf)	2.9
W_L (kgf)	9.2
W_{THN} (kgf)	32.8
d_{GA} (cm)	114.4
d_{GL} (cm)	52.1
d_{GTHN} (cm)	118.5
M_C (kgf.cm)	5509
d_W (cm)	96.6
d (cm)	95.9

Table PW5.4
Individual and group
results for d, d_W and
$d_W - d$

Subjects	h (cm)	W (kgf)	d (cm)	d^* (%)	d_W (cm)	d_W^* (%)	$d_W - d$ (cm)	$d_W - d^*$ (%)
Women								
1 Pamela	165.8	57	95.9	57.8	96.6	58.3	0.7	0.4
2 Jane	164.2	52	96.5	58.8	99	60.3	2.5	1.5
3 Susan	172	66	102.4	59.5	106.7	62	4.3	2.5
4 Sally	160.3	49	91.8	57.3	95.8	59.8	4	2.5
5 Fiona	155.5	55	90.4	58.1	91.1	58.6	0.7	0.5
Mean	163.6	55.8	95.4	58.3	97.8	59.8	2.4	1.5
SD	6.2	6.5	4.7	0.9	5.7	1.5	1.7	1
Men								
1 Stuart	169.3	68.5	91.7	54.2	96.3	56.9	4.6	2.7
2 Paul	176.5	77	103	58.4	108.9	61.7	5.9	3.3
3 Alastair	170.2	71	99.6	58.5	100.4	59	0.8	0.5
4 Graeme	184.8	79.5	102.9	55.7	109.2	59.1	6.3	3.4
5 Richard	181.3	76	109.2	60.2	111.9	61.7	2.7	1.5
Mean	176.4	74.4	101.3	57.4	105.3	59.7	4.1	2.3
SD	6.8	4.5	6.4	2.4	6.6	2	2.3	1.2

$*$ = % of h

Practical Worksheet **6**

Measurement of the moment of inertia of the human body

Objective

To measure the moment of inertia and radius of gyration of the human body about a vertical axis while in a seated position.

Location

Motion analysis laboratory.

Apparatus and equipment

1. A turntable with a radial pointer extending from the turntable.
2. A stool that can be placed on the turntable with the vertical axis through the centre of the stool in line with the spindle of the turntable.
3. A pulley-based gravitational load system to apply an angular impulse to the turntable.
4. A timer linked to two sets of photo cells to record the duration of the angular impulse (time for the load to descend from its starting point to the floor).
5. A timer linked to two sets of photo cells defining an arc of one radian within the field of the pointer.
6. A set of weighing scales.

Method

Subject's clothing
Shorts, shirt and training shoes.

Data collection
1. Record the mass (kg) of the subject in Table PW6.1.
2. With the stool resting on the turntable and the whole system at rest, a load is allowed to descend from its starting point to the floor. As the

Figure PW6.1
Diagram of turntable and pulley-based gravitational load system

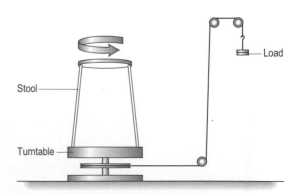

load descends, it applies, via the pulley system, an angular impulse to the turntable and stool about the vertical axis a_Y through the spindle of the turntable. The angular impulse generates a certain amount of angular momentum of the turntable and stool about a_Y, i.e.

$M.t = I.\omega$ (Eq. 3.20 where $\omega_1 = 0$)   Eq. PW6.1

where

F = load (N)
d = moment arm (m) of F about a_Y
$M = F.d$ = moment (N.m) exerted on turntable and stool about a_Y
t = duration (s) of the angular impulse
I = moment of inertia (kg.m^2) of turntable and stool about a_Y
ω = angular velocity (rad/s) of the turntable and stool about a_Y resulting from the angular impulse.

3. The duration of the angular impulse t_1 is the time taken for the load to descend from rest to the floor (over a distance of about 1 m; see Fig. PW6.1). After the load contacts the floor (at which point the string applying the load to the turntable disconnects from the turntable), the turntable and stool will continue to rotate about a_Y. If there was no friction around the spindle of the turntable, the turntable and stool would rotate with constant angular velocity, since angular momentum would be conserved. However, friction around the spindle will gradually reduce the speed of rotation. Consequently it is important to measure ω as soon as possible after the end of the angular impulse, i.e. after the load has contacted the floor. ω is measured from $\omega = 1/t_2$ where t_2 is the time for the pointer to sweep through the arc of one radian. Record t_1 and t_2 in Table PW6.1.

4. Record F and d in Table PW6.1. In the example results in Table PW6.3, $F = 4.905$ N (0.5 kgf) and $d = 0.235$ m.

5. Repeat steps 2–4 with the subject sitting on the stool.

Table PW6.1
Individual results

Name of subject:								
Mass of subject (kg):								
	F (N)	d (m)	M (N.m)	t_1 (s)	$M.t_1$ (N.m.s)	t_2 (s)	ω (rad/s)	I_1 and I_2 (kg.m^2/s)
Turntable and stool								
Turntable, stool and subject								
			I_3 (kg.m^2/s)				k (m)	
Subject								

Data analysis

1. Calculate the turning moment M and the impulse of the turning moment $M.t_1$ for the turntable and stool and for the turntable, stool and subject. Record the results in Table PW6.1.
2. Calculate $\omega = 1/t_2$ for the turntable and stool and for the turntable, stool and subject. Record the results in Table PW6.1.
3. Calculate the moment of inertia I_1 of the turntable and stool about a_Y and the moment of inertia I_2 of the turntable, stool and subject about a_Y from equation PW6.1, i.e. $I = (M.t_1)/\omega$. Record the results in Table PW6.1.
4. Calculate the moment of inertia I_3 of the subject about a_Y from $I_3 = I_2 - I_1$. Record the result in Table PW6.1.
5. Calculate the radius of gyration k of the subject about a_Y from $K = \sqrt{I_3/m}$ where $m =$ mass of the subject. Record the result in Table PW6.1.

Presentation of results

Your submission should consist of:

1. A completed copy of Table PW6.1 with your results.
2. A completed copy of Table PW6.2 showing the individual and group results for the subjects in your group.

Example results

Example data for a single male subject are shown in Table PW6.3. Table PW6.4 shows group mean results for 10 subjects (five women and five men). The group mean results for moment of inertia (I_3) and radius of gyration (k) are fairly similar for both groups, even though there is a considerable difference in the mean mass of the groups.

Table PW6.2
Individual and group results

Subjects	Mass (kg)	I_1 (kg.m²/s)	I_2 (kg.m²/s)	I_3 (kg.m²/s)	k (m)
Women					
1					
2					
3					
4					
5					
Mean					
SD					
Men					
1					
2					
3					
4					
5					
Mean					
SD					

Table PW6.3
Individual results

Name of subject: Dan								
Mass of subject (kg): 66.0								
	F (N)	d (m)	M (N.m)	t_1 (s)	$M.t_1$ (N.m.s)	t_2 (s)	ω (rad/s)	I_1 and I_2 (kg.m^2/s)
Turntable and stool	4.905	0.235	1.153	0.910	1.049	0.171	5.848	0.197
Turntable, stool and subject	4.905	0.235	1.153	3.751	4.325	0.826	1.210	3.574

	I_3 (kg.m^2/s)		k (m)	
Subject	3.377		0.226	

Table PW6.4
Individual and group results

Subjects	Mass (kg)	I_1 (kg.m^2/s)	I_2 (kg.m^2/s)	I_3 (kg.m^2/s)	k (m)
Women					
1. Fiona	52.2	0.197	3.336	3.139	0.245
2. Jennifer	63.9	0.197	3.347	3.150	0.222
3. Natalie	59.7	0.197	3.843	3.646	0.247
4. Lynne	68.2	0.197	3.641	3.444	0.245
5. Sarah	59.1	0.197	3.333	3.136	0.230
Mean	60.6	0.197	3.500	3.303	0.238
SD	5.96	0	0.232	0.232	0.011
Men					
1. Dan	66.0	0.197	3.574	3.377	0.226
2. Stuart	69.6	0.197	3.131	2.934	0.205
3. Richard	78.2	0.197	3.650	3.453	0.210
4. Paul	74.8	0.197	4.016	3.819	0.226
5. Ross	77.9	0.197	4.270	4.073	0.229
Mean	73.3	0.197	3.728	3.530	0.219
SD	5.35	0	0.437	0.437	0.011

Practical Worksheet 7

Determination of human power output in stair climbing and running up a slope

Objectives

To determine the external power output of the human body in stair climbing and running up a slope.

Location

Stair climbing

It is unlikely that a purpose-built stairway will be available, but any suitable stairway indoors or outdoors will suffice for the test. In the test, the subject is required to run up a stairway or part of a stairway as fast as possible. The time to complete a particular number of steps, involving a certain vertical displacement of the body, is measured by a timer linked to pressure mats placed on specific steps or photo cells placed at the sides of the stairway (Fig. PW7.1). The average external power output P_a of the body (rate of increase in gravitational potential energy) is given by $P_a = m.g.h/t$ where m = mass of the subject (kg), g = acceleration due to gravity, h = vertical displacement. For example, if $m = 70$ kg, the height of each step = 0.15 m and the time to complete four steps = 0.5 s then P_a is given by:

$$P_a = \frac{70\,\text{kg} \times 9.81\,\text{m/s}^2 \times 4 \times 0.15\,\text{m}}{0.5\,\text{s}} = 824\,\text{W} \qquad \text{Eq. PW7.1}$$

Fig. PW7.1
Location of photo cells in relation to stairway

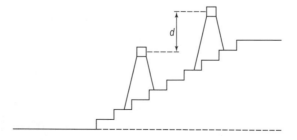

Fig. PW7.2
Location of photo
cells in relation
to slope

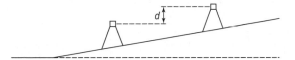

Running up a slope

Any even slope of approximately 25 m in length that is not too steep should be suitable for the test. In the test, the subject is required to run up the slope as fast as possible. The time to complete a particular distance up the slope, involving a certain vertical displacement of the body, is measured by a timer linked to photo cells placed at the sides of the runway (Fig. PW7.2). The subject begins his/her run about 5 m before the start of the test region and slows down after completing the test distance. The average external power output P_a of the body (rate of increase in gravitational potential energy) is measured in the same way as in the stair climbing test. For example, if the angle of the slope = 5° and the test distance up the slope = 10 m, then the vertical displacement = 0.87 m. If the mass of the subject m = 60 kg and the time to complete the test distance = 1.8 s, then P_a is given by:

$$P_a = \frac{60 \text{ kg} \times 9.81 \text{ m/s}^2 \times 0.87 \text{ m}}{1.8 \text{ s}} = 284.5 \text{ W} \qquad \text{Eq. PW7.2}$$

Method

Subjects' clothing
Shorts, shirt and trainers.

Data collection: stair climbing

1. Ensure that each set of photo cells is at the same height (approximately waist height) above the target steps.
2. Reset the timer.
3. Subject performs a trial, i.e. from a 5 m rolling start the subject runs up the stairs between the sets of photo cells (Fig. PW7.1) as quickly as possible.
4. Record the time for the trial in Table PW7.1.
5. Repeat stages 2–4 for five more trials.
6. Record the subject's mass (kg) in Table PW7.1.
7. Record the vertical displacement d between the photo cells in Table PW7.1.
8. Calculate the average external power P_a in each trial by using Equation PW7.1. Record P_a in Table PW7.1 in watts (W) and watts per kilogram of body mass (W/kg).
9. Calculate the mean and standard deviation of P_a and record the data in Table PW7.1.

Table PW7.1
Stair climbing test

Name of subject:			
Mass (kg):			
d (m):			
Trial	Time (s)	P_a (W)	P_a (W/kg)
1			
2			
3			
4			
5			
6			
Mean			
SD			

Data collection: running up a slope

1. Ensure that each set of photo cells is at the same height (approximately waist height) above the slope.
2. Reset the timer.
3. Subject performs a trial, i.e. from a 5 m rolling start the subject runs up the slope between the sets of photo cells (Fig. PW7.2) as quickly as possible.
4. Record the time for the trial in Table PW7.2.
5. Repeat stages 2–4 for five more trials.
6. Record the subject's mass (kg) in Table PW7.2.
7. Record the vertical displacement d between the photo cells in Table PW7.2.
8. Calculate the average external power P_a in each trial by using Equation PW7.2. Record P_a in Table PW7.2 in watts (W) and watts per kilogram of body mass (W/kg).
9. Calculate the mean and standard deviation of P_a and record the data in Table PW7.2.

Presentation of results

1. Calculate the group mean and standard deviation for P_a for the subjects in your group (based on their mean data) for both tests and record the results in Table PW7.3.
2. Present your individual results for both tests: Tables PW7.1 and PW7.2.
3. Present the group results for both tests: Table PW7.3.

Example results

Example data are shown in Tables PW7.4–PW7.6.

Table PW7.2
Running test

Name of subject:			
Mass (kg):			
d (m):			
Trial	Time (s)	P_a (W)	P_a (W/kg)
1			
2			
3			
4			
5			
6			
Mean			
SD			

Table PW7.3
Group results

Name of subject:	Stair climbing test		Running test	
	P_a (W)	P_a (W/kg)	P_a (W)	P_a (W/kg)
1				
2				
3				
4				
5				
Mean				
SD				

Table PW7.4
Stair climbing test

Name of subject:	John		
Mass (kg):	61.7		
d (m):	0.6 m		
Trial	Time (s)	P_a (W)	P_a (W/kg)
1	0.528	687.8	11.14
2	0.491	739.3	11.98
3	0.453	801.3	12.98
4	0.471	770.7	12.49
5	0.484	750.0	12.15
6	0.469	774.0	12.54
Mean	0.483	753.8	12.21
SD	0.026	38.8	0.63

Height of each step = 0.15 m. Four steps $\times$ 0.15 m = 0.6 m.
Depth of each step = 0.2 m.

Table PW7.5
Running test

Name of subject:	John		
Mass (kg):	61.7		
d (m):	0.87		
Trial	Time (s)	P_a (W)	P_a (W/kg)
1	1.890	278.6	4.51
2	1.864	282.5	4.58
3	1.870	281.6	4.56
4	1.902	276.9	4.49
5	1.879	280.2	4.54
6	1.877	280.5	4.55
Mean	1.880	280.0	4.54
SD	0.014	2.03	0.03
10 m test distance on a 5° slope: vertical displacement = 0.87 m.			

Table PW7.6
Group results

Name of subject:	Stair climbing test		Running test	
	P_a (W)	P_a (W/kg)	P_a (W)	P_a (W/kg)
1 John	753.8	12.21	280.0	4.54
2 James	854.9	10.42	368.5	4.49
3 Stephen	784.7	10.89	351.0	4.88
4 Callum	891.8	12.74	330.2	4.71
5 David	945.1	13.89	326.0	4.79
Mean	846.0	12.03	331.1	4.68
SD	77.9	1.40	33.3	0.16

Answers to review questions

CHAPTER 1

6. From Table 1.2:
   1 m/s = 2.2369 mph, i.e. 150 m/s = 150 × 2.2369 mph = 335.5 mph
   1 mph = 1.609 34 km/h, i.e. 10 mph = 10 × 1.609 34 km/h = 16.0934 km/h
   1 km/h = 0.277 78 m/s, i.e. 25 km/h = 25 × 0.277 78 m/s = 6.94 m/s.

CHAPTER 2

Linear kinematics

3. **Table 2A.1:** Average speed in laps 1 and 2 and in the whole race

Lap	Time (s)	Distance (m)	Average speed (m/s)
1	56.0	400	7.14
2	52.0	400	7.69
Total time	108.0	800	7.41

4. **Table 2A.2:** Leg length and stride parameters at 3.5 m/s and 5.5 m/s

Leg length (m)	Speed (m/s)	Time for 10 strides (s)	Stride rate (strides/s)	Stride length (m/stride)	RSL
0.9	3.5	6.94	1.44	2.43	2.70
0.9	5.5	5.80	1.72	3.20	3.55

5.1 **Table 2A.3:** Distance, time and average speed for the winner of the women's race in different units (winner's time = 2 h 23 min 21 s)

Distance		Time		Average speed	
Miles (m)	26.219	Hours (h)	2.389	mph	10.974
Kilometres (km)	42.195	Hours (h)	2.389	km/h	17.662
Metres (m)	42.195	Seconds (s)	8601	m/s	4.905

Table 2A.4: Distance, time and average speed for the winner of the men's race in different units (winner's time = 2h 7min 56s)

Distance		Time		Average speed	
Miles (m)	26.219	Hours (h)	2.132	mph	12.298
Kilometres (km)	42.195	Hours (h)	2.132	km/h	19.791
Metres (m)	42195	Seconds (s)	7676	m/s	5.497

5.2 Average speed of the winner of women's race $V_w = 4.905$ m/s
Average speed of the winner of men's race $V_m = 5.497$ m/s
V_w as a percentage of $V_m = 89.23\%$ ($4.905/5.497 \times 100$).

5.3 Table 2A.5: Average time per mile and average time per kilometre for the winner of the women's race and the men's race

	Distance (miles)	Distance (km)	Winner's time (min)	Per mile (min)	Per km (min)
Women's race	26.219	42.195	143.35	5.47	3.40
Men's race	26.219	42.195	127.93	4.88	3.03

Linear impulse and linear momentum

6.

Variable	Units	Unit abbreviation
Force	newton	N
Time	seconds	s
Impulse	newton seconds	N.s
Mass	kilogram	kg
Velocity	metres per second	m/s or m.s^{-1}
Linear momentum	kilogram metres per second	kg.m/s or kg.m.s^{-1}

7. $m = 0.35$ kg, $v_1 = 0$, $v_2 = 42$ m/s, $t = 0.05$ s
F = average force exerted on ball
$F = m(v - u)/t = 0.35 \times (42 - 0)/0.05$
$= 294$ N $= 29.97$ kgf $= 66.07$ lbf

8. $m = 0.06$ kg, $v_1 = 0$, $v_2 = 72$ m/s, $t = 0.0005$ s
F = average force exerted on ball
$F = m(v - u)/t = 0.06 \times (72 - 0)/0.0005$
$= 8640$ N $= 880.73$ kgf $= 1941.66$ lbf
$= 0.87$ tons

9. Impulse $F.t = 159.72$ N.s, $m = 7.26$ kg,
v = release velocity of shot
$F.t = m.v$, i.e. $v = F.t/m = 159.72/7.26 = 22$ m/s

10. It is necessary to adopt a convention for positive and negative, since the vertical component R of the braking force (vertical component of the ground reaction force) is in the opposite direction to that of the vertical component of the velocity v_1 of the gymnast on landing. Since it is necessary to calculate R, let upward be positive and downward negative.

R (acting upward) = average magnitude of the ground reaction force during landing, W = body weight (acting downward), $v_1 = 6.2$ m/s (downward), $v_2 = 0$, $t = 0.2$ s.

$F = m(v - u)/t$, where F is the resultant upward force acting on the body during landing

$F = R - W$

i.e. $R - W = m(v_2 - v_1)/t = 55 \times (0 - (-6.2))/0.2 = 55 \times 6.2/0.2 = 1705\,N$

i.e. $R = 1705\,N + W$

Since $W = 55\,kgf = 539.5\,N$

then $R = 1705\,N + 539.5\,N = 2244.5\,N$

$= 228.8\,kgf = 504.4\,lbf = 4.16\,BW$

Vectors

13. $a/c = \sin 40°$, i.e. $a = c.\sin 40°$
$= 20\,cm \times 0.643 = 12.86\,cm$
$b/c = \cos 40°$, i.e. $b = c.\cos 40°$
$= 20\,cm \times 0.766 = 15.32\,cm$

14. $A/F = \cos 40°$, i.e. $A = F.\cos 40°$
$= 200\,N \times 0.766 = 153.2\,N$
$B/F = \cos 50°$, i.e. $B = F.\cos 50°$
$= 200\,N \times 0.643 = 128.6\,N$

15. $T/B = \cos 30°$, i.e. $T = B.\cos 30°$
$= 100\,N \times 0.866 = 86.6\,N$
$S/B = \sin 30°$, i.e. $S = B.\sin 30°$
$= 100\,N \times 0.5 = 50.0\,N$

16. i. Magnitude of F_{xy}:
$F_{xy}^2 = F_x^2 + F_y^2 = 0.64 + 6.25 = 6.89$
i.e. $F_{xy} = 2.625\,BW$
Direction of F_{xy} with reference to horizontal: angle α:
$\cos \alpha = F_x/F_{xy} = 0.8/2.625 = 0.3047$
i.e. $\alpha = 72.2°$

ii. Magnitude of F_{yz}:
$F_{yz}^2 = F_y^2 + F_z^2 = 6.25 + 0.16 = 6.41$
i.e. $F_{yz} = 2.532\,BW$
Direction of F_{yz} with reference to horizontal: angle β:
$\cos \beta = F_z/F_{yz} = 0.4/2.532 = 0.1524$
i.e. $\beta = 80.9°$

iii. Magnitude of F_{xz}:
$F_{xz}^2 = F_x^2 + F_z^2 = 0.64 + 0.16 = 0.8$
i.e. $F_{xz} = 0.894\,BW$
Direction of F_{xz} with reference to F_z: angle θ:
$\cos \theta = F_z/F_{xz} = 0.4/0.894 = 0.4474$
i.e. $\theta = 63.4°$

iv. Magnitude of F:
$F^2 = F_y^2 + F_{xz}^2 = 6.25 + 0.7992 = 7.049$
i.e. $F = 2.655\,BW$
Direction of F with reference to F_{xz}: angle δ:
$\cos \delta = F_{xz}/F = 0.894/2.655 = 0.3367$
i.e. $\delta = 70.32°$

17. **Table 2A.6:** Magnitude and direction of F_x, F_y and F_{xy}

	Frame 2	Frame 4
F_x (BW)	−0.58	+0.42
F_y (BW)	+2.22	+2.7
F_{xy} (BW)	2.29	2.73
F_{xy} (°)	75.37	81.2

18. ii. L_V and L_H = vertical and horizontal components of L
F_V and F_H = vertical and horizontal components of F
M_V and M_H = vertical and horizontal components of M
All the vertical components are upward and therefore positive
Since horizontal components to the left will counteract horizontal components to the right, it is necessary to regard horizontal components to the left as negative and all horizontal components to the right as positive.
$L_V = L.\sin 70° = 50 \times 0.9396 = 46.98\,N$
$L_H = L.\cos 70° = 50 \times 0.342 = -17.10\,N$
$F_V = F.\sin 84° = 100 \times 0.9945 = 99.45\,N$
$F_H = F.\cos 84° = 100 \times 0.1045 = -10.45\,N$
$M_V = M.\sin 60° = 56.5 \times 0.866 = 48.93\,N$
$M_H = M.\cos 60° = 56.5 \times 0.5 = +28.25\,N$
Vertical component Q_V of the resultant quadriceps force Q
$= 46.98 + 99.45 + 48.93 = 195.36\,N$
Horizontal component Q_H of the resultant quadriceps force Q
$= -17.10 - 10.45 + 28.25 = +0.7\,N$
Resultant quadriceps force Q
$= 195.36\,N$ at an angle of $89.85°$
(upwards and slightly to the right in Fig. 2Q.6)

Ground reaction force

20. Table 2A.7: Analysis of the vertical component (F_y–time) of the ground reaction force acting on the right foot of a subject during contact time in running

Name of subject:		Mass (kg)		Weight (N)	
Mass of subject		70		686.7	
Key points on F_y–time graph		Time (s)	Force (N)	Force (BW)	
1. Heel contact (t_1, F_{y1})		0	0	0	
2. Impact force peak IFP (t_2, F_{y2})		0.0264	1022.4	1.489	
3. End of the passive phase (minimum force following IFP) (t_3, F_{y3})		0.0422	649.1	0.945	
4. End of absorption phase (t_4, F_{y4}) (when $F_y = 0$)		0.1217	1384.8	2.017	
5. Toe-off (t_5, F_{y5})		0.2650	0	0	
		Time (s)		Proportion of contact time (%)	
6. Contact time ($t_5 - t_1$)		0.2650		100	
7. Time to IFP ($t_2 - t_1$)		0.0264		9.96	
8. Duration of passive phase ($t_3 - t_1$)		0.0422		15.92	
9. Duration of absorption phase ($t_4 - t_1$)		0.1217		45.92	
10. Duration of propulsion phase ($t_5 - t_4$)		0.1433		54.08	
		L_R (N/s)		L_R (BW/s)	
Rate of loading (L_R) during impact ($F_{y2}/(t_2 - t_1)$)		38 727.2		56.40	

Uniformly accelerated motion

21. i. Vertical displacement of the centre of gravity from take-off to maximum height s_f:
Consider vertical motion from take-off to maximum height.

From $v^2 - u^2 = 2a.s$

where

u = vertical velocity at take-off = 4.2 m/s
v = vertical velocity at maximum height = 0
$a = -9.81$ m/s^2
$s = s_f$ = flight height

i.e.

$$s_f = (v_2 - u_2)/2a = \frac{(0 - 17.64)}{-19.62}$$
$$= 0.90 \text{ m}$$

 ii. Time from take-off to maximum height t_f
Consider vertical motion from take-off to maximum height.

From $v = u + a.t$
where
u = vertical velocity at take-off = 4.2 m/s
v = vertical velocity at maximum height = 0
$a = -9.81$ m/s^2
$t = t_f$ = time from take-off to maximum height

i.e.

$$t_f = (v - u)/a = \frac{(0 - 4.2)}{-9.81} = 0.43 \text{ s}$$

22. Consider vertical motion from take off to maximum height.
Step 1: Calculate take-off velocity v_0:
Impulse $I = mv - mu$
where $I = 246$ N.s
m = mass of jumper = 60 kg
u = upward velocity at the start of the propulsion phase = 0
$v = v_0$
i.e. $v_0 = I/m = 246/60 = 4.1$ m/s

Step 2: Calculate flight height s_f:

From $v^2 - u^2 = 2a.s$

where

$u = v_0 = 4.1$ m/s
$v =$ vertical velocity at maximum height $= 0$
$a = -9.81$ m/s^2
$s = s_f$

i.e. $s_f = (v^2 - u^2)/2a = \dfrac{(0 - 16.81)}{-19.62}$

$\qquad = 0.86$ m

23. Step 1: Calculate fall time t_d:

From $s = u.t + \dfrac{a.t^2}{2}$

where
$s =$ fall distance $= 150$ m
$u = 0$
$a = 9.81$ m/s^2
$t = t_d$

i.e. $150 = 0 + \dfrac{(9.81 \times t_d^2)}{2}$

$t_d^2 = 300/9.81 = 30.58$
$t_d = 5.53$ s

Step 2: Calculate the velocity of the stone on impact with the ground v_d:

From $v = u + a.t$
where
$u = 0$
$v = v_d$
$a = 9.81$ m/s^2
$t = 5.53$ s
i.e. $v_d = 0 + 9.81 \times 5.53 = 54.25$ m/s

24. Step 1: Calculate flight time t_f:
Flight time t_f can be found in three steps by finding the time from release to maximum height t_1, the vertical displacement from release to maximum height and the time from maximum height to landing t_2. $t_f = t_1 + t_2$. Flight time t_f can also be found in one step using
$s = u.t + a.t^2/2$
where
$s = -2$ m (the landing point is 2 m below the release point)
$u =$ release velocity $= 10$ m/s
$a = -9.81$ m/s^2
$t = t_f$

i.e. $-2 = 10 \times t_f - 4.905 \times t_f^2$

and

$4.905 \times t_f^2 - 10 \times t_f - 2 = 0$ \qquad Eq. 2A.1

This form of equation, $ax^2 + bx + c$, where a, b and c are constants and x is variable, is called a quadratic equation. A quadratic equation can be solved, i.e. the value of x can be found, by using the following formula:

$$x = \frac{-b \pm \sqrt{(b^2 - 4a.c)}}{2a}$$

In Equation 2A.1, $a = 4.905$, $b = -10$, $c = -2$
i.e.

$$t_f = \frac{-(-10) \pm \sqrt{(-10)^2 - 4 \times 4.905 \times (-2)}}{9.81}$$

$$t_f = \frac{10 \pm \sqrt{(100 + 39.24)}}{9.81} = \frac{10 \pm 11.8}{9.81}$$

Clearly, the negative alternative for the term 10 ± 11.8 (resulting in -1.8) cannot be correct. Consequently the positive alternative is taken, i.e. $10 + 11.8 = 21.8$

i.e. $t_f = \dfrac{21.8}{9.81} = 2.222$ s

Step 2: Calculate the velocity v_i of the ball at each time interval t_i:
Use $v = u + a.t_i$
where
$v = v_i =$ velocity at time t_i
$u = 10$ m/s
$a = -9.81$ m/s^2
$t = t_i$
For example, at $t_i = 0.2$ s
$v_i = 10 + ((-9.81) \times 0.2) = 10 - 1.962$
$\qquad = -8.038$ m/s
Similarly, for $t_i = 0.4$ s
$v_i = 10 + ((-9.81) \times 0.4) = 10 - 3.924$
$\qquad = -6.076$ m/s
and for $t_i = 2.222$ s (landing)
$v_i = 10 + ((-9.81) \times 2.222) = 10 - 21.799$
$\qquad = -11.799$ m/s
The velocity data are shown in Table 2A.8.

Table 2A.8:
Displacement and velocity of a ball thrown upward with a release velocity of 10 m/s from a release height of 2 m

Time into flight (s)	Velocity (m/s)	Displacement (m)
0	10.0	2.0
0.2	8.038	3.804
0.4	6.076	5.215
0.6	4.114	6.234
0.8	2.152	6.860
1.0	0.190	7.095
1.2	−1.772	6.937
1.4	−3.734	6.386
1.6	−5.696	5.443
1.8	−7.658	4.108
2.0	−9.620	2.380
2.2	−11.582	0.260
2.222	−11.799	0.003

Step 3: Calculate the displacement s_i of the ball at each time interval t_i:

At any point after release, the displacement of the stone s_i is given by $s_i = s_0 + s_r$, where

s_0 = vertical displacement at release = 2 m

s_r = displacement from the release point

s_r can be calculated by using $s = u.t + a.t^2/2$

For example, at $t_i = 0.2$ s, the displacement of the stone from the release point can be calculated as follows.

s_r = displacement of the stone from the release point

$u = 10$ m/s

$a = -9.81$ m/s^2

$t_i = 0.2$ s

i.e. $s_r = (10 \times 0.2) + \dfrac{(-9.81 \times 0.2^2)}{2}$

$\quad = 2 - 0.196 = 1.804$ m

As $s_i = s_0 + s_r$, then $s_i = 2$ m + 1.804 m

$\quad = 3.804$ m

Similarly, for $t_i = 0.4$ s

$s_r = (10 \times 0.4) + \dfrac{(-9.81 \times 0.4^2)}{2}$

$\quad = 4 - 0.785 = 3.215$ m

and $s_i = 2$ m + 3.215 m = 5.315 m

For $t_i = 2.222$ s (landing),

$s_r = (10 \times 2.222) + \dfrac{(-9.81 \times 2.222^2)}{2}$

$\quad = 22.22 - 24.217 = -1.997$ m

and $s_i = 2$ m + (−1.997) m = 0.003 m (i.e. at ground level)

The displacement data are shown in Table 2A.8.

25. Step 1: Calculate the vertical v_v and horizontal v_h components of release velocity v_0:

$v_v = v_0.\sin \alpha$ and $v_h = v_0.\cos \alpha$ where $v_0 = 12.5$ m/s and $\alpha = 38°$

i.e. $v_v = 7.69$ m/s and $v_h = 9.85$ m/s

Step 2: Calculate flight time t_f:

Consider vertical motion during flight:

$$s = u.t + \frac{a.t^2}{2}$$

where

$s = -2.1$ m (the landing point is 2.1 m below the release point)

$u = v_v = 7.69$ m/s

$a = -9.81$ m/s^2

$t = t_f$

i.e. $-2.1 = 7.69 \times t_f - 4.905 \times t_f^2$

i.e. $4.905 \times t_f^2 - 7.69 \times t_f - 2.1 = 0$

Calculate t_f by application of the formula for solving a quadratic equation, i.e. $x = \dfrac{-b \pm \sqrt{(b^2 - 4a.c)}}{2a}$

where $a = 4.905$, $b = -7.69$, $c = -2.1$

i.e.

$t_f = \dfrac{-(-7.69) \pm \sqrt{(-7.69)^2 - 4 \times 4.905 \times (-2.1)}}{9.81}$

$t_f = \dfrac{7.69 \pm \sqrt{(59.14 + 41.20)}}{9.81} = \dfrac{7.69 \pm 10.02}{9.81}$

Clearly, the negative alternative for the term 7.69 ± 10.02 (resulting in -2.33) cannot be correct. Consequently the positive alternative is taken, i.e. $7.69 + 10.02 = 17.71$,

i.e. $t_f = \dfrac{17.71}{9.81} = 1.805\,s$

Step 3: Calculate range s_r:
Consider horizontal motion during flight:

$s = u.t + \dfrac{a.t^2}{2}$

where
$s = s_r$
$u = v_h = 9.85\,m/s$
$t = 1.805\,s$
$a = 0$
i.e. range $s_r = (9.85 \times 1.805) + 0 = 17.78\,m$

Step 4: Calculate maximum height s_m:
Consider vertical motion from release to maximum height:
$s_m = s_0 + s_f$
where s_0 = release height = 2.1 m
and s_f = vertical displacement between release and maximum height.
From $v^2 - u^2 = 2a.s$

$s = \dfrac{(v^2 - u^2)}{2a}$

where
$s = s_f$
$u = v_v = 7.69\,m/s$
v = velocity at maximum height = 0
$a = -9.81\,m/s^2$
i.e. $s_f = (0 - 7.69^2)/-19.62 = 3.01\,m$
i.e. maximum height $s_m = s_0 + s_f = 2.1\,m + 3.01\,m = 5.11\,m$

Step 5: Calculate the impulse responsible for release velocity:
$I = mv - mu$
where
I = impulse
m = mass of shot = 7.26 kg
v = release velocity = 12.5 m/s
$u = 0$
i.e. impulse $I = (7.26 \times 12.5) - 0 = 90.75\,N.s$

CHAPTER 3

Moment of a force and levers

2. In equilibrium, CM = ACM, i.e. $W_B.d_B = W_A.d_A$
$W_B = (W_A.d_A)/d_B = (45\,kgf \times 3\,m)/3.75\,m$
$= 36\,kgf$

3. From Equation 3.5, $d = I \times (S_2 - S_1)/W_S$
$= 2.5\,m \times (42\,kgf - 10\,kgf)/80\,kgf = 1.0\,m$
$d/h = (1.0\,m/1.8\,m) \times 100 = 55.5\%$

4. In equilibrium, CM = ACM, i.e. $R.d_R = E.d_E$
$R = (E.d_E)/d_R = (20\,kgf \times 25\,cm)/7\,cm$
$= 71.4\,kgf$

5. In equilibrium, CM = ACM, i.e. $E.d_E = R.d_R$
$E = (R.d_R)/d_E = (40\,kgf \times 7\,cm)/25\,cm = 11.2\,kgf$
Minimum force required to lift lid further is
$E > 11.2\,kgf$

6. In equilibrium, CM = ACM, i.e. $A.d_A = W.d_W$
$A = (W.d_W)/d_A$, i.e. $A_1 = 16.9\,kgf$, $A_2 = 38.1\,kgf$,
$A_3 = 47.8\,kgf$

7. In equilibrium, CM = ACM, i.e. $W.d_W = F.d_F$
$F = (W.d_W)/d_F = (5\,kgf \times 2.5\,cm)/7.5\,cm$
$= 1.67\,kgf$
In equilibrium, $J - F - W = 0$
i.e. $J = F + W = 5\,kgf + 1.67\,kgf = 6.67\,kgf$

8. In equilibrium, CM = ACM, i.e. $W.d_W = F.d_F$
$F = (W.d_W)/d_F = (5\,kgf \times 4.5\,cm)/7.5\,cm = 3\,kgf$
In equilibrium: horizontal forces:
$J_H - F_H = 0$
$J_H = F_H$
$J_H = F.\cos 45° = 3\,kgf \times 0.7071 = 2.12\,kgf$

In equilibrium: vertical forces:

$J_V - F_V - W = 0$

$J_V = F_V + W$

$J_V = F.\sin 45° + W$

$J_V = 3\,kgf \times 0.7071 + 5\,kgf$

$J_V = 2.12\,kgf + 5\,kgf = 7.12\,kgf$

$J^2 = J_V^2 + J_H^2 = (7.12^2 + 2.12^2)kgf^2$

$J^2 = 55.19\,kgf^2$

$J = 7.43\,kgf$

If J makes an angle of θ with respect to the horizontal, then

$\tan \theta = J_V/J_H = 7.12/2.12 = 3.358$

$\theta = 73.4°$

9. In equilibrium, CM = ACM, i.e. $W.d_W = A.d_A$

$A = (W.d_W)/d_A = (60\,kgf \times 12\,cm)/7\,cm$

$\quad = 102.86\,kgf$

$A_H = A.\cos 80° = 17.86\,kgf$

$A_V = A.\sin 80° = 101.30\,kgf$

In equilibrium: horizontal forces:

$J_H - A_H = 0$

$J_H = A_H = 17.86\,kgf$

In equilibrium: vertical forces:

$J_V - A_V - W = 0$

$J_V = A_V + W = 161.3\,kgf$

$J = \sqrt{(J_V^2 + J_H^2)} = 162.3\,kgf$

If J makes an angle of θ with respect to the horizontal, then

$\tan \theta = J_V/J_H = 162.3/17.86 = 9.087$

$\theta = 83.7°$

10. In equilibrium, CM = ACM, i.e. $L.d_L = W.d_W$

$d_W = d.\cos 30° = 20\,cm \times 0.8660 = 17.32\,cm$

$L = (W.d_W)/d_L = (4.5\,kgf \times 17.32\,cm)/4\,cm$

$\quad = 19.48\,kgf$

$L_H = L.\cos 47° = 13.28\,kgf$

$L_V = L.\sin 47° = 14.25\,kgf$

In equilibrium: horizontal forces:

$L_H - T_H = 0$

$T_H = L_H = 13.28\,kgf$

In equilibrium: vertical forces:

$L_V - T_V - W = 0$

$T_V = L_V - W = 9.75\,kgf$

$T = \sqrt{(T_V^2 + T_H^2)} = 16.47\,kgf$

If T makes an angle of θ with respect to the horizontal, then

$\tan \theta = T_V/T_H = 9.75/13.28 = 0.7342$

$\theta = 36.3°$

11. i. Calculate the magnitude of P and L.

In equilibrium, CM = ACM about J

$R.d_R = A.d_A + L.d_L + P.d_P$

$P.d_P = R.d_R - A.d_A - L.d_L$

$P.d_P = R.d_R - A.d_A - 2P.d_L$

$P.d_P + 2P.d_L = R.d_R - A.d_A$

$P(d_P + 2d_L) = R.d_R - A.d_A$

$$P = \frac{R.d_R - A.d_A}{d_P + 2d_L} \qquad \text{Eq. 3A.1}$$

$d_R = d_3.\sin 80° = 60\,cm \times 0.9848$

$\quad = 59.09\,cm$

$d_A = d_2 = 29\,cm$

$d_P = d_1.\sin 20° = 10\,cm \times 0.3420 = 3.42\,cm$

$d_L = d_1.\sin 55° = 10\,cm \times 0.8191 = 8.19\,cm$

By substitution into Equation 3A.1

$$P = \frac{R.d_R - A.d_A}{d_P + 2d_L}$$

$$= \frac{(35.54\,kgf \times 59.09\,cm) - (3.5\,kgf \times 29\,cm)}{3.42\,cm + 16.38\,cm}$$

$$P = \frac{1999.1\,kgf.cm}{19.8\,cm} = 100.94\,kgf$$

Therefore $L = 201.88\,kgf$

ii. Resolve all forces into their horizontal and vertical components:

$R_V = R.\sin 80° = 35.0\,kgf$

$R_H = R.\cos 80° = 6.17\,kgf$

$A = 3.5\,kgf$

$P_V = P.\sin 20° = 34.52\,kgf$

$P_H = P.\cos 20° = 94.85\,kgf$

$L_V = L.\sin 55° = 165.37\,kgf$

$L_H = L.\cos 55° = 115.79\,kgf$

iii. Equate forces

In equilibrium: resultant vertical force = 0 i.e.

$R_V + S_V - A - P_V - L_V = 0$

$S_V = A + P_V + L_V - R_V$

$S_V = 3.5\,kgf + 34.52\,kgf + 165.37\,kgf$

$\quad - 35\,kgf$

$S_V = 168.39\,kgf$

In equilibrium: resultant horizontal force = 0, i.e.

$R_H + P_H + L_H - S_H = 0$

$S_H = R_H + P_H + L_H$

$S_H = 6.17\,kgf + 94.85\,kgf + 115.79\,kgf$

$S_H = 216.81\,kgf$

$S = \sqrt{(S_V^2 + S_H^2)} = 274.5\,kgf = 3.92\,BW$

If S makes an angle of θ with respect to the horizontal, then

$\tan \theta = S_V/S_H = 0.7767$

$\theta = 37.8°$

Segmental analysis

12. The solution is based on the method shown in Tables 3.3 and 3.4:

Table 3A.1: Coordinates of the segment end points and segment centres of gravity of the vaulter

Segment	Coordinates* (cm)		Length[†] (cm)	$CG_P{}^{\ddagger}$	$CG_S{}^{\S}$ (cm)	$CG_O{}^{\P}$ (cm)
	a	b			c	
Upper limb	Shoulder	Wrist				
x	3.1	2.3	−0.8	0.50	−0.4	2.70
y	6.9	2.9	−4.0	0.50	−2.0	4.90
Lower limb	Hip	Ankle				
x	6.9	9.3	2.4	0.436	1.05	7.95
y	6.4	1.5	−4.9	0.436	−2.14	4.26
Trunk, head & neck	Head	Hip				
x	0.7	6.9	6.2	0.566	3.51	4.21
y	7.7	6.4	−1.3	0.566	−0.74	6.96

* x and y coordinates of segment end points a and b. [†] Length of segment in the dimension = b − a. [‡] Position of segmental centre of gravity as a proportion of segment length in direction a to b (from Table 3.1). [§] Position of segmental centre of gravity in the dimension in relation to a. [¶] Coordinate of the position of the centre of gravity of the segment = a + c.

Table 3A.2: Coordinates of the segment centres of gravity and whole-body centre of gravity (determined by the principle of moments) of the vaulter

Segment	Coordinates* (cm)		Weight[†]	Weight[‡] (N)	Moment $X^{\S}$ (N.cm)	Moment $Y^{\P}$ (N.cm)
	x	y				
Upper limb	2.70	4.90	0.0577	39.62	106.97	194.14
Lower limb	7.95	4.26	0.1668	114.54	910.59	487.94
Trunk, head & neck	4.21	6.96	0.5510	378.37	1592.94	2633.45
Totals[∥]				686.70	3628.06	3997.61
Coordinates of CG**	5.28	5.82				

* x and y coordinates of the segmental centres of gravity from Table 3A.1(cm). [†] Weight of segments as a proportion of total body weight (from Table 3.1). [‡] Weight of segments in newtons (total body weight = 70 kgf = 686.7 N). [§] Moments of the segmental weights about z axis with respect to x dimension. [¶] Moments of the segmental weights about z axis with respect to y dimension. [∥] Total moment includes both upper limbs and both lower limbs. ** Moment of body weight = sum of moments of segments, i.e. $W.x_G$ = sum of Moment X, where W = body weight = 686.7 N and x_G = x coordinate of CG, i.e.

$$x_G = \frac{\text{sum of Moment X}}{W} = \frac{3628.06 \, \text{N.cm}}{686.7 \, \text{N}} = 5.28 \, \text{cm}.$$

Similarly,

$$y_G = \frac{\text{sum of Moment Y}}{W} = \frac{3997.61 \, \text{N.cm}}{686.7 \, \text{N}} = 5.82 \, \text{cm}.$$

Angular displacement, angular velocity and angular acceleration

14. i. $\theta_C = 125° = 2.181$ rad
$\theta_E = 240° = 4.188$ rad
   ii. $\omega = (\theta_D - \theta_B)/t = 400°/s = 6.98$ rad/s
   iii. $\alpha = (\omega_D - \omega_B)/t = 8$ rad/s$^2 = 458.4°/s^2$
   iv. $v_B = r.\omega_B = 3.1$ m/s, $v_D = r.\omega_D = 5.5$ m/s
   v. $a_B = r.\alpha_B = 7.1$ m/s^2, $a_D = r.\alpha_D$
$= 9.3$ m/s^2

15. From Equation 3.16, $F_C = (m_H.v_H^2)/r_H = 3084.5$ N
From Equation 318, $r_T = (m_H.r_H)/m_T = 0.129$ m

16. From Equation 3.16, $F_C = (m_C.v_C^2)/r_C = 364.5$ N
From Equation 3.19, $\tan\theta = F_C/F_V$ where
F_V = weight of cyclist and bike = 686.7 N;
$\theta = 27.9°$

Angular impulse and angular momentum

17.

Variable	Units	Unit abbreviation
Moment of a force	newton metres	N.m
Time	seconds	s
Angular impulse	newton metre seconds	N.m.s
Moment of inertia	kilogram metres squared	kg.m^2
Angular velocity	radians per second	rad/s
Angular momentum	kilogram metres squared per second	kg.m^2/s

18. i. Using Pythagoras' theorem, calculate the distances between a_G and the parallel axes through the centres of gravity of each upper limb, each lower limb and the trunk, head and neck. Distance scale: 1 cm on the figure $\equiv$ 0.132 m (Table 3A.3).
   ii. Use $I_z = m.k_z^2$ to calculate the moment of inertia of each segment about the mediolateral axis a_z through its centre of gravity parallel to a_G (columns 1–7 of Table 3A.4).
   iii. Use the parallel axis theorem to calculate the moment of inertia of each segment about a_G (columns 7–9 of Table 3A.4).
   iv. Sum the total moment of inertia about a_G (column 10 of Table 3A.4).

19. $\omega_{Z1} = 4.3$ rad/s, $\omega_{Z5} = 13$ rad/s.

Table 3A.3: x and y coordinates (cm) of the whole-body centre of gravity and the centres of gravity of each upper limb, each lower limb and the trunk, head and neck

	x	y
Whole body	5.28	5.82
Upper limb	2.70	4.90
Lower limb	7.95	4.26
Trunk, head & neck	4.21	6.96

d_A = distance between a_G and centre of gravity of each upper limb = 2.74 cm $\equiv$ 0.36 m; d_L = distance between a_G and centre of gravity of each lower limb = 3.09 cm $\equiv$ 0.41 m; d_T = distance between a_G and centre of gravity of the trunk, head and neck = 1.56 cm $\equiv$ 0.20 m.

Table 3A.4:
Determination of the moment of inertia of the vaulter about the mediolateral axis through his centre of gravity

		1 m (%)	2 m (kg)	3 Length (m)	4 k_z (%)	5 k_z (m)	6 I_z (kg.m²)	7 d (m)	8 $m.d^2$ (kg.m²)	9 I_G (kg.m²)	10 I_G (kg.m²)
UL		5.77	4.04	0.54	0.368	0.20	0.1616	0.36	0.5236	0.6852	1.3704
THN		55.1	38.6	0.50	0.503	0.25	2.4125	0.20	1.5440	3.9565	3.9565
LL		16.7	11.7	0.72	0.326	0.23	0.6189	0.41	1.9667	2.5857	5.1713
Total											10.4982

Whole body mass = 70 kg.

m% = mass of segment as a percentage of whole-body mass; UL = upper arm, forearm and hand; THN = trunk, head and neck; LL = thigh, shank and foot; Length = length of segment; a_G = mediolateral axis through the centre of gravity of the vaulter; k_z = radius of gyration of the segment about the mediolateral axis a_z through its centre of gravity as a percentage of segment length; I_z = moment of inertia of the segment about a_z; d = distance from a_G to the centre of gravity of the segment; I_G = moment of inertia of the segment about a_G; I_G = moment of inertia of both arms, both legs and the trunk, head and neck about a_G and the total moment of inertia about a_G.

CHAPTER 4

2. Mass of ball $m = 0.45$ kg, linear velocity of the ball after the kick $v = 25$ m/s, contact distance between ball and foot $d = 0.3$ m.
   i. Work done on the ball $W = F.d$ where
      F = average force exerted on the ball
      $W = F.d = m.v^2/2 = (0.45 \text{ kg} \times (25 \text{ m/s})^2)/2$
         $= 140.6$ J
      $F = 140.6 \text{ J}/0.3 \text{ m} = 468.7$ N
   ii. Calculate the contact time t between the ball and the kicker's foot.
      From Newton's second law of motion
      $F.t = m.v - m.u$, i.e.
      $F.t = m.v$ (as $u = 0$)
      $t = m.v/F = (0.45 \text{ kg} \times 25 \text{ m/s})/468.7$ N
         $= 0.024$ s
      Average power of the impact P_a
         $= 140.6 \text{ J}/0.024 \text{ s} = 5858.3$ W

3. Mass of hammer $m = 2.25$ kg, TKE of the hammer at impact $= 7$ J, distance travelled by the hammer before coming to rest $d = 0.03$ m.
   i. Work done on the wall $W = F.d = \text{TKE} = 7$ J
      where F = average force exerted on the wall,
      i.e. $F = 7 \text{ J}/0.03 \text{ m} = 233.3$ N
   ii. Calculate the contact time t of the impact.
      From Newton's second law of motion
      $F.t = m.v - m.u$ where $u = v_i$ = velocity of the hammer at impact and $v = 0$ = velocity of the hammer after the impact

$m.v_i^2/2 = 7$ J
i.e. $v_i = \sqrt{(14/2.25)}$ m/s $= 2.49$ m/s $- F.t$
   $= - m.v_i$
$t = m.v_i/F = (0.45 \text{ kg} \times 2.49 \text{ m/s})/233.3$ N
   $= 0.0048$ s
Average power of the impact P_a
   $= 7 \text{ J}/0.0048 \text{ s} = 1458.3$ W

4. Mass of box $m = 20$ kg, $\mu = 0.4$, $d = 3$ m,
   $F = \mu.R$ where F = friction between the box and the floor and R = normal reaction = weight of the box, i.e. $F = 0.4 \times 20 \text{ kg} \times 9.81 \text{ m/s}^2 = 78.5$ N.
   Work done on the box W is the work needed to overcome F, i.e.
   $W = F.d = 78.5 \text{ N} \times 3 \text{ m} = 235.5$ J

5. Slope $= 15°$, mass of the box $m = 20$ kg, weight of the box $B = 196.2$ N, $\mu = 0.4$, $d = 5$ m.
   i. $F = \mu.R$ where F = friction between the box and the floor and R = normal reaction = component of the weight of the box perpendicular to the slope $= B.\cos 15° = 189.5$ N, i.e. $F = 0.4 \times 189.5 \text{ N} = 75.8$ N
   ii. The work W required to push the box up the slope is the sum of the work required to overcome friction and the increase in the gravitational potential energy of the box, i.e.
      $W = F.d + m.g.h$ where h = vertical displacement of the box $= d.\sin 15°$
      $= 1.29$ m, i.e.

$W = (75.8 \, \text{N} \times 5 \, \text{m})$
$\quad + (20 \, \text{kg} \times 9.81 \, \text{m/s}^2 \times 1.29 \, \text{m})$
$\quad = 379 \, \text{J} + 253 \, \text{J} = 632 \, \text{J}$

iii. Average force = work/distance
$\quad = 632 \, \text{J/5 m} = 126.4 \, \text{N}$

6. Mass of ball $m = 7.26 \, \text{kg}$

   i. If the ball falls from a height of 1.5 m and comes to rest 0.04 m below the ground, its total mechanical energy before it is dropped = $m.g.h$ where $h = 1.54 \, \text{m}$, i.e.
   $m.g.h = 109.7 \, \text{J}$
   The work done by the ground on the ball $F.d = 109.7 \, \text{J}$ where F = average force exerted on the ball and d = distance travelled by the ball before coming to rest after hitting the ground = 0.04 m, i.e.
   $F = 109.7 \, \text{J/0.04 m} = 2742.5 \, \text{N}$

   ii. When $d = 0.01 \, \text{m}$, $m.g.h = 107.5 \, \text{J}$ ($h = 1.51 \, \text{m}$) and $F = 107.5 \, \text{J/0.01 m} = 10750 \, \text{N}$

7. Mass of the ball $m = 0.25 \, \text{kg}$, $h_1 = 1.2 \, \text{m}$, $h_2 = 0.8 \, \text{m}$

   i. Total mechanical energy of the ball before it is dropped = $m.g.h_1$ and the total mechanical energy of the ball at the top of its bounce = $m.g.h_2$, i.e. energy dissipated during the impact = $m.g.h_1 - m.g.h_2 = m.g \, (h_1 - h_2) = 0.25 \, \text{kg} \times 9.81 \, \text{m/s}^2 \times 0.4 \, \text{m} = 0.98 \, \text{J}$

   ii. Resilience of the ball = $(m.g.h_2/m.g.h_1) \times 100 = (h_2/h_1) \times 100 = 66.7\%$

8. Mass of the arrow $m = 0.015 \, \text{kg}$, linear velocity $v = 60 \, \text{m/s}$

   i. $F.d = m.v^2/2$ where F = average force exerted by the bowstring on the arrow and $d = 0.70 \, \text{m}$, i.e. $F.d = m.v^2/2 = (0.015 \, \text{kg} \times (60 \, \text{m/s})^2)/2 = 27 \, \text{J}$ and $F = 27 \, \text{J/0.70 m} = 38.6 \, \text{N}$

   ii. TKE of the arrow at impact with the target = 27 J
   $F_1.d_1$ = work done on arrow by the target where F_1 = average force exerted by the target on the arrow and $d_1 = 0.04 \, \text{m}$, i.e. $F_1.d_1 = 27 \, \text{J}$ and $F_1 = 27 \, \text{J/0.04 m} = 675 \, \text{N}$

9. Pedal frequency = 50 rev/min, distance moved by a point on the rim of the flywheel = 6 m/rev
   Work rate $P = W/t$ where W = work done against the friction F between the belt and the flywheel in time t
   $W = F.d$ where d = distance moved by a point on the rim of the flywheel in time t
   $d/\text{min} = 50 \, \text{rev/min} \times 6 \, \text{m/rev} = 300 \, \text{m/min}$
   $W/\text{min} = P = F \times d/\text{min} = 2 \, \text{kgf} \times 300 \, \text{m/min} = 19.62 \, \text{N} \times 300 \, \text{m/min} = 5886 \, \text{J/min} = 98.1 \, \text{J/s} = 98.1 \, \text{W}$

10. Mass of the vaulter = 70 kg, $h_1 = 1.1 \, \text{m}$, $v_1 = 9.1 \, \text{m/s}$, $v_2 = 1.0 \, \text{m/s}$

    i. Mechanical energy at take-off
    $= m.g.h_1 + m.v_1^2/2$
    Mechanical energy at maximum height
    $= m.g.h_2 + m.v_2^2/2$
    If mechanical energy is conserved, then
    $m.g.h_1 + m.v_1^2/2 = m.g.h_2 + m.v_2^2/2$, i.e.
    $h_2 - h_1 = (v_1^2 - v_2^2)/2g = 4.17 \, \text{m}$

    ii. $h_1 + 4.17 \, \text{m} = 5.27 \, \text{m}$

CHAPTER 5

2. $V = 1000 \, \text{m}^3$, $W_E = 50 \, \text{kgf}$, $\rho_o = 1.25 \, \text{kgf/m}^3$, $\rho_i = 1.10 \, \text{kgf/m}^3$
   The balloon will float if $B = W_E + W_H + W_L$ where B = the buoyancy force, W_E = weight of the balloon envelope, W_H = weight of the hot air inside the balloon and W_L = weight of the load
   $B = V.\rho_o = 1000 \, \text{m}^3 \times 1.25 \, \text{kgf/m}^3 = 1250 \, \text{kgf}$
   $W_E = 50 \, \text{kgf}$
   $W_H = V.\rho_i = 1000 \, \text{m}^3 \times 1.10 \, \text{kgf/m}^3 = 1100 \, \text{kgf}$
   i.e. the maximum load W_L that the balloon can carry and just float is given by
   $W_L = B - W_E - W_H$
   $\quad = 1250 \, \text{kgf} - 50 \, \text{kgf} - 1100 \, \text{kgf} = 100 \, \text{kgf}$

3. $\rho_w = 1025 \, \text{kgf/m}^3$, $V = 1.5 \, \text{m}^3$
   The weight of the boat W_B is equal to the weight of the water W_W that the boat displaces when it is floating, i.e. $W_B = W_W = V.\rho_w$
   $\quad = 1025 \, \text{kgf/m}^3 \times 1.5 \, \text{m}^3 = 1537.5 \, \text{kgf}$

4. $v = 3.5 \, \text{m/s}$, $\eta = 0.010 \, 02 \, \text{Pl}$, $\rho = 1000 \, \text{kg/m}^3$, $A_S = 1.8 \, \text{m}^2$, $v/h = 1.75/\text{s}$, $C_D = 0.2$, $A_P = 0.06 \, \text{m}^2$, $m = 70 \, \text{kg}$
   i. From Equation 5.8, viscous drag $F_V = \eta.A_S.v/h$, i.e.
   $F_V = 0.010 \, 02 \, \text{Pl} \times 1.8 \, \text{m}^2 \times 1.75/\text{s} = 0.0316 \, \text{N}$
   From Equation 5.9, pressure drag $F_P = C_D.A_P.\rho.v^2/2$, i.e.

$F_P = (0.2 \times 0.06\,m^2 \times 1000\,kg/m^3$
$\times (3.5\,m/s)^2)/2 = 73.5\,N$

ii. Total drag $= F_V + F_P = 0.0316\,N + 73.5\,N$
= 73.5316 N. From $F = m.a$, the
instantaneous acceleration $a = F/m =$
$-73.5316\,N/70\,kg = -1.05\,m/s^2$

5. $v = 22.35\,m/s$, $\eta = 0.000\,18$ Pl, $\rho = 1.25\,kg/m^3$,
$A_S = 0.152\,m^2$, $v/h = 2/s$, $C_D = 0.2$, $A_P = 0.04\,m^2$
   i. From Equation 5.8, viscous drag $F_V = \eta.A_S.v/h$,
   i.e.
   $F_V = 0.000\,18\,Pl \times 0.152\,m^2 \times 2/s$
   $= 0.000\,055\,N$
   From Equation 5.9, pressure drag $F_P =$
   $C_D.A_P.\rho.v^2/2$, i.e.
   $F_P = (0.2 \times 0.04\,m^2 \times 1.25\,kg/m^3$
   $\times (22.35\,m/s)^2)/2 = 2.5\,N$

   ii. Total drag $= F_V + F_P = 0.000\,055\,N + 2.5\,N$
   = 2.5 N. From $F = m.a$, the instantaneous
   acceleration $a = F/m = -2.5\,N/0.45\,kg$
   $= -5.55\,m/s^2$

6. $\theta = 5°$, $m = 390\,kg$, $\mu = 0.03$, $C_D = 0.45$,
$A = 0.413\,m^2$
The resultant force acting on the sleigh down the
slope (positive down) is given by
$R = W_P - F - D = m.a$ (Eq. 5.10), where W_P is
the component of the weight of m parallel to the
slope, F is the frictional force and $D =$ drag force.
Terminal velocity occurs when $R = W_P - F - D$
= 0, i.e. when
$W.\sin\theta - \mu.W.\cos\theta - C_D.A.\rho.v^2/2 = 0$ (Eq. 5.11),
where

$W_P = W.\sin\theta = 390\,kg \times 9.81\,m/s^2 \times 0.0871$
= 333.45 N
$F = \mu.W.\cos\theta = 0.03 \times 390\,kg \times 9.81\,m/s^2$
$\times 0.9962 = 114.34\,N$
$D = C_D.A.\rho.v^2/2 = (0.45 \times 0.413\,m^2$
$\times 1.25\,kg/m^3 \times v^2)2 = 0.116v^2\,N$, i.e.
333.45 N $-$ 114.34 N $-$ 0.116v^2N = 0

$v = \sqrt{219.11/0.116} = 43.46\,m/s$
$= 97.2\,mph$

7. $m = 0.45\,kg$, $r = 0.11\,m$, $t = 1\,s$
   i. Atmospheric pressure P_A at ground
   level is approximately 101 325 Pa =
   10.13 N/cm^2
   ii. The cross-sectional area of the ball $A = \pi.r^2$
   = 0.038 m^2 = 380 cm^2
   iii. If there was no sideways pressure differential on
   the ball, i.e. if the atmospheric pressure on each
   side of the ball was the same, the force F on
   each side of the ball would be given by $F =$
   $P_A.A = 10.13\,N/cm^2 \times 380\,cm^2 = 3849.4\,N$
   iv. A pressure differential of 0.1% would result
   in a force differential $F = 0.001 \times$
   3849.4 N = 3.85 N
   v. The sideways acceleration of the ball
   $a = F/m = 3.85\,N/0.45\,kg = 8.55\,m/s^2$
   vi. The sideways distance s moved by the ball
   (assuming constant acceleration of 8.55 m/s^2)
   in one second is given by $s = u.t + a.t^2/2$
   where $u = 0$, $a = 8.55\,m/s^2$ and $t = 1\,s$
   i.e. s = 4.3 m.

Glossary

Acceleration: the rate of change of speed, i.e. change in speed divided by change in time.

Active load: any external load (other than body weight) that is completely controlled by conscious muscular activity.

Aerofoil: an object that is designed to produce hydrodynamic lift by asymmetrical shape.

Anatomical frame of reference: a three-dimensional spatial reference system used to describe the location of body parts with respect to the anatomical position.

Anatomical position: a reference posture for the human body in which the body is upright with the arms by the sides and palms of the hands facing forward.

Angle of attack: the angle that the axis of an aerofoil makes with respect to the linear velocity of the aerofoil.

Angular momentum: the product of the moment of inertia of an object about a particular axis and the angular velocity of the object about the axis.

Angular motion: angular motion, also referred to as rotation, occurs when a body or part of a body moves in a circle or part of a circle about a particular line in space, referred to as the axis of rotation, such that all parts of the body move through the same angle in the same direction in the same time.

Archimedes' principle: an object that is partially or completely immersed in a fluid will experience a buoyancy force that is equal to the weight of the fluid displaced.

Atmosphere: the layer of gas surrounding any planet or star.

Atmospheric pressure: the pressure exerted by the atmosphere.

Attraction force: a force exerted between two bodies that tends to make the bodies move toward each other if they are apart and to maintain contact with each other after contact is made.

Bernoulli's principle: when a fluid flows over a surface, the pressure exerted by the fluid on the surface is inversely proportional to the speed of flow.

Biomechanics: the study of the forces that act on and within living organisms and the effect of the forces on the size, shape, structure and movement of the organisms.

Boundary layer: the layer of fluid adjacent to the surface of an object when a fluid flows over it.

Buoyancy force: the upthrust experienced by an object immersed or partially immersed in a fluid.

Calorie (cal): 1 calorie is the energy required to raise the temperature of 1 g (gram) of water by 1°C. 1 cal = 4.186 J.

Centre of buoyancy: the point of application of the buoyancy force. The centre of buoyancy is the centre of gravity of the displaced fluid.

Centre of gravity: the point at which the whole weight of an object can be considered to act.

Centre of pressure: the point at which the ground reaction force can be considered to act.

Centrifugal force: the reaction exerted by a rotating object to the centripetal force; it is due to the inertia of the object, which resists a change in direction.

Centripetal force: the force acting on a body that causes it to move on a curved path. The centripetal (centre-seeking) force is directed toward the centre of curvature, i.e. the centre of the circle on which the object is instantaneously moving. The centre of curvature of an object moving in a circle is the centre of the circle.

Coefficient of drag: a dimensionless number that reflects the effect of the surface texture and shape of an object on the drag force experienced by the object when moving through a fluid.

Coefficient of lift: a dimensionless number that reflects the effect of the surface texture and shape of an object on the hydrodynamic lift force experienced by the object when moving through a fluid.

Concentric force: a force whose line of action passes through the centre of gravity of the object on which it acts; a concentric force produces or tends to produce rectilinear translation.

Conservation of angular momentum: if the resultant moment acting on a rotating object is zero, the angular momentum of the object will remain constant; a change in the moment of inertia of the object will result in a simultaneous change in angular velocity so that angular momentum is conserved.

Conservation of linear momentum: if no external force acts on a system of colliding objects, the total amount of linear momentum in the system remains constant, i.e. the sum of the linear momentum of the colliding objects remains constant.

Conservation of mechanical energy: the effect of a conservative force (*see* Conservative force); there are no conservative force systems in nature since the movement of objects is always resisted to a certain extent by friction and/or fluid (air, water) resistance.

Conservative force: a force acting on an object that changes the proportions of the different forms of mechanical energy of the object but does not change the total amount of mechanical energy of the object.

Contact force: a force exerted on a body that is due to physical contact with its environment.

Coronal plane (or frontal plane): the vertical plane perpendicular to the median plane that divides the body into anterior and posterior portions.

Couple: a system of two parallel, equal and opposite forces, one concentric and one eccentric or both eccentric, that tend to rotate an object in the same direction about a particular axis. A couple produces or tends to produce rotation without translation. Rotation of any object about a fixed axis is the result of a couple.

Curvilinear motion: linear movement that follows a curved path (*see* Linear motion).

Cycle length: the distance achieved in each cycle of movement (e.g. stride length, stroke length).

Cycle rate: the number of cycles of movement per unit of time (e.g. stride rate, stroke rate).

Damping: a low level of resilience; the lower the resilience the greater the damping.

Density: the amount of mass per unit volume.

Desired response (in movement analysis): the movement pattern that a teacher or coach expects to see in a performance of a particular movement.

Deterministic model: a model of the mechanical and anthropometric factors that determine performance of a particular movement.

Distance: (a) the length of the line between two points in three-dimensional space. (b) the length of the path followed by a body as it moves from one position to another in three-dimensional space.

Drag: the retarding force experienced by an object moving through a fluid. Drag acts in the opposite direction to the movement of the object.

Dynamics: the subdiscipline of mechanics that is concerned with the study of bodies under the action of unbalanced forces.

Eccentric force: a force whose line of action does not pass through the centre of gravity of the object on which it acts; an eccentric force produces or tends to produce simultaneous rectilinear translation and rotation of the object about an axis that passes through the centre of gravity of the object and is perpendicular to the eccentric force.

Energy: the capacity to do work.

Entropy: energy that is transformed into forms that cannot be recovered to do work.

Equilibrium: with regard to linear motion, an object is in equilibrium when the resultant force acting on the object is zero. With regard to angular motion, an object is in equilibrium when the resultant moment acting on the object is zero.

External force: in biomechanical analysis of human movement, the forces that act on the body from external sources, such as body weight, ground reaction force, water resistance and air resistance, are referred to as external forces.

External work (W_E): the work done by the human body against external forces. External work consists of two components, the work done in changing the gravitational potential energy of the body (W_{Eg}) (weight is an external force) and the work done against other external forces (W_{Eo}). W_{Eo} comprises three main types of work: changes in the gravitational potential energy of other objects, changes in the kinetic energy of other objects, work done against external sources of friction.

Fineness ratio: the ratio of the length of an object to the diameter of the object with respect to the direction of fluid flow.

First law of thermodynamics (incorporates the principle of conservation of energy): the total amount of energy in a closed system is constant; the energy in a system cannot be created or destroyed, it can only be converted from one form to another.

Fluid mechanics: the study of the forces that act on bodies in fluids and the effects of the forces on the movement of the bodies.

Fluid: a substance that has a natural tendency to flow or change shape.

Force: that which alters or tends to alter a body's state of rest or type of movement.

Frame of reference: *see* Newtonian frame of reference and Anatomical frame of reference.

Free body diagram: a diagram showing all the forces acting on an object.

Friction: when one object moves or tends to move across the surface of another there will be a force parallel to the surfaces in contact that will oppose the movement or tendency to move; this force is called friction.

Fully turbulent flow: when the whole of the boundary layer of a fluid flowing over an object becomes turbulent.

Gravitational potential energy: the energy possessed by an object by virtue of its height above any particular reference position, usually ground level.

Gravity: the acceleration experienced by a body due to the force of attraction (weight of the body) exerted on the body by the earth.

Ground reaction force: the force exerted by the ground on the body.

Hydrodynamic lift: the movement of an object resulting from hydrodynamic lift force.

Hydrodynamic lift force: the force acting on an object at right angles to the drag force that results from differences in the speed of fluid flow and, therefore, differences in pressure on the opposite sides of the object.

Hydrostatic pressure: the pressure exerted by a fluid on an object immersed or partially immersed in the fluid.

Hysteresis loop: the loop on a load–deformation curve defined by the loading and unloading phases; the loop defines the amount of strain energy dissipated between the end of the loading phase and the end of the unloading phase.

Impact: a collision, usually of short duration, between two bodies.

Impact force peak: the peak force during the passive phase of impact of the human body with another body or object.

Impulse of a force: the product of the magnitude of a force and the duration of the force.

Impulse of a turning moment: the product of the average resultant turning moment and the duration of the turning moment.

Impulse–momentum relationship: the relationship between (a) the impulse of a force and the resulting change in linear momentum and (b) the impulse of the moment of a force and the resulting change in angular momentum.

Inertia: the resistance/reluctance of a body to start moving if it is stationary or to change its speed and/or direction if it is already moving.

Internal force: in biomechanical analysis of human movement, the forces generated and transmitted by the musculoskeletal system are referred to as internal forces.

Internal work: the work done by the human body in changing the kinetic energy of the body segments.

Joint reaction forces: the equal and opposite forces exerted by the articular surfaces on each other in a joint.

Joule (J): the work done by a force of 1 newton (N) when it moves its point of application a distance of 1 metre (m) in the direction of the force. The units of energy, mechanical work and moment of a force consist of the same combination of base units, $kg.m^2/s^2$. To distinguish these quantities, the unit for energy and mechanical work is the joule (J) and the unit for moment of a force is the newton metre (N.m).

Kinematics: the branch of dynamics that describes the movement of bodies in relation to space and time.

Kinetic energy: the energy an object possesses by virtue of its movement.

Kinetics: the branch of dynamics that describes the forces acting on bodies, i.e. the cause of the observed kinematics.

Laminar flow (streamlined flow): when a fluid flows over an object without producing turbulence.

Lever: a rigid or quasi-rigid object that can be made to rotate about a fulcrum in order to exert a force on another object.

Linear momentum: the product of mass and linear velocity.

Linear motion: also referred to as translation, occurs when all parts of a body move the same distance in the same direction in the same time (*see* Rectilinear *and* Curvilinear motion).

Load: any force or combination of forces applied to an object.

Magnus effect: the production of hydrodynamic lift due to spin.

Mass: the amount of matter (physical substance) that comprises a body. The mass of a body is a measure of the inertia of the body.

Mechanical advantage: a measure of the efficiency of a lever system; the ratio of the resistance force to the effort force or the ratio of the moment arm of the effort force to the moment arm of the resistance force.

Mechanical approach (in movement analysis): a desired response that is based on the mechanical requirements of the movement.

Mechanical efficiency of the human body: the ratio of the mechanical work done by the body during a particular period of time to the corresponding metabolic energy expenditure, usually expressed as a percentage.

Mechanical energy: the energy of an object by virtue of its height above a particular reference point (gravitational potential energy) and its movement (kinetic energy).

Mechanical power: the rate at which energy is transformed in the form of work.

Mechanics: the study of the forces that act on bodies and the effects of the forces on the size, shape, structure and movement of the bodies.

Mechanics of materials: the subdiscipline of mechanics that is concerned with the study of the mechanical properties of materials.

Median plane: the vertical plane that divides the body down the middle into more or less symmetrical left and right portions.

Moment of a force: the product of the magnitude of the force and the perpendicular distance between the axis of rotation and the line of action of the force.

Moment of inertia: the reluctance or resistance of an object to change its angular motion.

Movement pattern: the way that the body as a whole moves in relation to its spatial environment (the movement of the whole body centre of gravity) and the way that the body segments move in relation to each other.

Movement sequence: a sequence of discrete movements involving static and dynamic postures that are performed one after the other.

Muscle latency: the time that a muscle takes to respond to changes in external loading.

Musculoskeletal system function: the mechanical function of the musculoskeletal system is to generate and transmit internal forces to counteract the effects of gravity and create the ground reaction forces (and propulsion forces in water) necessary to maintain upright posture, transport the body and manipulate objects, often simultaneously.

Newton: a newton is the unit of force in the SI system of units. A newton is defined as the force acting on a mass of 1 kg that accelerates it at $1 \, \text{m/s}^2$.

Newton's first law of motion: the resultant force acting on a body at rest or moving with uniform linear velocity is zero and the body will remain at rest or continue to move with uniform linear velocity unless the resultant force acting on it becomes greater than zero.

Newton's law of gravitation: every body attracts every other body with a force that varies directly with the product of the masses of the two bodies and inversely with the square of the distance between them.

Newton's second law of motion: when a force (resultant force greater than zero) acts on a body, the change in momentum experienced by the body takes place in the direction of the force and is directly proportional to the magnitude of the force and the length of time that the force acts.

Newton's third law of motion: whenever one body A exerts a force on another body B, body B simultaneously exerts an equal and opposite force on body A.

Newtonian frame of reference: a three-dimensional spatial reference system consisting of three orthogonal axes that intersect at a point called the origin.

Paddle propulsion (drag propulsion): propulsion due to the production of drag.

Parallel axis theorem: the equation that relates the moment of inertia I_A of an object about an axis A that does not pass through the centre of gravity of the object, to the moment of inertia I_G of the object about a parallel axis that does pass through the centre of gravity of the object. $I_A = I_G + m_t.d^2$ where m_t = total mass of the object and d = distance between the parallel axes.

Parallelogram of vectors: the method of determining the resultant of two component vectors by constructing a parallelogram in which the two component vectors arise from the same point and form two adjacent sides of the parallelogram.

Partially turbulent flow: when the fluid flowing over an object produces a turbulent wake.

Passive load: any change in external load that occurs within the latency period of the muscles.

Poise (P): a poise is the centimetre–gram–second system unit of viscosity. $1 \, \text{P} = 1 \, \text{g/(cm.s)} = 1 \, \text{g.cm}^{-1}.\text{s}^{-1}$. $1 \, \text{P} = 0.1 \, \text{Pl}$.

Poiseuille (Pl): a poiseuille is the SI unit of viscosity. $1 \, \text{Pl} = 1 \, \text{kg/(m.s)} = 1 \, \text{kg.m}^{-1}.\text{s}^{-1}$.

Potential energy: stored energy.

Power: the rate of transformation of energy from one form to another.

Pressure: force per unit area; 1 atm (1 atmosphere) is defined as a pressure of 101 325 Pa.

Pressure drag (profile drag, form drag): the retarding force exerted on an object moving through a fluid that is due to turbulence.

Principle of conservation of energy: the total amount of energy in a closed system is constant.

Principle of moments: the moment of the resultant of any number of forces about any axis is equal to the algebraic sum of the moments of the individual forces about the same axis.

Qualitative analysis of movement: analysis based on observation.

Quantitative analysis of movement: analysis based on measurements of the variables that determine performance.

Radian: a radian (rad) is the angle subtended at the centre of a circle by an arc of the circle that is the same length as the radius of the circle. 1 rad = 57.3°.

Radius of gyration: the radius of curvature k of an object of mass m rotating about a particular axis such that $I = m.k^2$ where I is the moment of inertia of the object about the axis.

Rectilinear motion: linear motion in a straight line (*see* Linear motion).

Relative density: the ratio of the density of an object to the density of water.

Resilience: the amount of energy returned during unloading as a percentage of the amount of energy absorbed during loading.

Resolution of a vector: the process of replacing a vector by two or more component vectors.

Right-handed axis system: The newtonian frame of reference in which positive X is forward, positive Y is upward and positive Z is to the right.

Rotational kinetic energy: the energy possessed by an object by virtue of its angular motion.

Running economy: the rate of energy expenditure for a given submaximal running speed.

Scalar quantity: a quantity that can be completely specified by its magnitude (size).

Screw propulsion: propulsion due to the production of hydrodynamic lift force.

Second law of thermodynamics: in any transformation of energy there is always entropy, i.e. energy that is transformed into forms that cannot be recovered to do work.

Sequential approach (in movement analysis): a desired response that is based on a mental checklist of body configurations during the performance of a movement.

Slipstream: the region of turbulence at the rear of an object moving through a fluid.

Slipstreaming: In sport, the practice of moving (running and cycling in particular) in the slipstream of another participant in order to reduce pressure drag.

Somersault: one complete rotation of the body about the mediolateral (Z) axis passing through the centre of gravity of the body.

Specific gravity: the ratio of the weight of an object to the weight of an equal volume of water.

Speed: the rate of change of position, i.e. distance moved divided by the time taken to move the distance.

Stability: with respect to a particular base of support, an object is stable when the line of action of its weight intersects the plane of the base of support and unstable when it does not.

Stall: the dramatic decrease in hydrodynamic lift and forward movement of an aerofoil that occurs when the angle of attack reaches a certain size.

Statics: the subdiscipline of mechanics that is concerned with the study of bodies under the action of balanced forces.

Stiffness: the resistance of a material to deformation.

Strain: in mechanics, the deformation of an object that occurs in response to a load is referred to as strain.

Strain energy: the energy stored in an object as a result of being strained.

Streamlined shape: rounded at the front and tapering to a point at the rear.

Strength of a material: the amount of force required to break the material.

Stress: the resistance of the intermolecular bonds of an object to the strain caused by a load.

Synovial bursa: a closed sac composed of synovial membrane containing synovial fluid that is interposed between different tissues that slide on each other to prevent friction.

Synovial membrane: a highly specialized form of connective tissue that lines the capsule in a synovial joint. The synovial membrane produces synovial fluid that lubricates and nourishes the articular cartilage.

Synovial sheath: a closed flattened sac composed of synovial membrane containing a capillary film of synovial fluid. A synovial sheath forms a protective sleeve around a tendon or ligament to prevent friction with adjacent tissue.

Thermodynamics: the branch of physics concerning the nature of heat and its association with other forms of energy (*see* First law of thermodynamics *and* Second law of thermodynamics).

Transfer of angular momentum: when an object is rotating with constant angular momentum, any change in the angular momentum of one or more parts of the object as a result of internal forces will simultaneously result in a change in the angular momentum of one or more of the other parts of the body so that the angular momentum of the object is conserved.

Translational kinetic energy: the energy possessed by an object by virtue of its linear motion.

Transverse plane: A horizontal plane, perpendicular to both the median and coronal planes, that divides the body into upper and lower portions.

Trigonometry: the branch of mathematics that deals with the relationships between the lengths of the sides and the sizes of the angles in a triangle.

Twisting: rotation of the human body about the vertical (Y) axis passing through the centre of gravity of the body.

Vector chain: the method of determining the resultant of a number of component vectors by joining the component vectors together in a chain.

Vector quantity: a quantity that requires specification in both magnitude and direction.

Velocity gradient of a fluid: the shear strain rate of a fluid in response to a given shear stress.

Viscosity: a fluid's resistance to flow.

Viscous drag (friction drag, surface drag): the retarding force exerted on an object moving through a fluid that is due to the viscosity of the fluid.

Volume: the amount of space that a mass occupies.

Watt: 1 watt is the work rate of 1 joule per second (J/s).

Wave drag: the retarding force exerted on an object by the wave of fluid created by the object when moving though the boundary between two different fluids.

Weight of a body: the force of attraction exerted on a body by the earth.

Work of a force: the product of a force and the distance moved by the point of application of the force in the direction of the force.

Work of the moment of a force: the product of a moment of force and the angular distance in radians moved by the object in the direction of the moment of force.

Work–energy relationship: the relationship between (a) the work done by a force and the resulting change in translational kinetic energy and (b) the work done by the moment of a force and the resulting change in rotational kinetic energy.

Index